ARTIFICIAL PARTS, PRACTICAL LIVES

T0260654

Edited by KATHERINE OTT,
DAVID SERLIN, and STEPHEN MIHM

ARTIFICIAL PARTS, PRACTICAL LIVES

Modern Histories of Prosthetics

New York University Press • *New York and London*

To Akela, Brian, Karen, and Kay Jin'E

NEW YORK UNIVERSITY PRESS
New York and London

© 2002 by New York University
All rights reserved

Library of Congress Cataloging-in-Publication Data
Artificial parts, practical lives : modern histories of prosthetics / edited
by Katherine Ott, David Serlin, and Stephen Mihm.
p.   cm.
Includes bibliographic references and index.
ISBN 0-8147-6197-6 (cloth : alk. paper) — ISBN 0-8147-6198-4 (pbk. :
alk. paper) 1. Prosthesis—History.   I. Ott, Katherine. II. Serlin,
David. III. Mihm, Stephen.
RD130 .A784 2002
617'.9—dc21   2001006460

New York University Press books are printed on acid-free paper,
and their binding materials are chosen for strength and durability.

Manufactured in the United States of America

10 9 8 7 6 5 4 3 2 1

Contents

III: Use and Representation

The Sum of Its Parts

An Introduction to Modern Histories of Prosthetics

Katherine Ott

HISTORIES OF PROSTHETICS are probably better written by playwrights than by historians. The stories are full of contradiction, emotion, creativity, intrigue, and myth, gestures that are fraught with meaning, and sometimes improbable (but more often than not, tedious) events. There is the young woman, a double leg amputee, deciding what height she would like to be and her preferred shoe size as she is fitted with new legs. Another young woman, born without arms and legs, decides to forgo the use of any prosthetic limbs. Police in 1905 arrest a notorious woman who rides in public conveyances and uses artificial arms and hands seemingly to read a book, while her real hands pick the pockets of commuters seated beside her. In Tokyo, a *yakuza* decides to leave the gangster brotherhood but needs to replace the finger cut off during initiation. A 1930s housewife, recovering from cancer surgery, struggles to pay attention as her physician explains how to sew an artificial breast. A twelve-year-old wunderkind cellist inadvertently leaves her custom-made arm in a New York City taxicab. Soldiers in 1865, 1898, 1918, 1945, 1953, and 1968 wait for the government paperwork that will pay for their prostheses. What ties all these people together, besides visible bodily difference, is that each person enlists and integrates artificial parts in the practical details of daily living.[1]

The characters in this anthology are not cyborgs or bionic beings. Nor are they merely metaphors for empire, nationhood, or modernist anomie. Prostheses can certainly fill all those roles. In scholarly literature, prostheses usually perform cultural work unrelated to the

I

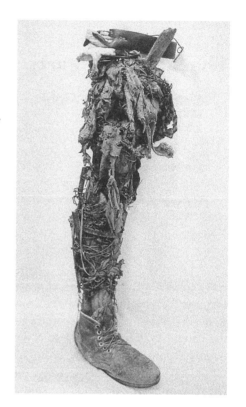

FIG. I.I. This late-20th-century leg, made and worn for fifteen years by Deroy Hill of South Carolina, captures the serendipity and opportunism in the lives of many prosthesis wearers. In self-reliant, do-it-yourself fashion, Hill framed his leg with wire and steel and kept it stuffed with cloth scraps as needed. Similarly, until the 1970s, it was common for women to sew their own breast prostheses. Although little else is known about Hill, his individuality and personality are strongly evident in his leg. Courtesy of the National Museum of American History, Smithsonian Institution.

practicalities of everyday life. One does not need real people to do a deep metaphorical analysis of symbolic forms; in many cases, putting real people into these scenarios would subvert or nullify the analysis. Prosthetic devices, as social objects with a complex set of meanings in the daily lives of people, have rarely, if ever, been understood as part of vernacular material life.

The essays in this anthology propose a historical perspective in order to provide a corrective to the vogue for prosthetics as found in psychoanalytic theory and contemporary cultural studies. Many scholars use the term "prosthesis" regularly, and often reductively, as a synonym for common forms of body-machine interface. This occurs most explicitly in discussions of the cyborg, especially as introduced by scholars of science and technology studies like Donna Haraway.[2] Books such as Celia Lury's *Prosthetic Culture* or Gabriel Brahm and Mark Driscoll's anthology *Prosthetic Territories* use prostheses metaphorically to discuss artificial objects that mediate human relations.[3] In these studies, which owe much to the critical work on technologies of self making proposed by Michel Foucault, any machine or technology that intervenes on human subjectivity, such as a telephone, a computer, or a sexual device, can be said to be prosthetic.[4] As Kathy Woodward has written, "[T]echnology serves fundamentally as a prosthesis of the human body, one that ultimately displaces the material body."[5] Such assertions, while intellectually provocative and culturally insightful, hardly begin to comprehend the complex historical and social origins of prosthetics. Cyborg theorists who use the term "prosthesis" to describe cars and tennis rackets rarely consider the rehabilitative dimension of prosthetics, or the amputees who use them. To a certain extent, prostheses do illustrate a type of body-machine interface emblematic of modern culture. What, after all, could be a greater expression of modern anomie than the worker or soldier who, after losing his or her arm to modern warfare or an industrial accident, gets a replacement limb fabricated of synthetic materials?

Analysis and interpretation of prostheses have also come from psychoanalytic theory. Thinkers as diverse as Sigmund Freud, Jacques Lacan, and Kaja Silverman have scrutinized the concept of the prosthesis in order to discuss somatic or cognitive dissonance between the natural body and an artificial appendage, fetish, or object.[6] Male injury, for example, is assuredly a symbolic emasculation but, in certain places, it is also a manly badge of courage.[7] Although none of the essays in this volume are overtly psychoanalytic, they do include numerous examples of prostheses as a literal symbol of more complex issues. The people in the history this volume chronicles were too busy living to be restrained by our post-structuralist worries over the cultural contingencies of what they did or who they were.

Rather than theorizing a post-structuralist body or using prosthetics as metaphors for other things, the contributors to this anthology take a material culture approach to their subject. It is certainly necessary to ask of prosthetics, "But what else is it?" and the influence of Donna Haraway and her students is undeniably profound. But such explorations tend to ignore the preexisting historical complexities. The material and social tales of prosthetics provide a more intimate and compelling history of embodied technology than any postmodern cyborg can account for: from the ivory, leather, and vulcanized rubber in Victorian artificial limbs, to the acrylic parts and power-assisted controls

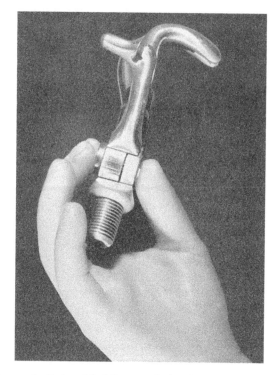

FIG. I.2. This prosthetic hand holding a split-hook prosthesis defies any one interpretation. The image not only illustrates the body-machine interface, it also fools the eye by presenting a peculiar kinship among machines. From Bess Furman, *Progress in Prosthetics* (Washington, DC: U.S. Department of Health, Education, and Welfare, 1962).

used in limbs of the 1950s and 1960s, to the CAD-CAM–designed prostheses of the twenty-first century, which, like many automated processes, threaten to eliminate the role of the prosthetist in the production of artificial limbs.[8]

All the essays in this collection focus on the materiality of the body, not only or exclusively its abstract and metaphoric meanings. Keeping prostheses attached to people limits the kinds of claims and interpretive leaps a writer can make. But more important, it excites new narratives and produces unconventional knowledge. Whereas some work, such as that of Judith Butler or David Wills, abstracts the body by elegantly theorizing it, historical studies, such as those of David Rothman or Joanne

Meyerowitz, depend primarily on uncritical accretion of detail or voyeuristic reduction.[9] Following in the footsteps of Michel Foucault, other scholars have examined the cultural dimensions of technologies associated with bodily surveillance, regulation, and control.[10] But their work tends to cast technology as the instrument of some ill-defined and diffuse set of power relations that, more often than not, obscures the identity and experience of individual historical actors. Scholars interested in the intersection of hardware and human tissue often find themselves trapped by the discursive model of the cyborg, which tracks analysis into a bland critique of contemporary culture, leaving history to an occasional footnote.

Instead, this collection interweaves theory with history, bringing to this combination the critical nuances of a social constructionist perspective so as not to lose track of the material body. Even though it critiques, historicizes, and theorizes prosthetics, this volume lays out a balanced and complex picture of its subject, and avoids either vilifying or celebrating the merger of the flesh and the machine.[11] The resulting essays demonstrate that the relationship between the body and technology cannot be understood simply in terms of domination, much less as the inexorable integration of human beings and machines. Instead, the peculiar history of prosthetic devices reveals the extent to which the evolution and design of technologies of the body are intertwined with the subjective and practical needs of people. It is the material "stuff" that most clearly conveys ideologies of body ideals, body politics, and culture and illuminates the relationship between technological change and the "civilizing process" of modernity.

It is also important to note that the essays in this volume look not so much at how "impairment" is a historically changing category but at how attempts to alter the effects of impairment are historically bound—tied as they are to the political and economic needs of nations. The authors indirectly (and sometimes, directly) examine the containment of cultures through artificial limbs. This involves such things as the shift in venues where information is represented—the 1893 Chicago World's Columbian Exposition versus a ninety-second spot on the nightly news. The mode and location of presentation of a prosthesis are significant especially because most people gain knowledge of prostheses through exhibition—whether in a Victorian Arts and Industry extravaganza, its modern incarnation on the Discovery Channel, or a museum showcase.

As is evident in nearly every life decision that entails thoughtful discrimination, from what we eat to how we speak, the aesthetics of representation are class-bound. Similarly, elaboration of the body has been profoundly shaped by capitalism. The economic politics of who owns one's self and therefore who has the power to make decisions about one's self have continuously influenced prosthetics making and wearing. Historians such as Barbara Duden have written about the European premodern body, which was owned by God or his surrogate, the king.[12] Individuals submitted their will and being to the sovereignty of a higher authority. In the second half of the eighteenth century, ownership of one's body shifted. Political thinkers formulated the concept of autonomy over one's own body. The individual gained responsibility and possession of his (women were still civilly dead for most purposes) own body and could be said to "have" a body in the modern sense. The rise of the possessive individual brought increased freedom to make choices, which in turn affected the aesthetics of consumption. A rough-hewn peg leg, good enough for the eighteenth-century laborer, became a relic in the nineteenth century. And in the late twentieth century, a cosmetic skin glove of polyvinyl chloride chastened the clumsy and rigid hand of 1890. Yet bourgeois values of order, control, and regulated work can reach only so far into consumer culture, as Raman Srinivasan illustrates in his essay on the low-tech, inexpensive Jaipur foot and its integration into Indian aesthetics.

As in the case of the Jaipur foot, homemade or simply made goods oppose consumer culture at the same time they participate in it. Kirsten E. Gardner writes that until the 1970s it was acceptable for women to make their own breast prosthesis, and medical aftercare included explanations of how to do it. Limb prosthesis wearers have always rigged customized devices to accommodate their needs, from terminal devices with Velcro for playing musical instruments to waterproofing for swimming. And the prosthesis is always altered to suit the anatomy of the owner. Wherever they occur, homemade limbs are highly individualized and carry the personality of the maker in ways that no commercially produced prosthesis does.

The aesthetics of capitalism are visible throughout the design history of prosthetics. Once function has been produced, everything that comes after it is value-added flourish. The cosmetic outer skin and the pigmentation added to it, toes and fingers, the iris, pupil, and scleral veins added to an artificial eye are all surplus. Overdesigned and -decorated technology, epitomized by the big chrome of the 1957 Buick, may be less gaudy when found on prostheses, but it is equally superfluous. Under capitalism, prosthesis wearers are the ultimate entrepreneurs, forced to adapt to ever changing economies both within their own bodies and in external bureaucracies of representation, assistance, and ideology.

There are many issues important to the history of prostheses that are not part of this volume. The history of prosthetics is largely unexplored; much research needs to be done before the intersections of such critical categories as race, ethnicity, and region can be understood. At present, there are few scholars working in this area. This anthology is intended to stimulate research and critical inquiry into questions about, for example, the gender dynamics of prostheses. Why is the best amputee the male amputee? In what way do female amputees fit into the dominant aesthetic paradigms? Why do limbs comprise the bulk of historical analysis in the field of prosthetics? Other prostheses in need of their Boswell include dentures, dental implants, assistive technologies, toupees, the artificial larynx, silastic penile prostheses for sexual impotence, artificial ears, noses, and hands. There are also devices that straddle the fence with orthotics, such as the iron lung, the cochlear implant, vibrators, eyeglasses, contact lenses, the intraoral obturator, and the wheelchair. Because this volume places the prosthetic boundary at the threshold of tissue—notwithstanding Alex Faulkner's essay on artificial hips and Elizabeth Haiken's on cosmetic implants—it excludes potential prosthetics such as blood substitutes, artificial organs, and other implants.[13] We also have not included essays on the current boom in high-tech, "gee-whiz" technologies under development and featured every week in awed infomercials and news stories.[14] Absent are essays on popular culture spin-offs such as Inspector Gadget, go-bots, comic book characters, television's enthusiastic expansion of the realm of prosthetics with lip-syncing rock stars, and the *Knight Rider* adventures of Kit the car.

The history of prosthetics has an intellectual "limb" in several fields of endeavor. Disability studies, histories of the body, medicine, and rehabilitation, histories of technology and engineering, and material culture studies all lay claim to this subject. The works in this anthology reflect those alliances. The book is deliberately interdisciplinary, with authors from fields as diverse as sociology, anthropology, American studies, science and technology studies, history, and gender and queer studies.

This anthology is deeply indebted to the work of scholars in disability studies, despite the fact that most of its authors do not think of themselves as working within that area of study. The authors come from several fields and have differing relationships to the topic, as makers, wearers, critics, and reluctant voyeurs. Yet all struggle with how to understand and situate prostheses. Without the foundation created by the vigorous work of disability scholars like Lennard Davis, Simi Linton, Paul Longmore, and Rosemarie Garland Thomson, a volume such as this could not have been conceptualized or published.[15]

Scholars in disability studies have produced complex critiques of the concepts of "normalcy" and beauty by challenging assumptions about self-definition, discrimination, equality, civil rights, citizenship, community, and the valorization of autonomy and independence. In this way, disability as an analytical category has much in common with the more familiar interpretive structures of race, class, and gender. These macro-concepts influence the creation and deployment of cultural processes related to politics, religion, sexuality, economics, fashion, leisure, and every other aspect of life. Yet disability often trumps race, class, and gender because it both consumes those categories and exists within them.

Disability studies scholars also offer powerful critiques of medical practice. In Western culture, popular and intellectual understanding of disability has been based on a medical model for over a hundred years. Just as having sex, eating meat, and drinking liquor have become medically related activities, so is understanding of the size, shape, and behavior of one's body. This means that for certain people, the nature of their difference is noticed according to a particular set of "noticing" rules that are vernacular versions of medical diagnosis. Diagnosis defines bodily difference as pathology. The process of diagnosis, formal or informal, whether employed by a medical practitioner or a personnel manager, places difference within organizational categories of loss and inadequacy. This act of diagnosis is fundamental to the medical model of understanding life. It seeks out difference and prioritizes impairment. This is inevitable because that is what medical diagnosis and its social counterpart are for: to a person with a hammer, everything looks like a nail.

Furthermore, the medical model assumes dependency, whether on a health care system or the kindness of strangers and family. This means that a person must have her or his difference reclassified as disability or

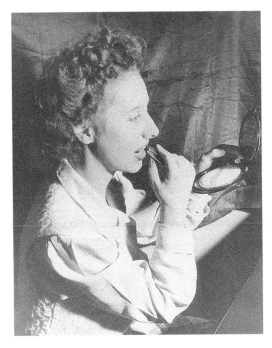

FIG. I.3. One indication of a prosthesis's success, mentioned throughout the professional literature on prostheses, is that the wearer be able to participate in courtship rituals, such as dancing and dating; the ultimate accomplishment is marriage. This woman, in a 1940s Science Service photograph, uses a hand that is imperceptibly prosthetic in applying lipstick. Courtesy of the Collections of the National Museum of American History, Smithsonian Institution.

impairment and validated by the health care system. Without that expert validation or corroboration, there is no access to basic goods and services necessary for living safely. Health insurance companies require prescriptions for clients in need of prosthetics and wheelchairs. These items, including artificial eyes, are classified along with hospital furniture as durable goods. David Serlin addresses some of this in describing the psychological "care industry" surrounding World War II veterans, though Serlin focuses more on the links between American masculinity and the engineering of prosthetics in the postwar era.

In the medical model, intrinsic to the high-speed track over which American culture clatters, impairment is equated with illness or pathology. Impairment and disability are something to be cured and treated,

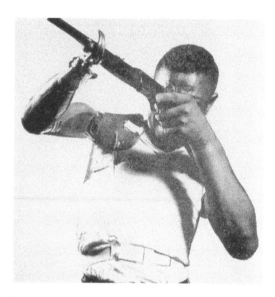

FIG. I.4. Masculinity, as represented with prostheses, often entails not so much "passing" for nondisabled as acting hypermasculine. The original caption for this image explained that the man's multiple-action shoulder unit permitted rifle shooting. In an image such as this, both manhood and disability are redeemed and even esteemed through the deployment of a prosthesis. From Leonard Bender, *Prostheses and Rehabilitation after Arm Amputation* (Springfield, IL: Charles C. Thomas, 1974).

changed and altered. Hence the familiar, stigmatizing terms that mark the relationship to medical cure, such as "cripple," "handicapped," "physically challenged," "retarded," as well as the stereotype of the heroic individual who cheerfully and doggedly overcomes obstacles despite medicine's failure to cure. Widespread acceptance of the medical model pressures the diagnosed disabled to achieve a degree of "normalcy" in which the individual performs or participates in normalcy, or tries to pass for normal. The norm, of course, is indeterminate and episodic, fluctuating between a twenty-year-old white male athlete during Olympic seasons and the current *GQ* cover model, the wife of the president, or a theme Barbie doll.[16]

Rituals of normalcy often necessitate the evocation of pity to stimulate emotion about disability. Doctors and rehabilitation workers present the wearing of a prosthesis as a strategy for avoiding pity and unwanted stares and questions.[17] These familiar rites are enacted in telethons and popular magazines and on the floor of Congress, where bodily difference is seen alternately as a threat, a tragedy, and an inspiration. Historical documents related to prosthetics are rife with visual narratives that chronicle the revocation of and return to normalcy.[18] These historical narratives include at least two graphics, a "before" and "after" image, and an explanation of the circumstances of the injury, in the form of personal or medical testimony. Until recently, in these graphic representations of heroic domination, it was the male body that was paraded, not the female. Although the disabled female body appears occasionally in medical textbooks, rarely does an image occur elsewhere. Conventions of female modesty, as well as ignorance about and public reluctance to discuss female anatomy, account for this historical lacuna. Additionally, since men more often than women worked in heavy industry and as soldiers, more men sustained disabling injuries.

While the human body in these graphic images is reducible to fragmented parts, such ideas are also common in medical doctrines.[19] Practitioners of traditional Western biomedicine assume that one can re-

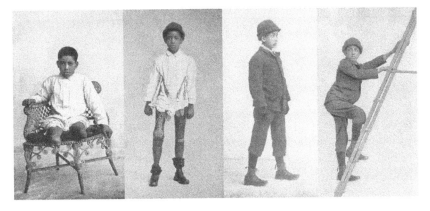

FIG. I.5. Visual narratives, such as this one about fourteen-year-old Johnnie Briggs, isolated prosthesis wearers and suspended them in time and place. The dramatic performance also required intimacy, represented by the boy's dependent and semi-naked state, which could be contrasted with a more public "cure" as Johnnie, now fully clothed, triumphantly climbed the ladder. From A. Condell, *Condell's Improved, Lifelike Artificial Legs and Arms* (New York: A. Condell, 1897).

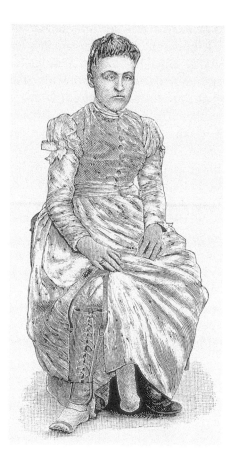

FIG. I.6. "Miss L. N., Newark, NJ, after Syme's amputation" is one of the few nineteenth-century images of women amputees. The discreet and genteel viewer was permitted to examine the prosthesis in its entirety, but only the ankle of Miss L. N. From A. Condell, *Condell's Improved, Lifelike Artificial Legs and Arms* (New York: A. Condell, 1897).

move, substitute, and alter parts of the body without altering the identity or integrity of the person. Examples from the history of prosthetics problematize this premise and challenge the cultural politics underneath the managerial approach to health care that require a segmented and decontextualized human body. The history of the last two hundred years chronicles the attrition of craft aspects and substitution of industrial processes rationalized for mass production, although some aspects of artificial body parts are still custom-made. Commercial ovens, compressors, and tasks broken into production line–oriented units have gradually become part of the fabrication process. The result is a method of small-scale production of artificial body parts that mirrors large-scale production of automobiles, refrigerators, and computers. Corporate health care budgets that group artificial eyes with invalid beds are practicing sound business under industrial capitalism. A plethora of artificial body parts with interchangeable components exist in commercial medicine and produce the illusion of abundance and consumer choice.[20]

Developments in medicine, of course, have had a far-reaching influence on the history of prosthetics.[21] Medical practitioners figure throughout as benevolent plunderers or bedeviled saints, but never as benign innocents. The push and pull of industrial capitalism is too well mapped throughout modern history for medicine to be able to claim a grounding in objective science (that hoary concept shorn of mystique by feminist science scholars) as a way to avoid engaging with the messiness of culture. Large and small shifts in medical practice have displaced fixed ideas about health and the wholeness of bodies. The use of antisepsis and disinfection after the 1870s meant that far more people survived surgery.[22] In the mid-nineteenth century, use of anesthesia such as ether and chloroform allowed for new amputation techniques, since a surgeon had more time to operate without an awake and writhing patient under the saw. A more carefully sutured skin flap over a stump resulted in a better fit in prosthetics. Before World War I, there was little or no coordination between the surgeon and the limb maker. This meant that many surgeons were unaware of the need to situate bones with a padding of tissue. Patients' follow-up by physicians came only when their stumps became infected, and then patients seldom went to the original surgeon for aid.

Consequently, the historical influence of amputation technique on prosthesis design is uneven.[23] This is illustrated by the history of Syme's operation. The surgeon James Syme published a description of his procedure for amputation at the ankle joint in 1843.[24] His operation was advantageous for the patient because the resection was farther from vital organs and kept more of the limb intact. In the decades after its introduction, physicians found that Syme's patients experienced fewer complications from cardiovascular disease, for example, than those who had amputations performed higher up the leg. Syme's amputees walked with less fatigue and had more mobility. The problem with the procedure, even today, is that prosthetists have found it nearly impossible to design an ankle joint piece that is durable enough to fit into the small area available and still function. Since the biomechanics of the human foot and ankle cannot be replicated with a prosthesis, amputation at the ankle joint is not often done.[25] Surgeons must take care to leave a padded stump, otherwise the leg bones will make walking painful when the person's weight forces down on the prosthesis. The stump will rub, become infected and inflamed, and cause medical complications for the amputee. Before widespread use of antisepsis, amputation often ended in death. During the Civil War, for example, a surgeon might use the same knife all day, wiping his hands and blade on his apron between patients. Soldiers had a macabre joke that, given a choice, they would rather have a limb shot off than cut off by a surgeon.

Historically, and even today, most amputations are of the lower extremities. The ratio of leg to arm amputation is four to one. In the West, leg amputation is usually performed on elderly patients and often necessitated by vascular deficiencies that accompany diabetes and heart disease. Unfortunately, civil wars worldwide and their land mine aftermath have produced many thousands of children and adults in need of both upper- and lower-extremity prostheses. Events in countries such as Angola, Thailand, Afghanistan, Cambodia, Bosnia, and Sierra Leone have fueled an international movement to ban the use of land mines as well as create grassroots programs to fabricate prosthetics from inexpensive, local materials. The Jaipur foot, which Raman Srinivasan writes about in this volume, is a low-tech device that costs less than a pair of Indian shoes.[26]

The fortunes of amputation are also related to the evolution of skin grafting and the repair of large areas of damaged skin. Modern skin graft and plastic techniques date from the 1820s, with the work of Johann Diffenbach, C. F. von Gräfe, Eduard Zeis, and others early in the nineteenth century.[27] Plastic surgery relied on transplantation of skin and successful suturing of tissue flaps, both critical to amputation and other reparative surgical techniques. Surviving battle injuries could depend as much on skin grafts as on bone cutting, especially if the wound involved expanses of soft tissue. In the late nineteenth century, surgeons performed split-thickness grafts with razor blades. They succeeded with mesh grafts around 1908 and fifteen years later were using mechanical dermatomes, which permitted cutting of uniform and predetermined thicknesses of skin. Skin grafting and plastic surgery advanced rapidly with each war, reaching professional maturation as a specialty in the 1920s.[28] Elizabeth Haiken's essay traces how cosmetic surgery and implanted prostheses became intertwined. In the twentieth century, understanding of blood groups, management of infection, discovery of penicillin and the commercial manufacture of its derivatives, along with sulfa drugs and insulin, increased the survival chances of persons with deep wounds and trauma, the precursors to amputation. Later, microsurgery brought improved vascularization to wounds and better outcomes in plastic surgery. Beginning in the 1960s and 1970s, surgeons could use extremely delicate instruments in vascular and nerve anastomes, the creation of channels between tiny vessels.

Rehabilitation medicine is the other medical specialty with obvious kinship with prostheses. Rehabilitation, as distinct from general nursing and postoperative care, is a relatively recent addition to medical practice. It originated in the specialty of electrotherapy, the application of mild electrical charges to the body, which began in the eighteenth century and was considered quackery until the late nineteenth century, when physicians employed it for its soporific effect, even though they could not explain how or why it worked. After the discovery of X-rays in 1895, many "electrical" physicians enthusiastically embraced the therapeutic use of the rays. Physicians who defected to radiology greatly thinned the ranks of electrotherapists and, around the time of World War I, the group expanded its definition to include physical therapists and other similar specialists. These early rehabilitation experts were also encouraged by states that were beginning to pass worker's compensation laws. As a result of the accretion of knowledge, the care provided for disabled World War I soldiers was markedly different from that given to injured soldiers in earlier conflicts. The Veterans Administration (VA) managed amputation centers for a while after World War I, and an artificial limb lab was established at Walter Reed Hospital in 1918. By the 1930s, the practice of rehabilitation medicine had matured sufficiently to support the specialty called physiatry. Physiatrists preferred mechanical adjustment and ultraviolet ray and heat treatments to drugs and surgery. World War II was a watershed period for rehabilitation medicine. Only four hundred men paralyzed from the waist down had survived World War I, but two thousand paraplegic men survived World War II. It was during World War II that the term "rehabilitation" came into common use, as standardization of devices and treatment protocols began in earnest.[29] Howard Rusk at New York University Medical Center, Henry Kessler in New Jersey, Mary E. Switzer in the Rehabilitation Services Administration, and Henry Betts in Chicago were among the most influential figures in shaping rehabilitation medicine in the postwar era. They participated, both formally and informally, in all the major research and development projects. In the 1950s and 1960s, rehabilitation centers became the primary locations for people in need of prosthetics, as care and treatment moved into the clinic and hospital.

If the histories of medicine, the body, and rehabilitation constitute the intellectual skin of the prosthesis, then surely technology contributes the scaffolding.[30] The writers in this anthology, coming from different disciplines, address technology in different ways by providing numerous examples of how a prosthesis is a tool a person intentionally uses for his or her own purposes. It can be simple or complex, homemade or mass-produced, mechanically engineered or high-tech. Nor is a prosthesis, as is true of every technology, hardware alone. It can serve as a prop or an accessory, a means to accomplish work, indicate gender, and so on. Historians of technology, such as Steven Lubar, David Landes, Carroll Pursell, and Ruth Schwartz Cowan, have established that technology is ideologically bound.[31] To understand technology, they argue, one needs to comprehend more than the sum of its hardware. Objects and devices are meaningless without their social and cultural context: railroad engines, barbed wire, and smart bombs, for just three examples, symbolize ideas about freedom, self-determination, and republicanism. And just as technologies are ideological tools, prosthetic technologies are no different. They are systems of power and economics that converge within the mainframe of technology, ideology, and the human body.[32]

Examination of the ideas and cultural circumstances that shape the material culture of prosthetic devices often reveals important disjunctions between the field of technology proper and its medical subsets. For example, the measure of success of an automobile engine is whether it gets the automobile (and you) safely to your destination. How should we determine the success of a kidney machine or an artificial limb? Medicine judges success by cure. But what of instances where medical cure cannot be achieved? Increasingly, in areas of medical measurement and assessment, effective use of a technology substitutes for successful medicine.[33] Or from another direction, as Sander Gilman and others have noted, if disease represents a loss of control, then technology is a powerful means for regaining it. In this arena, where prosthetics (and orthotics) exist, success is not about cure, but about technique. In the history of technology and medicine, the human body is a design and engineering project. In this narrative, prosthetists apply themselves to solving basic problems with materials, mechanics, and hardware. For legs, materials are needed that can bear weight and force. Limb joints have always posed engineering challenges. In the nineteenth century, using wood and metal increased the strength of joints but also made them too heavy for extended wear. Lighter shaft materials, such as celluloid, emitted a foul odor over time. A leather socket was flexible, but sweat made it stink with use. And in every era, the improper fit of a prosthesis—whether a limb, an eye, or an ear—can result in skin disorders and infection, and compromise the function of the device. Consequently, hygiene is critically important to both the wearer and the device, which must be of a design and composition that can withstand the chemistry of both cleaning fluids and bodily secretions. The use of molded plastics in early-twentieth-century manufacturing and acrylics and silicone after World War II brought solutions to many of these issues.

Makers spend long and frustrating Rotwang-like hours on elements related to retention and activation of prostheses.[34] The earliest described devices, explained by the surgeon Ambrose Pare in the 1560s, employed simple retention systems. The artificial eye, ear, or nose was held in place by a wire or strap that circled the head. Limbs fastened in a similar manner, with leather lacings and belts.[35] In the nineteenth and twentieth centuries, wearers frequently attached their facial prostheses to eyeglass frames. Others glued their prostheses in place and prayed for cool, dry weather. Mechanical and adhesive retention were joined by the Brånemark implant system in the 1970s and 1980s. P. I. Brånemark, a Scandinavian surgeon, figured out a method of securing screws in the bone of the jaw, cheek, skull, or elsewhere, depending on the prosthesis, which supported a thin bar. A silicone prosthesis was clipped to the bar via companion posts embedded in the artificial part. Called an osseo-integrated implant, the buried titanium post resided peacefully in the bone as tissue grew and bonded around it. Dental surgeons and prosthodontists were the first to use osseo-integrated implants in replacing teeth. From there, prosthetists adapted the technique to other maxillo-facial and head devices.[36] So far, the engineering problems in attaching a prosthetic limb directly to the bone have proved insurmountable. In the late 1940s, German and American researchers experimented with a tibia attachment for below-the-knee amputees, but

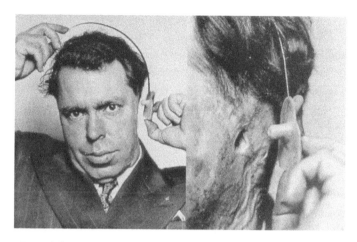

FIG. I.7. One of the most important design issues has been how to attach the prosthesis to the body. This mechanical retention device used a segment of a spiral clock spring to attach the prosthetic ear. From Arthur Bulbulian, *Facial Prosthesis* (Philadelphia: W. B. Saunders, 1945). Courtesy of Charles C. Thomas, Publisher, Ltd., Springfield, Illinois.

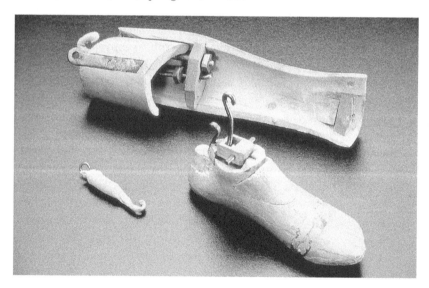

FIG. I.8. Government contracts for prosthetics for military veterans have been one of the most influential forces in stimulating new designs. This 1863 patent model of a leg, taken apart to show its joint mechanism, was part of the brisk market in prosthetics during the American Civil War. Courtesy of the Collections of the National Museum of American History, Smithsonian Institution.

they had little success.[37] Alex Faulkner, in his essay on artificial hips, offers another example of attachment mechanisms as he describes the design and materials for an internal environment.

Activating a prosthesis that requires functional movement entails other design solutions. A lower-limb prosthesis, for example, has one basic function—locomotion. Movement of an upper-extremity prosthesis, by contrast, is more complicated than a leg. A cable and shoulder harness device for activating arms and hands became popular during World War II and remains the most common body-powered method in use. In this appliance, a shoulder harness delivers movement through a cable mechanism as the wearer arches and relaxes his or her back. The postwar era also brought a number of improvements in upper-extremity limb design, such as multiplier lever systems and improved cable designs. Fabricators began to use magnesium, which is very light, to hollow cast artificial fingers. The use of plastic laminate for stump sockets dramatically improved fit and comfort for wearers. Northrup Aircraft, under a government contract, was among the first makers to successfully replace the older socket style of wood, leather, and metal with laminate plastic.[38]

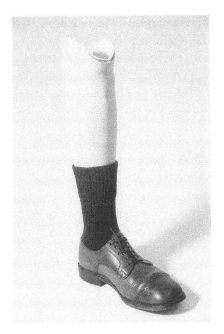

FIG. I.9. The use of plastics in limb fabrication brought a level of verisimilitude to prosthetics. This late-20th-century commercially made plastic leg with sock and shoe was contemporaneous with the home-made leg shown in figure I.1. Comparison of these two legs also illustrates class differentials in access to both medical care and consumer culture. Courtesy of the Collections of the National Museum of American History, Smithsonian Institution.

Earlier arm and hand designs provided little movement. Hands were designed for a single activity. The client had a hand made to suit his or her most frequent activity, such as holding cards, grasping a pen, gripping a knife or pistol, or remaining rigid.[39] A hand had no variable tension or pinch—only hold and release functions, activated by a button. Because of their mechanical nature, prostheses with joint mechanisms were often made by locksmiths and clock makers.[40] A more complicated and expensive control system increasingly in use since World War II is the myoelectric appliance. Myoelectric activation occurs when the prosthesis wearer contracts a designated muscle. The muscle signal is amplified and then relayed to a battery control, which in turn operates the hook or hand. Myoelectric limbs have yet to reach an engineering level that makes them commercially viable on a large scale.[41]

The emphasis on engineering fluid and elegant movement in prostheses reflected similar aesthetics found in other human contrivances. Hillel Schwartz has described the kinesthetic of natural motion that pervaded late-nineteenth- and most of twentieth-century aesthetics. Citing numerous inventions and innovations, such as modern dance, escalators, movies, the Ford assembly line, zippers, and the philosophy of children's play, Schwartz recorded the context in which engineers became captivated by the concept of torque in their search for strategies to integrate muscle and nerve with inanimate objects.[42] Torque, first used by electrical engineers, referred to the path and force of a twisting movement, such as torsion and rotation, around an axis. In prosthetics, the search for fluid movement sustained development of such innovations as cineplasty, popular in the 1950s, and the Seattle foot. In use since 1982, the Seattle foot employed an internal spring mechanism that gave the wearer added propulsion.[43]

Once nineteenth-century engineers and fabricators designed mechanisms to lessen the telltale joint snap or clapping sound when a foot hit the ground or clip as the shoulder cable released, they turned their attention to other issues. Archaic descriptions of prostheses as "anatomical machinery" gradually gave way to new formulations in the mid-twentieth century.[44] Some engineers took up careers with NASA in the U.S. space program. These engineers and biotechnicians looked to robotics and cybernetics for solutions to the physical limitations humans would encounter in outer space. Others became caught up in the thrill of using neuronal implants and nanotechnology to increase the efficiency of human function.

Since the 1960s, bionics and cybernetic organisms, or cyborgs, have overtaken more conventional prosthetic devices as the popular symbol of human-machine hybrids.[45] Since prosthetic devices are an embodied technology that predates cyborgs and cyberculture, prosthetic and cyborg aesthetics markedly differ. They diverge in the valence each carries in relation to a person who has become "machined-up." Cyberpunks and 'borgs can draw a crowd to a Web site or a Hollywood movie. On Madison Avenue and in *Wired* magazine, a high-tech human is sexy. Painters and performance artists like Matthew Barney and Stelarc, who play with categories of the artificial and natural, are esteemed as maverick visionaries. Voluntary bionics can be very desirable. But when the wearer has less of a choice, or when the technology references disability and not glamour, the attraction of engineered beauty fades. Rehabilitation technology is not worshiped in popular culture. A dusting of disability on the technology ends the beauty pageant. Cyborgs are divorced from disability and are commissioned by needs other than physiological.

The differences between prosthetics and cyborgs are reasonably clear, but the line between assistive and prosthetic technology is more like a hyphen. Assistive technology is a variation of traditional prostheses; both assist with independent living and access to life- and work-related activities. Since all useful technology is assistive, it is peculiar that we stipulate that some devices are assistive while others need no qualification. Besides serving to stigmatize and segregate a benign and inanimate entity—a device or appliance—the term "assistive technology" also needlessly complicates understanding of the devices so designated. Identifying telecaptioning decoders or voice recognition software as assistive technologies both reinforces outmoded categories of dependency and victimhood for those who use them, and tracks the technologies into professional and consumer groups where few people will find out about or benefit from them. The designation creates a technological ghetto at the margins of consumer and political culture. It also produces an odd logic. When is a widely used device such as the horseshoe-shaped neck pillow, insisted on by many long-distance airplane travelers and bedtime readers, merely a luxury item, and when does it become stigmatized as an assistive technology? Whose comfort is taken for granted and whose warrants qualification and justification? The same questions can be asked of such "assistive" technologies as sticky keys and zoom-text features on computers, or picture-based keyboards. In this sense, then, what do we say about typewriters and telephone headsets, or larger work site technologies like wheelbarrows and backhoes?

Devices to aid in daily activities have always existed, from Velcro to stirrups, from magnifying lenses to Ben Franklin's mechanical "Long Arm" as described by David Waldstreicher in this volume.[46] As Jennifer Davis McDaid and Heather R. Perry discuss in their essays, the kinds of devices that have come to be known as assistive technologies have their direct origins in institutions and programs organized for the rehabilitation of disabled soldiers and industrial workers. The Vocational Rehabilitation Act of 1918 and the Smith-Fess Act of 1920 funded vocational rehabilitation, which necessitated the creation of physical aids for daily tasks and work. The Social Security Act, subsequent amendments to it, and the Vocational Rehabilitation Act underwrote the maturation of the field, such that by the 1950s, assistive technology was well established. As a category of IT (information technology) devices, assistive technology was legislated into being by the U.S. government in the 1950s and 1960s. Engineers and physiatrists studied the new concepts coming out of ergonomics and human factors research and applied them to their clients. Section 504 of the Rehabilitation Act of 1973 went even further in pushing for technologies to facilitate access to public spaces and information, placing access within a civil rights framework.

During the 1960s, 1970s, and 1980s, numerous pieces of legislation required equal access to education, transportation, employment, and other public services. Each law brought more people into the community. As the population of people with disabilities grew and became more articulate, they pushed for and demanded universally designed facilities and products. The 1990 Americans with Disabilities Act built on this foundation. This modern disability rights movement, led by people with disabilities and supported by families, friends, and federal law, fueled the market for assistive technologies.[47]

One consequence of the channeling of government resources into development and fabrication of prostheses has been the amassing of vast visual and material stockpiles of ephemera. Every veterans hospital and VA clinic has old devices, photographs, and manuals related to rehabilitation. The quantity of prostheses and rehab equipment depicted in propaganda produced by the Veterans Administration, the National Institute on Disability and Rehabilitation Research (NIDRR), and other government-funded projects was intended to educate consumers as well as give the illusion of limitless possibility

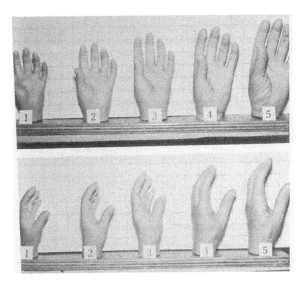

FIG. I.10. Part of the attraction of and interest in prosthetics for many people, especially those who do not wear one, is that they offer the utopian prospect of infinite choices and endless replacement of damaged or aging body parts. From Bess Furman, *Progress in Prosthetics* (Washington, DC: U.S. Department of Health, Education, and Welfare, 1962).

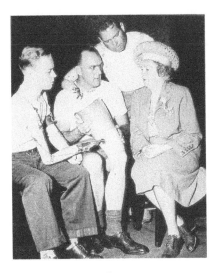

FIG. I.11. This photograph of a group of amputee veterans with a U.S. congresswoman was typical of postwar government propaganda intended to reassure families that injured soldiers received superior care. From Bess Furman, *Progress in Prosthetics* (Washington, DC: U.S. Department of Health, Education, and Welfare, 1962).

and opportunity thanks to federal agencies mobilized to meet the needs of its citizens.

As the wealth of the visual evidence demonstrates, the history of prosthetics is full of contradictions. One of the great design conundrums Stephen Mihm addresses in his essay is exactly why it took so many centuries—the existence of capitalism notwithstanding—for human-looking legs to replace the peg, stump, and crutch that dominated Western culture from Lazarus to Lincoln. Although the simulacra were not very lifelike—try as the builders might, they were heavy, noisy, stiff, dirty, and difficult to control—the Victorians were the ones who persisted with prosthesis designs that resembled real limbs. Their insistence cannot be explained as technological determinatism—that materials and technology made it possible—although a version of Thomas Hughes's theory of technological momentum may be at work in keeping the cultural dynamic of mimicry strong.[48] Certainly in our own time, an artificial leg that mimics a real one is the ideal, despite the fact that the easiest and most efficient design to use may not be one that is cosmetically acceptable. For example, a split hook hand is easier for the wearer to manipulate, but less real-looking. The circumstances that explain why function gave way to aesthetics need more scholarship.

David Serlin, Heather R. Perry, and Stephen Mihm describe how the enunciation and acceptance of a prosthesis by an individual represent a bourgeois commitment to a certain kind of productive citizenship. That is, the felicitous and smooth adaptation to an artificial limb at once proves the "rightness" of the capitalist-democratic mission and simultaneously asserts the individual's legitimate right to join the rest of us at the trough—whether it is Mihm's late nineteenth century, Perry's post–World War I Germany, or Serlin's 1950s. In the United States, Oliver Wendell Holmes and postwar-era engineers celebrated prosthetic technology in the belief that American exceptionalism inevitably leads to global dominance. For many, the second course in the wall of American greatness is laid by "Homo Faber," the legendary science and technology geek who can design Trident missiles for deterrence, as well as luxury cars and prosthetic limbs.

The 1990s brought a new influence in prosthetics design. Runner's legs, made for Aimee Mullins and other competitive athletes, imitated the flexion of the cheetah's leg and resembled the suspension band in a pickup truck more than a familiar articulated leg. This design trajectory of a technology—from mimicry to modification and then to disassocia-

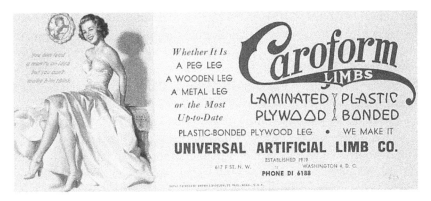

FIG. I.12. This ad for Caroform limbs depicts a glamorous woman with beautiful legs seated beneath a framed portrait of Cupid and the motto, "You can lead a man to an idea but you can't make him think." In this example of the cheesecake aesthetic typical of 1950s advertising, the (male) consumer is encouraged to associate the company's prosthetic limbs with desire and sexual potency. Courtesy of the author.

tion with the original—has happened many times in history. The first movable type resembled written script. Initially, railroad cars looked like horse-drawn coaches, and were pulled by horses along wooden and iron tracks. Early automobiles, the familiar horseless carriages, imitated buggies in design and suspension. Artisans of these technologies have long since abandoned any allegiance to their precursors. Following a similar course, many prosthesis makers in the late twentieth century took a turn into visionary engineering, where parts replicated neither form nor function of the human body. Engineers who believe that nature's way may not always be the best way continue to toy with and tease evolution. Engineering students are already at work on a generation of hand prostheses incorporating sensors that will communicate with computers and bypass the keyboard hardware.[49] Are prostheses, then, like bicycles and typewriters or like mechanical lipsticks? Is an artificial leg more like an antitoxin or an iron lung? Or maybe a hemostat or the elegant pin tumbler Yale lock? The answer depends on who does the asking.

If the history of prosthetics is about the history of medicine and technology, it is also about learning strategies to live with one's own body and adapt to circumstances, learning to understand other people's bodies. This is true whether you are a prosthesis maker, as Steven Kurzman recounts in this volume, or you are a fellow human with expectations about health, body appearances, and body functions. These intimate aspects of the history of prostheses lie buried in the compost of cultural events such as wars, economic shifts, and political changes.

Nothing has affected how we understand the integrity of the human body more than war and its aftermath of injured soldiers, civilian casualties, and the sequelae of generations dwelling with land mines and other live ordnance. Ethnic cleansings by machete and ax are as destructive to the human body as are bullets and bombs. The Civil War in the United States and the Napoleonic Wars in Europe initiated the first large-scale attention to prosthetics and their design and use. Jennifer Davis McDaid, in this volume, describes the experiences of Confederate veterans in petitioning the state of Virginia for limbs. As a result of the Civil War, federal, state, and local governments entered the business of providing limbs, made by contractors, for the thirty-five thousand amputee soldiers who survived. An 1862 federal law granted one artificial limb to each honorably discharged soldier and sailor. A. A. Marks and J. E. Hanger outbid competitors for lucrative contracts in supplying replacement limbs. The prospect of government contracts accelerated limb making, and competition spurred design. By 1895 the U.S. government had granted 144 patents for legs and in 1917, as the United States entered World War I, there were 200 artificial limb manufacturers in the country. Heather R. Perry, Elspeth Brown, and David Serlin look at war and its effect on limb making. Perry and Brown note the influence of scientific management in Germany and the United States in conceptualizing limbs as machines that can carry the gospel of efficiency deeper into the workplace. With nearly every modern war, governments have quickly mobilized to repair the bodies of their soldier casualties. The manner in which this is done and the way the citizenry reacts to it are parts of a complicated story of the need for national regeneration of public sentiments and rehabilitation of popular conventions of manhood, prowess, and their symbolic importance as the foundation of empire and military vigor.[50] David Serlin describes the importance for cold warriors to showcase technological superiority at all levels, including that of the mundane limb prosthesis, as the United States pressed its claim to global dominance.

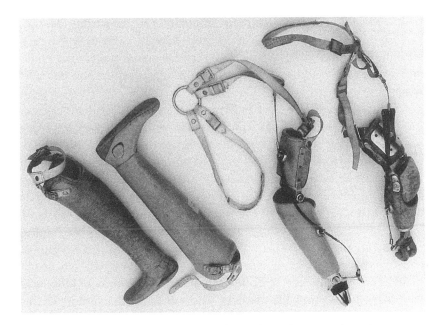

FIG. I.13. Although war injuries and industrial accidents are the primary reasons persons have need of prosthetics, other events have created prosthesis wearers too. These limbs from the 1960s were worn by a child whose mother had taken the sedative thalidomide during her pregnancy. Courtesy of the Collections of the National Museum of American History, Smithsonian Institution.

Sentimental references to war-wounded amputees abound in popular culture, from folklore about Antonio Lopez de Santa Ana's leg, lost at the 1838 Battle of Vera Cruz, to the dear departed arm of Stonewall Jackson, interred on a farm near Fredericksburg, Virginia, under a modest 1863 gravestone maintained by the National Park Service. Generations of soldiers have self-consciously forgone the wearing of prostheses, instead selecting eye patches and empty sleeves and trouser legs as the mark of courage, heroism, and manly sacrifice.[51] "Good-By, Old Arm," a popular 1865 parlor song, chronicles the supposedly true story of a young Union soldier who, upon awaking in the hospital tent to find his right arm amputated, called to have it brought to him for a tender and melodic farewell. The song also summarized why a pinned-up sleeve or pant leg played better in patriotic times: "O, Native land! O, hallowed soil! The birthplace of the free! Had I a dozen arms like this, I'd lose them all for thee." It was composed by the peripatetic evangelist Philip Phillips, who held singing services across the United States and around the world in India, Egypt, Australia, and the Sandwich Islands.[52]

Industrialization and urban living also created their share of prosthesis wearers. Factory work could be grim and dangerous, to both a seasoned worker and a new recruit more used to the pace and equipment of farm work than to that of three hundred-pound ingots, steam boilers, and belt-driven edge tools. Railroad wrecks, trolley accidents, and automobile crashes, as well as horse calamities, injured thousands of people, to say nothing of the pitfalls of unlit and unrepaired tenement stairs; wood, steam, and coal heating systems; mechanical reapers; dynamite; and misfiring rifles.[53] Stephen Mihm, in this volume, picks up this story in analyzing the importance to bourgeois citizens of maintaining the illusion of bodily wholeness in a world of industrial and domestic hazards. He presents, as do many of the authors in this volume, the dominant societal necessities of the nondisabled, who often understand disability as personal tragedy, shame, and loss. A. A. Marks, arguably the king of nineteenth-century prosthetics makers, explained to readers in nearly every catalog and pamphlet the need to "rescue the crippled from a life-long condition of dependence."[54] Marks explained to those undecided about wearing a prosthesis that not only was it natural to conceal physical defects, but also a conspicuous "deficiency of the body" attracted attention and invited sympathy, and such reactions from others were inimical to maintaining self-respect.[55] Physicians echoed these sentiments in their professional journals throughout the nineteenth and early twentieth centuries, in discussing the beneficial reasons for wearing a prosthesis. One doctor explained that a glass eye would deceive observers "by hiding a loathsome deformity, restoring personal appearance, and [be] the means of effecting a complete revolution in the worldly prospects of the wearer."[56]

Body aesthetics are too complicated to track through culture and across time or to present anything more than a few suggestive concepts in this introduction.[57] Modern worry over the boundary between humans and machines replaced medieval anxieties over the boundary between humans and animals.[58] Older fears of contamination of the human species through coupling with or possession by beasts, golems, and machines have been augmented by yet another identity-breaker.

The recent genetic manipulations of soybeans, tomatoes, corn, and other crops have produced trepidation over the potential ill effects of breaching species boundaries with insects and plants.[59] Elizabeth Haiken and Steven Kurzman, in this volume, examine some of the repercussions for human specificity, ableness, and subjectivity as a prosthesis wearer incorporates inorganic devices into personal identity.

In the seventeenth century, when disability was commonly interpreted as divine punishment for a moral or spiritual defect, some aesthetes thought it better not to walk at all, rather than to walk with a cumbersome gait and bring attention to one's failing. Note, too, that these Renaissance contour critics also invented the mouche, a patch of black plaster or a hanging curl of hair, deployed to cover a scar or blemish. In the eighteenth century, when men's fashions featured the leg with a flexed calf, commentators praised ballet-like walking and posture. By the nineteenth century, middle-class people felt peer pressure to use a prosthetic leg no matter how labored one's gait or hazardous to one's personal safety. Walking, whether with a prosthesis, crutch, or brace, was believed preferable to using a wheelchair or the even more stigmatizing knuckle-board associated with beggars and indigents. The premium placed on erect posture and mobility developed over time, from the eighteenth- and early-nineteenth-century emphasis on the spine and its alignment as the core for a fashionable clothing fit, to Europeans' mid-nineteenth-century proto-eugenical fears about racial decline and regression toward their ape ancestry, to the arrow-straight spine of the corseted Victorian ingenue.[60] Consequently, spinal alignment and a premium on erect posture figured in the artificial creation of gait with prostheses long before the science of ergonomics provided additional aesthetic imperatives.

One of the great themes of modernity has been how to make the everyday and the typical into something strange. Creators of film, photography, and other media, for example, portray typical experiences as exotic, dramatic, or ominous, in an effort to gain an audience. Medicine, too, has been indispensable in pathologizing the typical. Medical workers isolate fragments of bodies—which is what medical specialists spend their lives training to do—and interpret the fragments as flawed or broken or diseased as they place each disembodied piece along an arbitrary continuum. Scholars have tried to explain the modern fascination with the exotic or aberrant in various ways, by examining it through the lens of the search for authenticity in an alienating world,

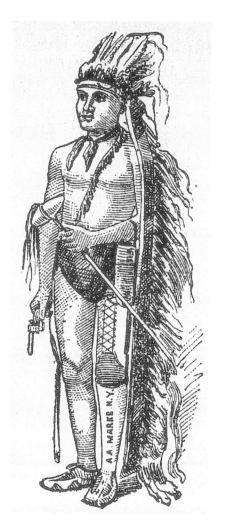

FIG. I.14. Graphic images of people
wearing prostheses have often incorporated elements of the strange or
bizarre, reflecting the modernist
need to make the everyday into
something exotic. From A. A. Marks,
Manual of Artificial Limbs (New York:
A. A. Marks, 1893).

the crisis of authority and waning of deference politics, the search for
the real thing, and the essentialist formulations of early anthropologists. Europeans and their descendants struggle with the mythic attraction of an uncensored experience and authentic consciousness that
are constantly obscured by the mirage of modern existence. The
search for authenticity pits contrived nature against an equally contrived artificiality, with the more prestigious nature understood as
what looks real.[61]

Histories of prosthetics enable us to ask about the body's limits, boundaries, and essence, as well as about authenticity and agency. Since the 1960s and 1970s, the most powerful force in redirecting and criticizing the conventional wisdom on bodily difference, next to feminist theory, has been the disability rights movement. The movement resulted from several historical processes. Beginning in the 1940s and 1950s, as a result of improved medical treatment and care, the life expectancy of people with disabilities dramatically increased. Men with paraplegia from war injuries, who ten years earlier would have died from urinary tract infections and other complications, survived and required assistance. Children who contracted polio survived and needed to attend school. Parents fought for education and other services for their children. Once those children grew to adulthood, many of them became incensed about the denial of their rights guaranteed under the U.S. Constitution. People with disabilities, who in other eras would have been isolated in their homes or in institutions, began to meet each other in centers for independent living and later over the Internet. They compared experiences and shared alternative ways to interpret their lives and organize their environments. The successes of the African American civil rights movement also inspired people and propelled them into action. As a result of all this, the community of consumers with disabilities expanded, and along with it, came criticism of concepts such as "normal," "perfect," and "beautiful."

In addition to advocating legislation and alterations to public space, disability rights activists challenged (and continue to question) the representation of people with disabilities. Academic activists have written extensively about issues of representation and interpretation of people with disabilities, aesthetics, and the cultural influences of politics, class, and gender.[62] All the essays in this volume are about representation in some way, since all are about cultural understanding of prostheses.

The shifting technological metaphors used to model human bodies show up in several essays. Stephen Mihm and Heather Perry articulate the body of the high mechanical age—when leather, wood, ivory, and rubber were used to approximate the mechanical behavior of joints, sockets, stumps, and muscles. David Serlin and Steven Kurzman show us how in the mid-twentieth century this model was replaced by an engineering or circuitry model, in which designers used electronic and chemical devices to imitate the brain and nervous system through my-

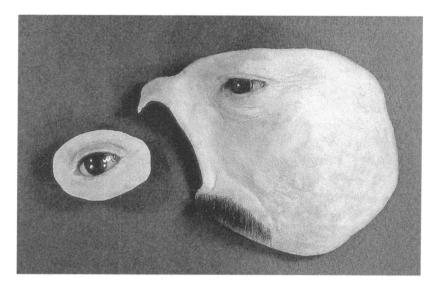

FIG. I.15. Facial restorations made of acrylic, from the 1970s. Courtesy of the Collections of the National Museum of American History, Smithsonian Institution.

oelectrics and cybernetics. Design of hearing aids also illustrates this shift: nineteenth-century aids increased sound collection and amplification in support of the mechanical work of the outer ear and tympanum. The cochlear implant, a late-twentieth-century device, works by direct electrical stimulation of the auditory nerve.

Elizabeth Haiken, Kirsten E. Gardner, and Katherine Ott describe yet another consequence of the shift in representation of the body. In the nineteenth century, "looking" and studied observation of the natural world became a primary activity of the middling classes. The education of the eye became an important life skill. This domestication of sight was simultaneous with an emphasis on "appearance" as crucial to comprehending everyday life. Sight was converted into vision, as seeing became equivalent to understanding.[63]

Finally, the essays in this anthology are loosely organized to reflect the chronological experience of a person who uses a prosthesis, through need, design, and use. David Serlin, Heather Perry, Kirsten Gardner, and Jennifer Davis McDaid analyze circumstances related to a need for an artificial part. Katherine Ott, Elizabeth Haiken, Alex Faulkner, and

Steven Kurzman discuss the cultural and individual pressures on the professionals who engineer the prosthesis. Elspeth Brown, Stephen Mihm, David Waldstreicher, and Raman Srinivasan discuss the relationship of prostheses to the practicalities of everyday life. All the essays gamely plunge into the relationship between the body and technology, a topic of increasing urgency in this era of high-tech capitalism.

NOTES

1. This anthology focuses on prosthetic devices. As editors, we somewhat arbitrarily define prosthetics as external appliances used either to restore function or for physiological cosmetic effect. Orthotics is closely related to prosthetics but not within the scope of this volume. Orthoses generally do not replace body parts, but instead support parts that have limited function. Orthoses typically include such things as braces, splints, elastic wrist bandages, custommade shoes, walkers, and crutches. Orthoses are more often used by people who have had polio, a stroke, or spinal cord injury rather than an amputation. For more on orthotics, see the American Academy of Orthopedic Surgeons, *Atlas of Orthotics: Biomechanical Principles and Application* (St. Louis: Mosby, 1985).

One further note about terminology. The authors use the terms "prosthesis," "prosthetic," and "prosthetic device" interchangeably. Additionally, although "epithesis" is the international term for facial prosthesis, to keep the language as free of jargon and complicated vocabulary as possible, we use the latter term wherever appropriate.

2. For some pertinent examples, see Donna Haraway, *Simians, Cyborgs, and Women: The Re-Invention of Nature* (New York: Routledge, 1991); Chris Hables Gray, ed., *The Cyborg Handbook* (New York: Routledge, 1995); Mark Seltzer, *Bodies and Machines* (New York: Routledge, 1992); and Hillel Schwartz, "Torque: The New Kinaesthetics," in Jonathan Crary and Sanford Kwinter, eds., *Incorporations: Fragments for a History of the Human Body* (New York: Zone Books, 1992).

3. Celia Lury, *Prosthetic Culture: Photography, Memory, and Identity* (New York: Routledge, 1998); and Gabriel Brahm Jr. and Mark Driscoll, eds., *Prosthetic Territories: Politics and Hypertechnologies* (Boulder: Westview, 1995).

4. See, for example, Luther H. Martin, Huck Gutman, and Patrick H. Hutton, eds., *Technologies of the Self: A Seminar with Michel Foucault* (Amherst: University of Massachusetts Press, 1988).

5. Kathleen Woodward, "From Virtual Cyborgs to Biological Time Bombs: Technocriticism and the Material Body," in Gretchen Bender and Timothy Druckery, eds., *Culture on the Brink: Ideologies of Technology* (Seattle: Bay Press, 1994), 50.

6. See, for example, Sigmund Freud, *The Four Fundamental Concepts of Psychoanalysis* (New York: Norton, 1998); Jacques Lacan, *Ecrits: A Selection* (New York: Norton, 1982); Kaja Silverman, *The Threshold of the Visible World* (New York: Routledge, 1995).

7. Roxanne Panchasi has shown, for example, how the scarred, maimed male bodies of World War I amputees in France became a fantasy site for dreams of national recuperation. See Roxanne Panchasi, "Reconstruction: Prosthetics and the Rehabilitation of the Male Body in World War I France," *differences: A Journal of Feminist Cultural Studies* 7.3 (1995): 109–40.

8. CAD-CAM stands for computer-assisted device, computer-assisted manufacture. The CAD-CAM process uses a scanner to image the body and also fabricate the replacement part.

9. See, for example, Judith Butler, *Bodies That Matter: On the Discursive Limits of "Sex"* (New York: Routledge, 1993); David Wills, *Prosthesis* (Stanford: Stanford University Press, 1995); David Rothman, *Medicine and Western Civilization* (New Brunswick: Rutgers University Press, 1995); Joanne Meyerowitz, "Sex Change and the Popular Press: Historical Notes on Transsexuality in the United States, 1930–1955," *Gay and Lesbian Quarterly*, spring 1998, 159–87.

10. Bryan Turner, *The Body and Society* (Oxford: Basil Blackwell, 1984); Seltzer, *Bodies and Machines*; Anson Rabinbach, *The Human Motor: Energy, Fatigue, and the Origins of Modernity* (New York: Basic Books, 1990); Haraway, *Simians, Cyborgs and Women*.

11. For an attack on machined bodies, see Nina Lykke and Rosi Braidotti, eds., *Between Monsters, Goddesses and Cyborgs: Feminist Confrontations with Science, Medicine, and Cyberspace* (New Jersey: Zed Books, 1996). For an enthusiastic embrace of cyborgs, see Donna Haraway, "A Manifesto for Cyborgs: Science, Technology and Socialist Feminism in the 1980s," *Socialist Review* 15 (1985): 65–107.

12. See, for example, Barbara Duden, *The Woman beneath the Skin: A Doctor's Patients in Eighteenth Century Germany* (Cambridge: Cambridge University Press, 1998); and Carolyn Bynum, *Fragmentation and Redemption: Essays on Gender and the Human Body in Medieval Religion* (New York: Zone Books, 1991).

13. For background on some of these excluded topics, see Wilfred Lynch, *Implants* (New York: Van Nostrand, 1982); Rachel Maines, *The Technology of Orgasm: The Vibrator and Women's Sexual Satisfaction* (Baltimore: Johns Hopkins University Press, 1999); Stuart Blume, "Histories of Cochlear Implantation," *Social Science and Medicine* 49 (1999): 1257–68; John Najarian and Richard Simmons, eds., *Transplantation* (Philadelphia: Lea and Febiger, 1972); Janice Cauwels, *The Body Shop: Bionic Revolutions in Medicine* (St. Louis: C. V. Mosby, 1986); Robert Shanks and James Shanks, "Laryngectomee Rehabilitation: Past and Present," *Speech and Language: Advances in Basic Research and Practice* 9 (1983): 103–52.

For an early description of obturators, a prosthesis used to close cleft palates, see James Snell, *Observations on the History, Use, and Construction of Obturators, or Artificial Palates* (London: Callow and Wilson, 1828).

14. For descriptions of this, see, for example, William Schwartz, *Life without Disease: The Pursuit of Medical Utopia* (Berkeley: University of California Press, 1998).

15. Disability studies is a thriving field. A selection of the most important works includes Lennard J. Davis, ed., *The Disability Studies Reader* (New York: Routledge, 1997); Gary Kiger, Stephen C. Hey, and J. Gary Linn, eds., *Disability Studies: Definitions and Diversity* (Salem, OR: Society for Disability Studies and Willamette University, 1994); Simi Linton, *Claiming Disability: Knowledge and Identity* (New York: New York University Press, 1998); Paul K. Longmore, "A Note on Language and the Social Identity of Disabled People," *American Behavioral Scientist* 28 (January–February 1985): 419–23; David T. Mitchell and Sharon L. Snyder, eds., *The Body and Physical Difference: Discourses of Disability* (Ann Arbor: University of Michigan Press, 1997); Rosemarie Garland Thomson, *Extraordinary Bodies: Figuring Physical Disability in American Culture and Literature* (New York: Columbia University Press, 1997); Rosemarie Garland Thomson, ed., *Freakery: Cultural Spectacles of the Extraordinary Body* (New York: New York University Press, 1996); Thomas G. Couser, *Recovering Bodies: Illness, Disability, and Lifewriting* (Madison: University of Wisconsin Press, 1997).

16. Among the works that analyze the production of normative knowledge, see Lennard J. Davis, *Enforcing Normalcy: Disability, Deafness and the Body* (New York: Verso, 1995); Georges Canguilhem, *The Normal and the Pathological*, trans. Carolyn Fawcett (New York: Zone Books, 1989); Carol Donley and Sheryl Buckley, eds., *The Tyranny of the Normal* (Kent: Kent State University Press, 1996); Sander Gilman, *Picturing Health and Illness: Images of Identity and Difference* (Baltimore: Johns Hopkins University Press, 1995).

17. See, for example, the prosthetist A. A. Marks's discussion, "Is It Profitable to Buy an Artificial Limb?" in A. A. Marks, *Manual of Artificial Limbs* (New York: A. A. Marks, 1905), 183–87.

18. Typical graphic stories about the redemption of the disabled through deployment of prosthetic devices can be found in Garrard Harris's appropriately titled book *The Redemption of the Disabled: A Study of Programmes of Rehabilitation for the Disabled of War and of Industry* (New York: D. Appleton, 1919). See also William Bainbridge, *Report on Medical and Surgical Developments of the War: U.S. Naval Medical Bulletin* (Washington, DC: Government Printing Office, 1919); Berton Blakeslee, ed., *The Limb-Deficient Child* (Berkeley: University of California Press, 1963).

19. The essays in this volume also integrate concepts developed by scholars working in the history of the body. This field addresses issues such as the role of capitalism in shaping strategies for bodily maintenance and health, and

the politics of the aesthetics of beauty and normalcy. Important works include Norbert Elias, *The Civilizing Process* (New York: Urizen Books, 1978); Mike Featherstone et al., eds., *The Body: Social Process and Cultural Theory* (London: Sage, 1995); Peter Freund, *The Civilized Body: Social Domination, Control and Health* (Philadelphia: Temple University Press, 1986); Hillel Schwartz, *Never Satisfied: A Cultural History of Diets, Fantasies and Fat* (New York: Free Press, 1986); David Lowe, *The Body in Late-Capitalist USA* (Durham: Duke University Press, 1995); Pasi Falk, *The Consuming Body* (London: Sage, 1994).

20. For more on the economics of modern medicine, see Rosemary Stevens, *American Medicine and the Public Interest: A History of Specialization* (Berkeley: University of California Press, 1998); Rosemary Stevens, *In Sickness and in Wealth: American Hospitals in the Twentieth Century* (New York: Basic Books, 1989); Marc Berg, *Rationalizing Medical Work: Decision-Support Techniques and Medical Practices* (Cambridge: MIT Press, 1997).

21. This book contributes to the growing literature that offers historical and cultural critiques of medicine and health care. Some of these include Katherine Ott, *Fevered Lives: Tuberculosis in American Culture since 1870* (Cambridge: Harvard University Press, 1996); Roger Cooter and John Pickstone, eds., Medicine in the Twentieth Century (Newark, NJ: Harwood Academics, 2000); Robert Aronowitz, *Making Sense of Illness: Science, Society, and Disease* (Cambridge: Cambridge University Press, 1998); Tera Ziporyn, *Nameless Diseases* (New Brunswick: Rutgers University Press, 1992); and John Harley Warner, *The Therapeutic Perspective* (Cambridge: Harvard University Press, 1989).

22. For this history, see Thomas Gariepy, "The Introduction and Acceptance of Listerian Antisepsis in the United States," *Journal of the History of Medicine and Applied Sciences* 49 (1994): 167–206; Jerry Gaw, *Time to Heal: The Diffusion of Listerism in Victorian Britain* (Philadelphia: American Philosophical Society, 1999).

23. For background on amputation during the Civil War, see, for example, Laurann Figg and Jane Farrell-Beck, "Amputation in the Civil War: Physical and Social Dimensions," *Journal of the History of Medicine and Allied Sciences* 48 (1993): 454–75.

24. James Syme, "Amputation at the Ankle Joint," *Monthly Journal of Medical Science* 3 (1843): 93.

25. For more on Syme's amputation, see Valarie Cottrell-Ikerd et al., "The Syme's Amputation: A Correlation of Surgical Technique and Prosthetic Management with an Historical Perspective," *Journal of Foot and Ankle Surgery* 33 (1994): 355–64.

26. For technical background on the foot, see Shri Gopal Kabra and Ramji Narayanan, *The Jaipur Ankle Foot Prosthesis: A Manual of Fabrication and Testing* (Jaipur, India: Rawat Publications, 1991).

The cost of a custom-made U.S. prosthesis has always been high. In 1889 George Tiemann and company sold a nose or ear for $50 to $100. A leg cost from $15 to $25 and an upper extremity, $75 to $150. In addition, yearly maintenance for a limb (in 1900) was anywhere from $5 to $50. In 1981 the Hanger Company sold a below-elbow prosthesis for about $870 and a hook for $155. A Hanger cosmetic hand and glove cost $181. In 1995 the cumulative five-year cost for a typical below-the-knee amputee was $6,200–$20,000. See Douglas Smith et al., "Prosthetic History, Prosthetic Charges, and Functional Outcome of the Isolated, Traumatic Below-Knee Amputee," *Journal of Trauma* 38 (1995): 44–47.

27. Although Gaspare Tagliacozzi in the sixteenth century and members of the potters' caste in eighteenth-century India performed nasal reconstructive surgery, there was not enough supporting knowledge to make plastic surgery a viable practice until well into the nineteenth century. The first textbook in plastic surgery, *Handbuch der plastischen Chirurgie*, was written by Eduard Zeis and published in Berlin in 1838.

28. For the history of reconstructive and plastic surgery, see Elizabeth Haiken, *Venus Envy* (Baltimore: Johns Hopkins University Press, 1997); Sander Gilman, *Creating Beauty to Cure the Soul: Race and Psychology in the Shaping of Aesthetic Surgery* (Durham: Duke University Press, 1998). Physicians' histories of the subject include Maxwell Maltz, *Evolution of Plastic Surgery* (New York: Froben Press, 1946); Blair Rogers, "A Chronologic History of Cosmetic Surgery," *Bulletin of the New York Academy of Medicine* 47.3 (March 1971): 265–302; B. K. Rank, "The Story of Plastic Surgery, 1868–1968," *Practitioner* 201 (1968): 114–21.

29. For the history of rehabilitation, see Roger Cooter, *Surgery and Society in Peace and War: Orthopaedics and the Organization of Modern Medicine, 1880–1948* (London: Macmillan, 1993); Glenn Gritzer and Arnold Arluke, *The Making of Rehabilitation: A Political Economy of Medical Specialization, 1890–1980* (Berkeley: University of California Press, 1985).

30. Several of the authors in this anthology directly engage the secondary literature on the development and use of medical technology. These include studies such as Ott, *Fevered Lives*; Cauwels, *The Body Shop*; Susan Bartlett Foote, *Managing the Medical Arms Race* (Berkeley: University of California Press, 1992); Joel Howell, *Technology in the Hospital: Transforming Patient Care in the Early Twentieth Century* (Baltimore: Johns Hopkins University Press, 1995); Andrew Kimbrell, *The Human Body Shop: Engineering and the Marketing of Life* (San Francisco: HarperSanFrancisco, 1993); Stanley Reiser, *Medicine and the Reign of Technology* (New York: Cambridge University Press, 1978); Sandra Tanenbaum, *Engineering Disability: Public Policy and Compensatory Technology* (Philadelphia: Temple University Press, 1993); John H. Knowles, ed., *Doing Better and Feeling Worse* (New York: Norton, 1977).

31. Works in the social history of technology that frame this volume include Ruth Schwartz Cowan, *Social History of American Technology* (New York: Oxford University Press, 1997); Steven Lubar and David Kingery, eds., *History from Things: Essays on Material Culture* (Washington, DC: Smithsonian Press, 1993); David Landes, *Revolution in Time* (Cambridge: Harvard University Press, 1983); David Noble, *America by Design* (Oxford: Oxford University Press, 1977); David Nye, *American Technological Sublime* (Cambridge: MIT Press, 1993); Carroll Pursell, *The Machine in America: A Social History of Technology* (Baltimore: Johns Hopkins University Press, 1995); Brooke Hindle, *Emulation and Invention* (New York: Norton, 1981); Adrian Forty, *Objects of Desire: Design and Society from Wedgewood to IBM* (New York: Pantheon, 1986); Thomas P. Hughes, *American Genesis* (New York: Viking, 1989); Wiebe Bijker et al., eds., *The Social Construction of Technological Systems: New Directions in the Sociology and History of Technology* (Cambridge: MIT Press, 1987).

32. Many writers have undertaken to explain the role of technology within political and economic power structures. See, for example, Michael Adas, *Machines as the Measure of Men: Science, Technology, and Ideologies of Western Dominence* (Ithaca: Cornell University Press, 1989); Bruno Latour, *Aramis, or The Love of Technology* (Cambridge: Harvard University Press, 1996); Arjun Apadura, *The Social Life of Things* (Cambridge: Cambridge University Press, 1996); Donald Norman, *The Design of Everyday Things* (New York: Doubleday, 1988).

33. Lewis Thomas has written about the use of "half-way technology." such as an iron lung, which does not cure, but stabilizes and supports the body through trauma and crisis. See Lewis Thomas, *The Medusa and the Snail* (New York: Viking, 1979).

34. The conceptual elements for limb design include the type of suspension for the appliance, type of control harness, type of terminal device (for legs for running, walking, swimming; hands for writing, tools, etc.), location of the amputation, and the contour of the stump. For more on technical aspects, see Paula Sauerborn, "Advances in Upper Extremity Prosthetics in the United States during World War II and Early Post–World War II Era," *Journal of Facial and Somato Prosthetics* 4.2 (1998): 93–104.

For typical manuals on the design and use of prostheses, see E. Muirhead Little, *Artificial Limbs and Amputation Stumps* (Philadelphia: P. Blakiston's Sons, 1922); Arthur Bulbulian, *Facial Prosthesis* (Philadelphia: W. B. Saunders, 1945); Bess Furman, *Progress in Prosthetics* (Washington, DC: U.S. Department of Health, Education, and Welfare, 1962); A. Bennett Wilson Jr., *Limb Prosthetics* (Huntington, New York: Robert E. Krieger, 1976). Rotwang was the obsessed inventor in Fritz Lang's 1926 classic film *Metropolis*.

35. For information on early devices, see Vittorio Putti, *Historic Artificial Limbs* (New York: Paul Hoeber, 1930).

36. Other osseointegration systems exist, such as the core-vent implant, introduced in 1982. The Brånemark system is well documented and the most commonly used in facial prostheses. For technical information on osseointegrated implants, see M. Gregory et al., "A Clinical Study of the Dental Implant System," *Journal of the British Dental Association* 168.1 (1990): 18–23; John Ismail and Hussein Zaki, "Osseointegration in Maxillofacial Prosthetics," *Dental Clinics of North America* 34.2 (1990): 327–41.

37. Eugene Murphy, "History and Philosophy of Attachment of Prostheses to the Musculo-Skeletal System and Passage through the Skin with Inert Materials," *Journal of Biomedical Materials Research Symposium* 7.4 (1973): 275–95.

38. See Sauerborn, "Advances in Upper Extremity Prosthetics;" Gilbert Motis, comp., *National Research Council Committee on Artificial Limbs . . .Contractor's Final Report* (Hawthorne, CA: Northrup Aircraft, 1951).

39. See, for example, Carl Geissler, "Description and Illustration of Artificial Hands and Arms," *Medical Progress in Technology* 2 (1974): 171–74.

40. Reed Benhamou, "The Artificial Limb in Preindustrial France," *Technology and Culture* 35 (1994): 835–45.

41. For technical data on the use of myoelectric arms, see Committee on Prosthetics Research and Development, "Report: Seventh Workshop Panel on Upper-Extremity Prosthetics of the Subcommittee on Design and Development; Externally Powered Devices" (Santa Monica, CA: Committee on Prosthetics Research and Development, 1969). The 1981 cost of a below-elbow prosthesis with a myoelectric hand was $3,500.

42. Schwartz, "Torque: The New Kinaesthetics." See also Rabinbach, *The Human Motor.*

43. For descriptions of the Seattle, SACH, and recent ankle and foot prostheses, see Joan Edelstein, "Prosthetic Feet: State of the Art," *Physical Therapy* 12 (1988): 1874–81. For cineplasty, see Henry Kessler, *Cineplasty* (Springfield, IL: Chas. C. Thomas, 1947).

44. An example of the nineteenth-century machinery approach is George Yerger and John Ord, *The United States Orthopedic Institute for the Application of Improved Anatomical Machinery to the Treatment of Every Variety of Deformity* (Philadelphia: George Yerger and John Ord, 1851).

45. For more on the rise of cyberculture, see Gray, *The Cyborg Handbook.*
A crucial difference between prosthetics and cyborgs is that the cyborg is a hybrid biological-mechanical machine that exceeds the limits of the organic human body. By contrast, the prosthesis wearer is a person who has adopted an appendage or organ to restore some component of able-bodied functioning. The concept of the cyborg applies to circumstances in which a prosthesis is used to transcend the organic boundaries of the human body.

46. For early descriptions of prosthetic devices designed to assist people with disabilities, see George Webb Derenzy, *Enchiridion, or A Hand for the*

One-Handed (London: T. and G. Underwood, 1822); "Man and His Machines," *World's Work* 36 (June 1918): 221–24.

47. Karen Fippo et al., *Assistive Technology: A Resource for School, Work, and Community* (Baltimore: Paul H. Brookes, 1995), 8–21. For background on the disability rights movement, see Fred Pelka, *The ABC-CLIO Companion to the Disability Rights Movement* (Santa Barbara, CA: ABC-CLIO, 1997); Paul Longmore and David Goldberger, "The League of the Physically Handicapped and the Great Depression: A Case Study in the New Disability History," *Journal of American History* 87 (2000): 888–922; and Joseph Shapiro, *No Pity: People with Disabilities Forging a New Civil Rights Movement* (New York: Random House, 1993).

48. Thomas Hughes, *Networks of Power: The Social Construction of Technological Systems* (Cambridge: MIT Press, 1987). See also Merritt Roe Smith and Leo Marx, eds., *Does Technology Drive History? The Dilemma of Technological Determinism* (Cambridge: MIT Press, 1994).

49. "Phantom Finger Control Possible for Those Born without Hands, Young Investigator Finds," *Biomedical Instrumentation and Technology*, March–April 1999, 138–39.

The relationship of engineering to cultural sensibilities is especially fraught in the fields of artificial organs and genetics. It remains to be seen whether prosthetics and biomedicine continue to follow a technological model or a humanities model as they develop. For more on the controversy over genetics, see Enzo Russo and David Cove, *Genetic Engineering, Dreams and Nightmares* (New York: Oxford University Press, 1998); Lily Kay, *Who Wrote the Book of Life? A History of the Genetic Code* (Stanford: Stanford University Press, 2000); Jeremy Rifkin, *The Biotech Century: Harnessing the Gene and Remaking the World* (New York: Putnam, 1999).

50. Others who have written about the intersection of war, disability, and prosthetics include Ansley Wegner, "Phantom Pain: Civil War Amputation and North Carolina's Maimed Veterans," *North Carolina Historical Review* 75 (1998): 277–88; Seth Koven, "Remembering and Dismemberment: Crippled Children, Wounded Soldiers, and the Great War in Great Britain," *American Historical Review* 99 (1994): 1167–1202; Lisa Herschbach, "Prosthetic Reconstructions: Making the Industry, Re-Making the Body, Modeling the Nation," *History Workshop Journal* 44 (1997): 23–57; Panchasi, "Reconstruction: Prosthetics and the Rehabilitation of the Male Body in World War I France"; Bill Brown, "Science Fiction, the World's Fair, and the Prosthetics of Empire, 1910–1915," in Amy Kaplan and Donald Pease, eds., *Cultures of United States Imperialism* (Durham: Duke University Press, 1993), 129–57.

51. For more discussion of this as it relates to Civil War soldiers, see Figg and Farrell-Beck, "Amputation in the Civil War." For eyewitness accounts that illustrate the sentimentality of the "empty sleeve," see Mary Livermore, *My Story of the War* (Hartford, CT: A. D. Worthington, 1889); Louisa May Alcott, *Hospital Sketches* (Boston: J. Redpath, 1863).

52. "Philip Phillips," in *National Cyclopaedia of American Biography*, vol. 7 (New York: James T. White, 1897), 530–31.

53. For more on this, see John Williams-Searle, "Courting Risk: Disability and Liability on Iowa's Railroad, 1868–1900," *Annals of Iowa* 58 (1999): 27–77; Erin O'Connor, "'Fractions of Men': Engendering Amputation in Victorian Culture," *Comparative Studies in Society and History* 39.4 (1997): 742–77; Roger Cooter and Bill Luckin, eds., *Accidents in History: Injuries, Fatalities and Social Relations* (Amsterdam: Editions Rodopi B.V., 1997). See also Tamara Ketabgian, "The Human Prosthesis: Workers and Machines in the Victorian Industrial Scene," *Critical Matrix* 11 (1997): 4–32.

54. For more on Marks, see "Amasa A. Marks," in *The National Cyclopaedia of American Biography*, vol. 11 (New York: James T. White, 1909), 386.

55. Marks, *Manual of Artificial Limbs*, 183–84.

56. "Artificial Eyes," *Medical Examiner*, n.s. 11 (1855): 569.

57. Numerous authors explore the iconography of the body and its relation to cultural events. See, for example, Thomson, *Freakery: Cultural Spectacles of the Extraordinary Body*; Tom Flynn, *The Body in Three Dimensions* (New York: Harry N. Abrams, 1998); Peter Stearns, *Fat History: Body and Beauty in the Modern West* (New York: New York University Press, 1999); Gilman, *Picturing Health and Illness*; Nicholas Mirzoeff, *Bodyscape: Art, Modernity and the Ideal Figure* (London: Routledge, 1995); T. J. Jackson Lears, "American Advertising and the Reconstruction of the Body, 1880–1930," in Kathryn Grover, ed., *Fitness in American Culture* (Amherst: University of Massachusetts Press, 1989) 48–66; John O'Neill, *Five Bodies: The Human Shape of Modern Society* (Ithaca: Cornell University Press, 1985); Susan Bordo, *Twilight Zones: The Hidden Life of Cultural Images from Plato to O.J.* (Berkeley: University of California Press, 1997).

58. For analysis of this, see Dorothy Yamamoto, *The Boundaries of the Human in Medieval English Literature* (London: Oxford University Press, 2000).

59. For one account of this, see Alan Shuldiner, "Molecular Medicine, Transgenic Animals," *New England Journal of Medicine* 334 (1996): 653–55.

60. Thanks to Claudia Kidwell, curator at the Smithsonian's National Museum of American History, for her insights about fashion and posture. For background on the shift to a more relaxed, casual aesthetic, see David Yosifon and Peter N. Stearns, "The Rise and Fall of American Posture," *American Historical Review* 103 (1998): 1057–95. For a typical period account of racial evolution and its inscription on the body, see Eugene Talbot, "Etiology of Face, Nose and Jaw Deformities," *Journal of the American Medical Association* 52 (1909): 1020–23.

61. For analysis of this, see Miles Orvell, *The Real Thing: Imitation and Authenticity in American Culture, 1880–1940* (Chapel Hill: University of North Carolina Press, 1989); T. Jackson Lears, *No Place of Grace* (New York: Pantheon, 1981); S. Elizabeth Bird, ed., *Dressing in Feathers: The Construction of the Indian in American Popular Culture* (New York: Westview, 1996); Elizabeth Edwards, ed.,

Anthropology and Photography, 1860–1920 (New Haven: Yale University Press, 1992).

62. See notes 16 and 47 for references.

63. For discussion of this shift, see, for example, Jonathan Crary, *Techniques of the Observer: On Vision and Modernity in the Nineteenth Century* (Cambridge: MIT Press, 1990); Hal Foster, *The Return of the Real: The Avant-Garde at the End of the Century* (Cambridge: Cambridge University Press, 1996).

PART I

NEED

I

Engineering Masculinity

Veterans and Prosthetics after World War Two

David Serlin

THE EVENTS OF World War Two straddled an uncomfortably unstable period in United States history between the desperate 1930s and the arrogant 1950s. Before the booming economy and unbridled prosperity normally associated with the mid-1950s Pax Americana, many Americans spent the first years of the postwar period recovering slowly from the disruption that wartime had generated in their daily lives.[1] The historian William Graebner has called the decade of the 1940s a "culture of contingency," a time when the chaos of daily life fueled social awkwardness in the face of mass death and destruction.[2] While this culture of contingency undoubtedly existed in earlier periods, especially right after World War One, no previous war had called upon so many mental and material resources to create so much technological power capable of so much death. Writing in the late 1950s, Norman Mailer accurately described the previous decade's sense of contingency as a form of existential anxiety: "Probably, we will never be able to determine the psychic havoc of the concentration camps and the atom bomb upon the unconscious mind of almost everyone alive in these years."[3] To a large degree, this sense of contingency or uncertainty experienced by survivors of the concentration camps and Hiroshima and Nagasaki was shared in the United States by the thousands of wounded, disfigured, and traumatized war veterans returning to civilian life after 1945.

Many disabled veterans who returned home after wartime service were amputees and, in many cases, also prosthesis wearers who worked hard to integrate these new artificial body parts into their civilian lives. One of the foremost concerns of the era was what effect trauma and disability would have on veterans' sense of self-worth, especially in a competitive economy defined by able-bodied men. Social workers, advice columnists, physical therapists, and policy makers during and after World War Two turned their attention to the perceived crisis of the American veteran, much as they had done after the Great War some thirty years earlier. As Susan Hartmann has written, "By 1944, as public attention began to focus on the postwar period, large numbers of writers and speakers . . . awakened readers to the social problems of demobilization, described the specific adjustments facing ex-servicemen, and prescribed appropriate behavior and attitudes for civilians."[4]

For many, the return of tens of thousands of male amputees and prosthesis wearers signaled an altogether different kind of social response. In the 1930s, conservative critics had already sounded a note of fear over what they perceived to be the erosion of masculinity among American men during the work shortages of the Great Depression. Similar anxieties about American manhood crystallized after the war effort began in 1941 with the new sexual divisions of labor that occurred on the civilian home front. The mobilization of hundreds of thousands of women in the wartime labor force, in combination with the prolonged absence of men from traditional positions of familial and community authority, gave a new shape to civilian domestic culture. In the best-selling *Generation of Vipers* (1942), for example, Philip Wylie coined the phrase "Momism" to describe what he perceived to be the emasculating effects of "aggressive" mothers and wives on the behavior of passive husbands and sons. Veterans of the war came back to a country where, among other changes they encountered, gender roles had been turned upside down. How, then, did postwar society make sense of veterans and their prostheses, given contemporary hostilities toward "aggressive" women, and given the cultural mandate to readjust veterans to become physically and psychologically "whole" men, made to assume the idealized stature of "real" American men?

This essay explores the significance of prostheses during the late 1940s and early 1950s in the context of the emphasis that postwar U.S. society placed on certain normative models of masculinity. In particular, the essay examines the design and representation of post–World War Two prostheses developed for veterans as neglected components of the historical reconstruction of gender roles and heterosexual male archetypes in early Cold War culture. Like artificial body parts created for victims of war and industrial accidents after the Civil War and World War One, prosthetics developed during the 1940s and 1950s were linked explicitly to the fragile politics of labor, employment, and self-worth for disabled veterans.[5] But discussions of prosthetics also reflected concomitant social and sexual anxieties that attended the public specter of the damaged male body.

As this essay will argue, the physical design and construction of prostheses help to distinguish the rehabilitation of veterans after World War Two from earlier periods of adjustment for veterans. Prosthetics research and development in the 1940s was catalyzed, to a great extent, by the mystique of scientific progress. The advent of new materials science and new bioengineering principles during the war and the application of these materials and principles to new prosthetic devices helped to transform prosthetics into its own biomedical subdiscipline. The convergence of these two different areas of research—making prostheses as physical objects and designing prosthetics as products of engineering science—offers important insights into the political and cultural dimensions of the early postwar period, especially in light of what we know about the social and economic restructuring of postwar society with the onset of the Cold War. By the mid-1950s the development of new materials and technologies for prostheses had become the consummate marriage of industrial engineering and domestic engineering.

Prostheses designed and built in the 1940s and 1950s were not merely symbolic or abstracted metaphors. For engineers and prosthetists, these artificial parts were biomedical tools designed and used for rehabilitating bodies and social identities. For doctors and patients, prosthetics were powerful anthropomorphic tools that refracted contemporary fantasies about ability and employment, heterosexual masculinity, and American citizenship. I describe prostheses as tools that enable rather than transcend the organic body, showing how they provided the material means through which individuals on both sides of the therapeutic divide imagined and negotiated the boundaries of what it meant to look like and behave as an able-bodied man in mid-twentieth-century American culture.

PATRIOTIC GORE

Long before World War Two ended in August 1945—the month that Japan officially surrendered to the United States after the bombing of Hiroshima and Nagasaki—images in the mass media of wounded soldiers convalescing or undergoing physical therapy treatments occupied a regular place in news reports and popular entertainment.[6] In John Cromwell's film *The Enchanted Cottage* (1945), for example, a young soldier played by Robert Young hides from society and his family in a remote honeymoon cottage after wartime injuries damage his handsome face.[7] *The Enchanted Cottage* updated and Americanized the substance of Sir Arthur Wing Pinero's 1925 play of the same title. Pinero's drama focused on a British veteran of World War One who symbolized the plight of facially disfigured veterans (sometimes called "les gueules cassés" by their countrymen) who were often considered social outcasts by an insensitive public.[8] In the 1945 North American production, as in the original, the cottage protects the mutilated soldier and his homely, unglamorous fiancée from parents and family members who cast aspersions on the couple for their seemingly "abnormal" physical differences. That both the play and film versions perceive her homeliness and his disfigurement as comparable social disabilities is a telling reminder—relevant in 1925, 1945, or 2002—that we must be vigilant in our continued effort to question the social basis of normative standards of appearance and behavior.

Amputees who returned from war to their homes, hometowns, and places of work—if they could find work—often suffered from lack of due respect, despite the best efforts of the federal agencies like the Veterans Administration to promote the needs of the disabled. Physicians, therapists, psychologists, and ordinary citizens alike often regarded veterans as men whose recent amputation was physical proof of emasculation or general incompetence, or else a kind of monstrous defamiliarization of the "normal" male body. Social policy advocates recommended that families and therapists apply positive psychological approaches to the rehabilitation process for amputees.[9] Too often, however, such approaches were geared toward making able-bodied people more comfortable with their innate biases so that they could "deal" with the disabled. This seemed to be a more familiar strategy than empowering the disabled themselves. In William Wyler's Academy Award–winning film *The Best Years of Our Lives* (1946), for example, real-life war veteran Harold Russell played Homer, a sensitive para-plegic who tries to challenge the stereotype of the ineffectual amputee while he and his loyal girlfriend cope valiantly with his two new split-hook, above-the-elbow prosthetic arms. Given the mixed reception of disabled veterans in the public sphere—simultaneous waves of pride and awkwardness—scriptwriters made Homer exhibit tenacious courage and resilience of spirit rather than show evidence of the vul-nerability or rage that visited many veteran amputees. As David Gerber has written, "[t]he culture and politics of the 1940s placed considerable pressure on men like Russell to find individual solutions, within a con-stricted range of emotions, to the problem of bearing a visible disability in a world of able-bodied people."[10] As a result, recurring images of dis-abled soldiers readjusting to civilian life became positive propaganda that tried to persuade able-bodied Americans that the convalescence of veterans was unproblematic. Such propaganda was to be expected in the patriotic aftermath of World War Two—and not surprising, either, given the War Department's decision during the early 1940s to expunge all painful images of wounded or dead soldiers from the popular media.[11]

The U.S. media were instrumental in concocting regular stories about amputees and the triumphant uses of their prostheses. The cir-culation of such optimistic and unduly cheery narratives of tolerance in the face of adversity implied a direct relationship between physical trauma—and the ability to survive such trauma—and patriotic duty. In the summer of 1944, for example, U.S. audiences were captivated by the story of Jimmy Wilson, an army private who had been the only sur-vivor of a ten-person plane crash in the Pacific Ocean. When he was found forty-four hours later amidst the plane's wreckage, army doctors were forced to amputate both of Wilson's arms and legs. After shipping him back to his hometown of Starke, Florida, surgeons outfitted Wilson with new prosthetic arms and legs, and he became a kind of poster boy for the plight of thousands of amputees who faced physical and psy-chological readjustment upon their imminent return to civilian life. In early 1945, the *Philadelphia Inquirer* initiated a national campaign to raise money for Wilson. By the end of the war in August, the *Inquirer* had raised over $50,000, collected from well-known philanthropists and ordinary citizens alike, such as a group of schoolchildren who raised $26 from selling scrap iron.[12] By the winter of 1945, Wilson's trust fund had grown to over $105,000, and he pledged to use the money to

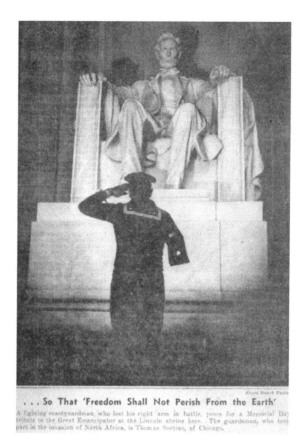

Coast Guard Photo

. . . So That 'Freedom Shall Not Perish From the Earth'

A fighting coastguardsman, who lost his right arm in battle, poses for a Memorial Day tribute to the Great Emancipator at the Lincoln shrine here. The guardsman, who took part in the invasion of North Africa, is Thomas Sortino, of Chicago.

FIG 1.1. This image of war veteran Thomas Sortino of Chicago conjures many historical associations, from the Civil War to World War Two, that link the public appearance of the amputee's body (especially in such a hallowed space) with patriotic devotion and national identity. From an unknown newspaper clipping (probably late 1945 or early 1946) in the Donald Canham Collection, Otis Historical Archives, courtesy of the Armed Forces Institute of Pathology, Walter Reed Army Medical Center, Washington, D.C.

get married, buy a house, and study law under the newly signed G.I. Bill. Wilson's celebrity status as a quadriplegic peaked when he posed with Bess Myerson, Miss America for 1945, in a brand-new Valiant, a car (whose name alone championed Wilson's patriotic reception) that General Motors designed specifically for above-ankle amputees.[13] Wilson learned how to operate the car by manipulating manual gas and brake pedals attached to the car's steering column. Demand for the Valiant was so great that, in September 1946, Congress allocated funds that provided ten thousand of these automobiles to needy veterans and amputees.[14]

If men like Jimmy Wilson were regularly celebrated as heroic and noble, it was because tales of their perseverance and resilience grew proportionately with the fervor of a growing Cold War mentality. In lieu of allowing them to speak for themselves, the media transformed amputees into powerful visual *and* rhetorical symbols through which war-related disability was identified with unequivocal heroism. In one photographic example published by the Coast Guard press corps in late 1945, the small body of Thomas Sortino of Chicago is framed deliberately against the Olympic-sized Abraham Lincoln (fig. 1.1). The caption underneath proclaims, "A fighting coastguardsman . . . poses for a Memorial Day tribute to the Great Emancipator at the Lincoln shrine here." The photograph uses Sortino's patriotic gesture to endorse the democratic ethos of sacrifice, as if his amputation had been nothing less, or more, than that which the government demanded of all its citizens during wartime: "pitching in," buying war bonds, maintaining victory gardens, and rationing consumer goods. Under Lincoln's attentive glare, the visual and verbal cues here invoke a nostalgia for the Civil War, which serves to reinforce the idea that those disabled during World War Two fought and won the war to preserve democracy. Two newspaper articles published around the same time in the Washington *Evening Star* confirm this theme. One, about the Quebec-born veteran amputee Fernand Le Clare, declares in a headline, "Canadian GI Proud to Be an American," while another, about the Hawaiian-born disabled veteran Kenneth T. Otagaki, assures us that "This Jap Is Justly Proud That He Is an American."[15] The particular brand of normative domestic politics expressed by these images and headlines is precisely what Tom Engelhardt has described as the "victory culture" of the late 1940s and early 1950s.[16]

The postwar media used images of amputees (with and without their prostheses) strategically to remind the public of the recent war, as well as to memorialize the war-honored dead and disabled. It was, after all, yet another postwar period to which all citizens would need to acclimate, another period that mandated massive social reconstruction, policy making, and productive transitions to civilian life for millions of people, both able-bodied and disabled, both veteran and civilian.

Moreover, amputee veterans were a significant part of the popular image of soldiering itself and of military culture in general. Their public presence blurred the techniques of physical rehabilitation with tacit forms of democratic participation and civic duty.[17] In 1951, for example, Senator Joe McCarthy antagonized secretary of state Dean Acheson (whom McCarthy believed to be a communist) at a congressional hearing by invoking the name of a recent veteran amputee of the Korean War, Bob Smith, to contest some of Acheson's recent foreign policy proposals. Seamlessly combining homophobic intolerance with anticommunist hysteria, McCarthy contrasted Smith's masculine resilience with Acheson's perceived effeminate and aristocratic stance. "I suggest that . . . when Bob Smith can walk," McCarthy asserted,

> when he gets his artificial limbs, he first walk over to the State Department and call upon the Secretary if he is still there. . . . He should say to Acheson: "You and your lace handkerchief crowd have never had to fight in the cold, so you cannot know its bitterness. . . . [Y]ou should not only resign from the State Department but you should remove yourself from this country and go to the nation for which you have been struggling and fighting so long."[18]

The ideological links forged between public exhibitions of disability and patriotic commitment—usually exercised in a less spectacular fashion than McCarthy's exploitation of Smith—were not new phenomena in the Cold War era. Since the 1860s, photographers had developed a sophisticated visual lexicon for displaying and representing able-bodied and disabled soldiers and veterans. Alan Trachtenberg, among others, has discussed how images of wounded amputees sitting graciously for portrait photographs were rhetorical expressions of extreme patriotism (for both northern and southern veterans) distilled into visual form.[19] For many of these disabled veterans of the Civil War, the amputation stump, the artificial limb, and other physical markings that proved sustained injury became visual shorthand *for* military service. Disability, then, became the permanent uniform worn by those who participated in the aftermath of civil warfare.

Yet medical photographs of amputees in the nineteenth century, as Kathy Newman has argued, were sophisticated enough to capture the subject's brutal amputations and yet polished enough to preserve the genteel conventions of Victorian portrait photography.[20] This must explain why, in such photographs, the male body often appears as both disabled spectacle and eroticized object. For those reading these photographs today, these portrait sittings of handsome young men with deep wounds, radical amputations, or artificial limbs become material reflections of the photographer's desire to recuperate the soldiers' putatively "lost" masculinity. Perhaps medical photographers believed that by using an "objective" science of surveillance, they could displace the potentially emasculating effects of the camera's penetrations into the intimate spaces of the amputee's physical body.

Through the public circulation of these images of veteran amputees, we begin to see the formation of arbitrary (though no less hierarchical) categories for thinking about disability itself. How differently, for example, does a society view disability that results from war injury or industrial accident, as opposed to disability that results from congenital deformity, acquired illness, or even self-mutilation? Part of this delineation relies on the perceived difference between disability induced by modern technology or warfare and hereditary disability, attitudes toward which were influenced by antiquated notions of a "monstrous birth" even as late as the 1950s.[21] In the former, disability is material proof that confirms one's service to warfare, to the modern state, to industrial capitalism: these help to preserve patriotic values and respectable citizenship. In the latter, disability is a material stigma that marks one's rejection from competent service to the society. Among men, such stigmas may confirm the male body as weak, effeminate, and inimical to normative heterosexual versions of manly competence. In the aftermath of war and the rise of the hyperpatriotic culture of the late 1940s, veteran male amputees constituted a superior category on an unspoken continuum of disabled bodies, suggesting that hierarchies of value are constructed even *within,* and sometimes *by,* groups of differently abled individuals.

MAKING MEN WHOLE, AGAIN

The social and political climate of the late 1940s changed the terms on which images of disability were disseminated in the public sphere. Images of amputees undergoing rehabilitation—learning to walk, eat, and perform other "normal" able-bodied activities—were often used in tandem with materials to promote the agendas of postwar science and technology. This was especially true after the National Security Council's 1947 commitment to the "containment" of communism, by any means necessary, increased exponentially the military aggression and technological competition already mounting between the United States and the Soviet Union. The National Academy of Sciences and the National Research Council were among the most prominent federal agencies that funded and supported advanced prosthetics research, especially at university and military laboratories. At large, well-funded research institutions with other government contracts—such as Case Institute of Technology, Massachusetts Institute of Technology, Michigan State University, New York University, University of California at Los Angeles, and Western Reserve University—the development of new prosthetic designs arose concomitantly with new technologies used to protect and defend national interests. Writing in 1954, Detlev Bronk, president of the National Academy of Sciences, made clear the patriotic responsibilities to nation and citizenry that were articulated through the relationship between military research and rehabilitation medicine:

> Those whom this committee first sought to aid were those who suffered loss of limb in battle where they were serving their fellows. In times of war scientists have fortified the courage of our defenders by applying science to the development of better weapons. They have done significantly more; during times when it was necessary to sacrifice human lives they marshaled the resources of science for the protection of health and life. . . . [The development of prostheses] is a vivid reminder that human values are a primary concern of the scientists of freedom-loving nations.[22]

This was not the first time new materials and techniques had been applied to the design and creation of new prosthetic parts for those wounded during war. Industrial processes in the nineteenth and twentieth centuries had enabled the production of materials for prostheses, such as vulcanized rubber, synthetic resins, and plastics. What made new prostheses different was how they represented the marriage of prosthetic design to military-industrial production. Both materials science and information science—hallmarks of military research and funding—figured prominently in experimental prosthetics developed in the late 1940s. According to Wilfred Lynch, "The development of dependable [prostheses] proceeded at a snail's pace until the emergence of 'exotic' new materials in answer to the needs of the military in World War Two. The subsequent aerospace program and the high volume of burgeoning new postwar industries made the commercial production of these unique materials practical."[23] Some of these new materials included staples of the military-industrial economy such as Plexiglas, Lucite, polyester, silicone, titanium, duraluminum, stainless steel, ceramics, and high-grade plastics. By the Fall of 1947, funding from Congress had made artificial limbs made from new, lightweight plastics available to over five thousand veterans. Furthermore, newly patented technologies used in later experimental prosthetic models, such as Velcro and Siemes servomotors, benefited from advances made during wartime research in materials science and miniaturization of solid-state electronics.[24]

For the first time, scientists attempted to apply engineering techniques derived from military-industrial research to veterans' artificial limbs. In late August 1945, just two weeks after the war ended, Paul E. Klopsteg, chairman of the National Research Council's Committee on Prosthetic Devices, announced a research program into "power-driven" artificial limbs that resembled the "real thing" by "introducing power, either hydraulic, pneumatic, or electric," to prosthetic limbs.[25] Engineering designs for the first myoelectric arm in the United States—a prosthesis that operates by electrified muscle control—are perfect examples of the scale and degree of cross-institutional interests involved in prosthetic research in the post-1945 period. Variously called the "Boston arm" and the "Liberty Limb," the myoelectric arm was developed in the early 1960s by the MIT mathematician Norbert Wiener in conjunction with the Harvard Medical School, and sponsored by the Liberty Mutual Insurance Company of Boston. Relying on the principle self-adjusting electronic feedback loops, Wiener helped to design and build a battery-operated amplifier that could magnify existing nerve impulses in an amputee's stump, thereby generating enough power to lift and move the arm.[26]

The association between amputees and state-of-the-art prosthetics research may have been an intentional strategy to link disabled veterans with the positive, futuristic aura surrounding military-industrial science. In 1943, for example, the War Department commissioned Milton Wirtz, a civilian dentist, to develop artificial eyes using the then new wonder material, acrylic.[27] Wirtz's expertise with acrylic derived from his use of the new material in forging dental prostheses for patients. It made him the ideal candidate to supply the armed forces with hundreds of prototype acrylic eyes, which proved to be more durable, lightweight, and even more realistic than glass eyes. Wirtz's kits provided low-skilled technicians at military hospitals with easy-to-follow charts for matching to the patient's eye color, and even contained red-brown threads for simulating optic nerves. In 1944, The Naval Graduate Dental Center in Annapolis, Maryland, developed a full complement of acrylic facial parts, including eye, nose, cheek, and ear prostheses. Surgeons in the field adapted these parts temporarily to the patient's face before the soldier was transferred to a military hospital for reconstructive surgery. The Naval Graduate Dental Center also built cases for holding these parts that resembled boxes of fishing tackle. Each case held a velvet-lined, candy box sampler of facial features, including a "Negro" ear and a "Caucasian" cheek. Despite this variety pack approach, prosthetists used a single mold from which to cast and paint each facial part. This process made fabrication of parts easy; at the same time, it may have had the effect of displacing, or even erasing, the perceived phenotypic differences between white and black facial characteristics. In some small way, such a technical feat of emergency medicine anticipated President Harry S Truman's desegregation of the U.S. military in 1948.

The postwar preoccupation with masculinity and productivity also bolstered and transformed prosthetics engineering and research for veteran amputees. Prosthetists and engineers working with amputees were directly influenced by, among other things, the fiercely heterosexual culture of postwar psychology, especially in its orthodox zeal to preserve the masculine status of disabled veterans. A 1957 rehabilitation manual developed by physical therapists at the University of California at Los Angeles, for example, explicitly correlated physical disability with the perceived heterosexual anxieties of the male amputee: "Will he be acceptable to wife or sweetheart? Can he live a normal sex-life? Will his children inherit anything as a result of his acquired physical defect? Can he hope to rejoin his social group? Must he give up having fun?"[28] This professional concern was concomitant with increasing panic about homosexuality, which predated the war but was formalized in the public imagination after the 1948 publication of Dr. Alfred Kinsey's *Sexual Behavior in the Human Male*. Among military and university researchers, this emphasis on rehabilitating the amputee's masculinity and his body was an artifact left over from the military's deep-seated and overt homophobia.[29] As Allan Bérubé has described in his book *Coming Out under Fire* (1990), the armed forces maintained statistics throughout World War Two on soldiers excused from military service for expressing perceived homosexual behavior or otherwise unmasculine psychological or physiological traits.[30] At New York University, rehabilitation therapists expected that prostheses would offer not only able-bodied activity for the wearer, but also positive self-esteem to those who participated in an experimental, technologically innovative laboratory study:

> [A] good prosthesis, provided in an atmosphere of understanding and interest by people who are looking to him as a *man*, a human being, and as an important cog in an experimental program fills two interwoven needs. He can feel a lessening of the threats against which he must continually arm himself and he can utilize the potentialities of the prosthesis to a much greater extent.[31]

Attitudes such as this, which equated heterosexual masculinity with independent activity in order to resist the potentially effeminizing interventions of family members, were hardly unique in postwar rehabilitation culture. Throughout the late 1940s and 1950s, physicians, psychologists, and engineers imagined amputees as potentially troubled and socially maladjusted. Most were not even expected to fulfill their routine daily chores, let alone their civic duties as sons, husbands, and citizens. For example, the physical therapists Donald Kerr and Signe Brunnstrom writing in 1956, encouraged amputees to reclaim their masculinity by repressing dependence on others and observing strict rules of self-reliance:

> From the time of surgery until he has returned to a normal life in the community, the amputee is beset by many doubts and fears. . . . The amputee must recognize that these attitudes are based on lack of knowledge, and he must not permit them to influence his own thinking. . . . [T]he family [should learn] to ignore the amputation and to expect and even require the amputee to take care of himself, to share in household duties, and to participate in social activities.[32]

In this institutional climate, prostheses were regarded not only as prescriptive tools for rehabilitating amputees but also as cultural tools

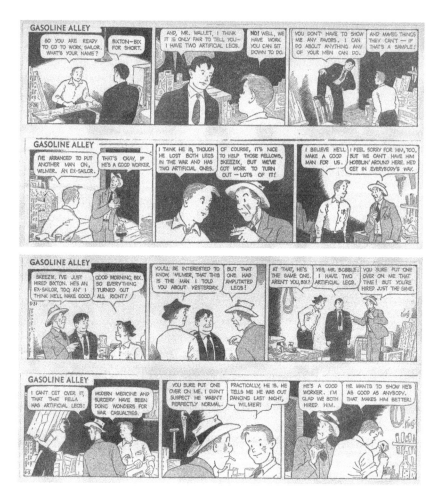

FIG. 1.2. Four-part series from the nationally syndicated cartoon *Gasoline Alley* about a below-the-knee amputee, Bix, whose prosthetic legs enable him to es-chew special treatment and pass as a regular American guy. Originally pub-lished May and June 1946. Reprinted with permission of Tribune Media Ser-vices, Inc. All rights reserved.

through which they might defend themselves against the onslaught of social criticism or the scrutinizing gaze of their male peers. For this rea-son, amputees also became embroiled in public discussions about the competency of veterans as American workers and providers. This, too, was not new: as K. Walter Hickel has argued, rehabilitation medicine after World War One was linked to larger questions about the needs of returning veterans and changes in domestic U.S. social policy.[33] Even while they were manipulated as symbols of American patriotism and stalwart defenders of national values, veterans and amputees often suffered explicit discrimination from employers in both white- and blue-collar industries. According to a 1947 interview with Fred Hetzel, director of the U.S. Employment Service for Washington, D.C., "During and immediately following World War I, employers were eager to help disabled men." The difference between these two postwar periods, Hetzel argued, was that "now that the labor market has tightened up, [employers] hire the physically fit applicant almost every time. They seem to want a Superman or a Tarzan—even though wartime experience showed that disabled men often turned in better work than those not handicapped."[34]

Hetzel's comments about the biases of the "tightened" labor market and Kerr and Brunnstrom's recommendations for self-sufficient living echoed a story line that was published in the comic strip *Gasoline Alley* in May and June 1946 (fig. 1.2). The comic ran at approximately the same moment that the media were saturated with stories about paraplegic Harold Russell and quadriplegic Jimmy Wilson. The comic focuses on the story of Bix, a veteran of World War Two who "lost both legs in the war and has two artificial ones," and the responses of able-bodied men who are impressed and won over by the display of Bix's normalcy.

In the brief narrative, Wilmer, the shop owner, protests foreman Skeezix's decision to hire Bix as a new employee on the warehouse floor. Wilmer tells Skeezix, "it's nice to help those fellows, but we've got work to turn out—lots of it!" When Wilmer hires an ex-sailor for the position, he is amazed to discover that the ex-sailor is the same paraplegic, Bix, that Skeezix hired the day before. The cartoon echoes the promotion of rehabilitation medicine as one of the perks of the postwar economy. Skeezix declares, parroting the rhetorical aplomb of medical miracles that saturated the postwar media, "Modern medicine and surgery have been doing wonders for war casualties. . . . [Bix] tells me he was out dancing last night!" By the social standards of the mid-1940s, what evidence was more reasonable assurance of an American man's fully restored able-bodiedness than his pursuit of Darwinian competition on the dance floor with other males? Apparently, Bix was not alone on the dance floor. In a 1946 autobiography, the writer Louise Baker observed that "[a] great wave of slick stories has pounced the public recently in which disabled soldiers bounce out of their beds, strap on artificial legs, and promptly dance off with pretty nurses. . . . [One nurse] not only affected a miraculous cure of the poor boy's complexes, she practically put blood and bones in his [prosthetic] leg."[35]

Artifacts of popular culture such as the *Gasoline Alley* comic strip suggest that sectors of the public were only too aware of the harsh standards by which amputees were judged. These were standardized versions of "normal," heterosexual masculinity with which few men, able-bodied or otherwise, could compete without fear of reprisal. That Bix is able to "pass" as an able-bodied, virile veteran—and is not immediately identified as a delicate or effeminized war casualty—is the comic's principal message. While watching Bix carrying an enormous carton across the shop, Wilmer declares, "You sure put one over on me. I didn't suspect [Bix] wasn't perfectly *normal*." Skeezix replies, "Practically he is. . . . He wants to show he's as good as anybody. That makes him better." These two quintessentially "American" expressions of masculine competence—the urgency of self-reliance and disdain for unequal treatment—were used by African-Americans to powerful rhetorical effect in the "I Am a Man" campaigns of the early civil rights movement of the mid-1950s.

As the *Gasoline Alley* comic demonstrated, preconceptions about amputees as maladjusted, fragile, or even neurotic were widespread and powerful. Yet such preconceptions did not disappear solely at the behest of cartoonists; they significantly influenced the way that prosthetics research was conducted—and consequently represented—during the 1950s. Such representations, in other words, were hardly the purview only of mass culture. A photograph taken at Walter Reed Army Hospital in March 1952, for example, was meant undoubtedly to capture the veteran amputee participating in a familiar, able-bodied activity: lighting and enjoying a cigarette (fig. 1.3). As usual, what was most at issue was not simply the vocational or domestic rehabilitation of the veteran, but the crucial preservation of his masculinity. The dramatic lighting and crisp graduated shapes of the amputee's body and pose, however, seem like a convention of iconography directly descended from fashion and celebrity photographers such as Cecil Beaton or George Platt Lynes. The photograph also suggests that the prosthesis will help the veteran, differently abled or not, preserve his male competence and self-reliant citizenship. Like other objects that celebrated

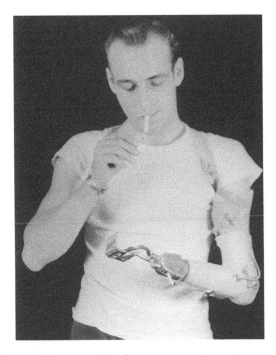

FIG. 1.3. Professional photographs of veteran amputees using new prosthetic devices to perform "normal" male activities—such as lighting and enjoying a cigarette—were deliberate attempts to challenge the reputation of the male amputee as ineffectual or effeminate. Taken March 1952. Courtesy of the Armed Forces Institute of Pathology, Walter Reed Army Medical Center, Washington, D.C.

the scientific and technological progress of postwar culture, such photographs taken at a military hospital known for its advanced prosthetics research were self-conscious attempts to illuminate and maintain the essential gestures of masculinity.[36] These familiar icons were circulated and disseminated throughout the world—not unlike Hollywood films, modern art, swing dancing, or phonograph records in decidedly American genres—as evidence of both domestic rehabilitation policies and the enduring legacies of American male toughness and resiliency.

Similarly, a photograph of an older veteran reading the newspaper taken at Walter Reed in 1949 challenges the notion that all amputees were young and virile objects of virtuous American character and identity (fig. 1.4). Difficult to discern—but no less poignant—in

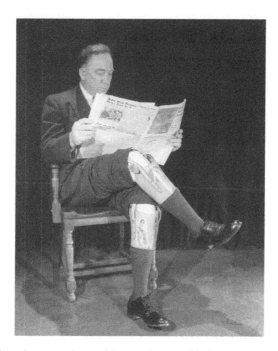

FIG. 1.4. In this photograph, an older professional below-the-knee double amputee nonchalantly reads the sports page of the Washington *Evening Star* while showing off new plastic prosthetic legs that have been customized with images of voluptuous pinup girls. The visual combination of these two "normal" heterosexual male accoutrements demonstrates how experts went out of their way to depict amputees who suffered no loss of masculine status. Taken 1949. Courtesy of the Armed Forces Institute of Pathology, Walter Reed Army Medical Center, Washington, D.C.

the photograph are images of pinup girls painted on the amputee's legs, icons more characteristic of the nose cones of airplanes or the back panels of bomber jackets than of the legs of older veterans. Such attempts to customize one's legs with figures reminiscent of Vargas calendar girls perpetuate the tradition of proudly decorating jeeps, tanks, airplanes, and other modes of military transportation.[37] Photographic images like these did double duty: first, as promotional materials for large rehabilitation centers, like Walter Reed, which could advertise their progress in prosthetics research. Such consciously crafted publicity images also served to assure the general public that amputees suffered no loss of ability, mobility, personality, or, most important, their manhood. Smoking, reading the sports section of the daily newspaper, and, in Bix's case, swing dancing were glorified almost matter-of-factly as "normal" and "American" expressions of heterosexual male desire. In the case of this older gentleman, perhaps pinup girls enabled him to take on the identity of a blue-collar worker. Appearing like rugged tattoos, these pinup images may have suggested that this veteran possessed a particular mechanical aptitude or technological competence that would have been denied to him if he were merely sitting at a desk all day. Such images indicate that the seductive lure of blue-collar accoutrements like tattoos for white-collar workers never disappeared but in fact expanded after the United States shifted its emphasis away from industry to a service economy in the 1950s. The singular image of the happy, efficient white-collar Organization Man in his postwar corporate office may have been, to a large degree, only a triumph of marketing, the genius of Madison Avenue.[38]

ENGINEERING THE POSTWAR WORKER-CITIZEN

The rapid development and diffusion of new prosthetic materials and technologies made it possible for thousands of veterans to return to existing jobs or pursue alternative careers. For engineering departments and rehabilitation centers, however, selecting which amputees would make good candidates for prostheses remained a matter of practical contention. Undoubtedly, the United States had a surfeit of veterans eager to participate in new programs at military and university hospitals—most notably those sponsored by the National Academy of Sciences, the Veterans Administration, and the National Research Council's Advanced Council on Artificial Limbs. Suspicions about the reliability of these veteran amputees, however, still lingered. Popular prejudices against veterans transformed professional discussions of veterans' social and psychological stability by focusing on the male amputee and his work competence, an especially potent mandate during a period when Freudian psychoanalysis, lobotomies, and shock therapy all held enormous medical authority. As Ellen Herman has described, psychologists in both military and civilian practice in the late 1940s and early 1950s emphasized social adjustment—or what the sociologist David Riesman described in his critique of the "outer-directed personality"—in endorsing manliness and self-reliance among veterans and amputees.[39] Prosthetic laboratories were no different. With the fate of large federally sponsored research contracts on the line, doctors and administrators made a concerted effort to choose just the right applicants for their research subjects.

For example, at New York University and the University of California at Los Angeles, engineers routinely gave potential prosthesis wearers a battery of psychological tests, all of which relied on expectations that amputees suffered from war-related neuroses. In 1957, amputees at the UCLA School of Medicine were given the California Test of Personality, "designed to identify and reveal the status of certain fundamental characteristics of human nature which are highly important in determining personal, social, or vocational relationships."[40] UCLA also asked potential prosthesis wearers to describe, in their own words, their personal concepts of "self reliance; sense of personal worth; sense of personal freedom; feeling of belonging; freedom from withdrawing tendencies; and freedom from nervous symptoms." These questions in the testing manual all fell under the ominous category "Personal Security." In 1953 clinical researchers at NYU's College of Engineering gave prospective prosthesis wearers the Ascendance Submission Reaction Study, a psychological test developed in the late 1930s "to discover the disposition of an individual to dominate his fellows (or be dominated by them) in various face-to-face relationships of everyday life."[41] This study examined the amputee according to his "[e]arly development—home setting; conforming or non-conforming behavior; neurotic character traits; attitude to parents; siblings; friends; cheerful or gloomy childhood; position of leadership; [and] attitude toward crippling." Through these examinations, engineers who built experimental prostheses believed that they could quickly estimate the amputees' psychological profile and citizenship values, including what the UCLA examiners called the test subjects' "social standards; social skills; freedom from anti-social tendencies; family relations; occupational relations; [and] community relations."

As we have already seen, this whirlwind of assumptions and connections between the amputee, his socialization, his personality, his masculinity, his work competence, and his mental state were hardly new associations. To a certain degree, the psychological dimension of rehabilitation medicine belonged to a much older historical discourse that exposed the traumatic effects of war on soldiers' and veterans' psyches.[42] After World War One, psychologists helped increasingly to develop training programs for the needs of industrial production and military regimentation. As Elspeth Brown has argued, the use of the human body as an industrial metaphor for the efficient, regulated machine was first applied to British and French (and, later, North American) factory workers in the late nineteenth century.[43] Routine job tasks performed by men on production lines were timed and measured so that work output could be made more efficient and productive under the philosophy of scientific management called Taylorism. European social scientists such as Jules Amar applied principles from industrial management to the rehabilitation of amputees and veterans in hospitals in Paris. For rehabilitation doctors and efficiency experts alike, the project of making the damaged male body productive was perhaps the greatest conceptual challenge to modern industrial capitalism. The early-twentieth-century call to enforce industrial efficiency in the workplace combined seamlessly with the mid-twentieth-century call to develop prostheses that would help to displace male work anxieties.

These two forces come to fruition in many of the new prosthetics designed during the 1940s and 1950s. The designer Henry Dreyfuss, whose work promoted the social and aesthetic benefits of ergonomic design, actually engineered and built a prosthetic hand for the Veterans Administration in 1955. One might say that Dreyfuss's work as industrial designer for the federal government marked the perfect cohesion of prosthetics as a tool of social engineering and as an apparatus of Cold War science. As he declared in his 1955 manifesto *Designing for People*, "the goal in [military projects] is a contribution to morale, the intangible force that impels soldiers to have confidence and pride in their weapons and therefore in themselves and that, in the long pull, wins battles and wars."[44] Dreyfuss had many experiences adapting his commercial designs to serve the needs of military-industrial science and technology.[45] In 1942, for example, Dreyfuss was contracted by the Coordinator of Information (COI) and the Office of Strategic Services (OSS) to design strategy rooms and conference rooms for the armed forces. Dreyfuss also designed war ordnance gun carriages for 105-millimeter and Howitzer rifles for the army, and ship habitats for the navy. Well into the 1950s, Dreyfuss's services were retained, and he designed missile launchers as well as the ergonomic interiors of the M46 and M95 tanks for the army. Completing the collaborative symbiosis between government and industry that so marks the Cold War period, Dreyfuss

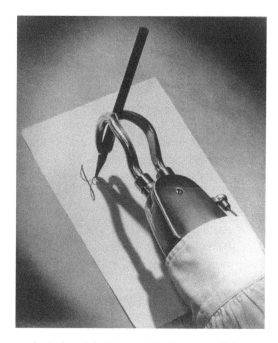

FIG. 1.5. This prosthetic hand, by Henry Dreyfuss in collaboration with the Veterans Administration in the early 1950s, was designed to satisfy the needs of below-the-elbow amputees who wanted white-collar jobs in the postwar service economy. It was a whole new hand for a whole new kind of work. Originally published in Henry Dreyfuss, *Designing for People* (New York: Simon and Schuster, 1955). Reproduced with permission of the Cooper-Hewitt National Design Museum, Smithsonian Institution/Art Resource, NY.

served as a consultant for Chrysler's confidential missile branch between 1954 and 1956. Just after the war, however, between 1948 and 1950, Dreyfuss served as a consultant to the National Research Council's Advanced Council on Artificial Limbs.

A photograph of Dreyfuss Associates' prosthetic hand, designed for the Veterans Administration's Human Engineering Division (fig. 1.5), was published in *Designing for People*. Appearing alongside images of familiar Dreyfuss objects, such as the round Honeywell thermostat and the black Bell telephone, the photography shows an intentionally elegant, sophisticated version of the prosthetic. Images such as this would have been a noticeable departure from visual illustrations of artificial arms—let alone legs, hands, or facial parts—advertised by nineteenth- and twentieth-century prosthesis manufacturers. As Stephen Mihm has argued, late-nineteenth-century catalogues by esteemed prosthetics manufacturers such as A. A. Marks routinely included images of working men using threshers, farming tools, and other heavy machines. Such images demonstrated the viability of an artificial arm that in no way compromised either the worker's masculinity or his ability to earn a living.[46] As one A. A. Marks catalogue declared in 1908, "The wholesome effect an [artificial] arm has on the stump, that of keeping it in a healthy and vigorous condition, protecting it from injuries, forcing it into healthful activity, together with its ornamental aspect, are sufficient reasons for wearing one, even if utility is totally ignored."[47]

The Dreyfuss hand would have been a self-conscious alternative to these types of photographic images and manufacturers' endorsements. Moreover, the Dreyfuss photograph would have "civilized" the otherwise painful and traumatic representations of amputees and prosthesis wearers that were displayed in public, especially those involved in blue-collar work, such as Bix from *Gasoline Alley*. As one can see in the photograph, Dreyfuss's hands for above-elbow amputees were shiny, rounded, stainless steel hooks that imitated the curve of fingers. Beginning a signature in beautiful longhand, and hidden tastefully by a crisp Oxford cloth shirtsleeve, the gleaming steel hand twinkles underneath the glow of a well-lit and expertly framed composition. Clearly, Dreyfuss was concerned with aspects of the hand that would not have provoked much interest, or comment, among prosthetists and amputees fifty years earlier. Dreyfuss commented in *Designing for People* that

> [i]f "feel" is of importance to the housewife at her ironing board, imagine how infinitely more important it is in the artificial limbs of an amputee. We learned a great deal about this in our work for the Veterans Administration. To understand the plight of the amputee, members of our staff had artificial limbs strapped to them.[48]

Dreyfuss's interest in "feel" was certainly not a conceptual category of design that was especially useful or even recognizable by many early manufacturers of prostheses. Even by the 1950s, the typical goal for prosthetists was to make the worker as productive and efficient as possible, not discounting necessary provisions for physical comfort and daily utility. "Feel" would have stimulated the interest only of an industrial designer, especially one concerned with the appearance and "feel" of American home and business environments. The Dreyfuss hand may have harkened back to the industrially managed body of the early twentieth century, but its aesthetic details were unequivocally *moderne*, a certain product of the design-conscious mid-1950s. The Dreyfuss hand was completely compatible with the objectives of an industrial designer whose goal was to package all consumer objects according to aesthetic criteria governed by beauty, harmony, and use-value. Dreyfuss was, after all, not only the man who shaped twentieth-century commercial design but the man who designed window displays for Marshall Field's in Chicago, Macy's in New York, and theatrical spaces at the 1939–40 New York World's Fair. For someone of such catholic tastes, designing a prosthetic hand provided similar aesthetic and ergonomic challenges. In Dreyfuss's hand, mechanical hardware was hidden either by the stainless steel casing or by the long-sleeve shirt, thus obeying his own strict design platitudes: no visible screws, single housing, no exposed seams or joints, no distracting colors or patterns. Indeed, as this photograph indicated, Dreyfuss's prosthetic hand was a mark of solidity and sophistication.

To whom, then, were these new Dreyfuss hands pitched? As we have seen from representations of amputees engaged in what appear to be "normal," able-bodied activities, images of men performing as men in familiar, and recognizably masculine, endeavors both individually and collectively were an extremely important part of the rehabilitation process. In the Dreyfuss photograph, however, we see historical evidence of industrial designers and commercial photographers grappling not with images of factory workers or G.I. amputees but with the postwar period's growing desire for a new model of American manhood. Such an image, ideally, would accommodate the growing army of corporate white-collar workers, not to mention those blue-collar workers encouraged—or forced—to make the professional transition to a service economy.[49] For this reason, the functionalist imperative in the Dreyfuss hand became a way of understanding how able-bodied function could be normalized for, and sold to, amputees who had professional aspirations that did not necessarily include assembly-line work. An amputated arm or leg may have provoked possible associations between anatomical dysfunction and a lack of reliability, sturdiness, fortitude, or commitment. But the utterly functionalist, aesthetically integrated, and mass-produced Dreyfuss hand would offer social prestige, not unlike a set of golf clubs or a Cadillac convertible. Perhaps this is why the white-collar sophistication that Dreyfuss's design team attempted to impart through both product and marketing reflected not the contents of contemporary rehabilitation manuals, but instead period magazines like *Playboy* and *Esquire* whose advertisements regularly featured high-tech appliances or multifunction Herman Miller furniture.[50]

The Dreyfuss hand may have promised to restore anatomical function and neutralize emasculation, but it could also confer self-esteem and cultural capital. It could be a proud new consumer item that reflected a profound new sense of prosperity, as predicted by economic theorists and carried out by service economy workers. Undoubtedly, many believed that the Dreyfuss hand would be the wave of the future. It was a whole new hand for a whole new kind of work.

NOTES

Early versions of this essay were presented at Drexel University, MIT, Pratt Institute, Rensselaer Polytechnic Institute, and UCLA. Thanks to all for inviting me to share my work. Special thanks to Jill Bloomer at the Cooper-Hewitt National Design Museum, Michael Rhode at the Otis Historical Archives of the Armed Forces Institute of Pathology at Walter Reed Army Medical Center, and Mark Santangelo, my research assistant in Washington, D.C. For encouragement and superb close readings of early drafts, thanks to Amanda Bailey, Carol Magary Carpenter, Ross Lewin, Sina Najafi, Niko Pfund, Andrew Ross, Alice Joan Saab, Rosemarie Garland Thomson, Danny Walkowitz, and, as ever, Brian Selznick.

1. For a discussion of these themes, see John Morton Blum, *V Was for Victory: Politics and American Culture during World War II* (New York: Harcourt Brace Jovanovich, 1976); Paul Boyer, *By the Bomb's Early Light: The Atomic Bomb in American Thought and Culture,* 2d ed. (Chapel Hill: University of North Carolina Press, 1994 [1986]); and Lewis Erenberg, ed., *The War in American Culture* (Chicago: University of Chicago Press, 1995).

2. See William Graebner, *The Age of Doubt: American Thought and Culture in the 1940s* (Boston: Twayne, 1991), 19–39.

3. Norman Mailer, "The White Negro" (1957), in *The Portable Beat Reader,* ed. Ann Charters (New York: Penguin, 1991), 520.

4. See Susan Hartmann, "Prescriptions for Penelope: Literature on Women's Obligations to Returning World War Two Veterans," *Women's Studies* 5 (1978): 224.

5. For historical studies of prosthetics in a U.S. context in the nineteenth century, see Erin O'Connor, "Fractions of Men: Engendering Amputation in Victorian Culture," *Comparative Studies in Society and History* 39.4 (October 1997): 736–71; and Lisa Herschbach, "Prosthetic Reconstructions: Making the Industry, Re-Making the Body, Modeling the Nation," *History Workshop Journal* 44 (autumn 1997): 23–57. On prosthetics and amputation with reference to British society after World War One, see Seth Koven, "Remembering and Dismemberment: Crippled Children, Wounded Soldiers, and the Great War in Great Britain," *American Historical Review* 99.4 (October 1994): 1167–1202; and Joanne Bourke, *Dismembering the Male: Men's Bodies, Britain, and the Great War* (Chicago: University of Chicago Press, 1996). For French and German responses to soldiers after World War One, see Roxanne Panchasi, "Reconstruction: Prosthetics and the Rehabilitation of the Male Body in World War I France," *differences: A Journal of Feminist Cultural Studies* 7.3 (1995): 109–40; Anson Rabinbach, *The Human Motor: Energy, Fatigue, and the Origins of Modernity* (Berkeley: University of California Press, 1992); and Heather R. Perry's essay, "Re-Arming the Disabled Veteran: Artificially Rebuilding State and Society in World War One Germany," in this volume.

6. See Glenn Gritzer and Arnold Arluke, *The Making of Rehabilitation: A Political Economy of Medical Specialization, 1890–1980* (Berkeley: University of California Press, 1985); and Jafi Alyssa Lipson, "Celluloid Therapy: Rehabilitating Veteran Amputees and American Society through Film in the 1940s," (unpublished senior thesis, Harvard University, 1995), author's collection.

7. More than half a century after the film's release, *The Enchanted Cottage* is still seen as a cautionary tale about narcissism, which reduces the content of the film to its most ahistorical form. According to one online movie review service, the film is about "[t]wo people [who] are thrown together and find love in their mutual unhappiness. Sensitive, touching romantic drama."

8. See Sir Arthur Wing Pinero, *The Enchanted Cottage: A Fable in Three Acts* (Boston: Baker, 1925).

9. For contemporary examples of this literature, see United States Veterans Administration, *Manual of Advisement and Guidance* (Washington, DC: Government Printing Office, 1945); and James Bedford, *The Veteran and His Future Job: A Guide-Book for the Veteran* (Los Angeles: Society for Occupational Research, 1946).

10. David Gerber, "Anger and Affability: The Rise and Representation of a Repertory of Self-Presentation Skills in a World War II Disabled Veteran," *Journal of Social History* (Fall 1993): 6. For more about the film, see Gerber, "Heroes and Misfits: The Troubled Social Reintegration of Disabled Veterans in *The Best Years of Our Lives*," *American Quarterly* 46.4 (December 1994): 545–74.

11. See George Roeder Jr., *The Censored War: American Visual Experience during World War Two* (New Haven: Yale University Press, 1993).

12. "50,000 Mark Passed in Drive to Aid Army Multiple Amputee," *Washington (D.C.) Evening Star,* August 30, 1945.

13. See photograph of Wilson and Myerson, *Washington (D.C.) Times-Herald,* January 31, 1946. See also material on Wilson in Bess Furman *Progress in Prosthetics* (Washington, DC: Department of Health, Education, and Welfare, 1962).

14. Arthur Edison, "Iwo Jima Vet First to Get Amputee Car," *New York Times-Herald,* September 5, 1946.

15. Newspaper clippings from the *Washington (D.C.) Evening Star,* probably 1947. From the scrapbooks of the Donald Canham Collection, Otis Historical Archives, Armed Forces Institute of Pathology, Walter Reed Army Medical Center.

16. See Tom Engelhardt, *The End of Victory Culture: Cold War America and the Disillusioning of a Generation* (New York: Basic Books, 1995).

17. See Matthew Naythons, *The Face of Mercy: A Photographic History of Medicine at War* (New York: Random House, 1993).

18. *Congressional Record,* 1951, p. 5579, quoted in David M. Oshinsky, *A Conspiracy So Immense: The World of Joe McCarthy* (New York: Free Press, 1983), 196.

19. See Alan Trachtenberg, *Reading American Photographs: Images as History from Matthew Brady to Walker Evans* (New York: Noonday, 1989). See also Michael Rhode, *Index to Photographs of Surgical Cases and Specimens and Surgical Photographs,* 3d ed. (Washington, DC: Otis Historical Archives, Armed Forces Institute of Pathology, Walter Reed Army Medical Center, 1996).

20. Kathy Newman, "Wounds and Wounding in the American Civil War: A Visual History," *Yale Journal of Criticism* 6.2 (1993): 63–86.

21. For examples of scholarship in this area, see Leslie Fiedler, *Freaks: Myths and Images of the Secret Self* (New York: Simon and Schuster, 1978); Robert Bogdan, *Freak Show: Presenting Human Oddities for Amusement and Profit* (Chicago: University of Chicago Press, 1987); Rosemarie Garland Thomson, ed., *Freakery: Cultural Spectacles of the Extraordinary Body* (New York: New York University Press, 1996); and Rosamond Purcell, *Special Cases: Natural Anomalies and Historical Monsters* (San Francisco: Chronicle Books, 1997).

22. Detlev W. Bronk, foreword to *Human Limbs and Their Substitutes* (New York: Hafner, 1968 [1954]), iv.

23. Wilfred Lynch, *Implants: Reconstructing the Human Body* (New York: Van Nostrand Reinhold, 1982), 1.

24. For more about the uses of new products developed in tandem with postwar materials science, see *Proceedings of the International Symposium on the Application of Automatic Control in Prosthetic Design* (Belgrade, Yugoslavia, 1962).

25. Cornelia Ball, "New Artificial Limbs to Be Power-Driven," *Washington (D.C.) Daily News,* August 27, 1945.

26. For further information about Norbert Wiener's involvement in the development of the "Boston arm," see David Serlin, *Replaceable You: Engineering the American Body after World War Two* (Chicago: University of Chicago Press, forthcoming). For further exploration, see Peter Galison's important essay "The Ontology of the Enemy: Norbert Wiener and the Cybernetic Vision," *Critical Inquiry* 21 (autumn 1994): 228–66.

27. All material on Milton Wirtz and the Naval Graduate Dental Center from collections of the Division of Science, Medicine, and Society, National Museum of American History, Smithsonian Institution, Washington, DC.

28. Miles Anderson and Raymond Sollars, *Manual of Above-Knee Prosthesis for Physicians and Therapists* (Los Angeles: University of California School of Medicine Program, 1957), 40.

29. Army psychologists who feared that one bad apple could convert the whole bunch taunted recruits with effeminate mannerisms and "code words" perceived to be the performative gestures and underground lingo of a vast homosexual conspiracy. The military also administered urine tests to determine which soldiers' bodies had appropriate levels of testosterone, and rejected those with too much estrogen. See "Homosexuals in Uniform," *Newsweek,* June 9, 1947, reprinted in Larry Gross and James Woods, eds., *The Lesbian and Gay Reader in Media, Society, and Politics* (New York: Columbia University Press, 1999), 78.

30. Allan Bérubé, *Coming Out under Fire: The History of Gay Men and Women in World War Two* (New York: Free Press, 1990).

31. New York University College of Engineering Research Division, *The Function and Psychological Suitability of an Experimental Hydraulic Prosthesis for Above-the-Knee Amputees* National Research Council Report 115.15, (New York: NYU/Advisory Committee on Artificial Limbs, 1953), 48, emphasis mine.

32. Donald Kerr and Signe Brunnstrom, *Training of the Lower Extremity Amputee* (Springfield, IL: C. C. Thomas, 1956), vii, 3–4.

33. See K. Walter Hickel, "Medicine, Bureaucracy, and Social Welfare: The Politics of Disability Compensation for American Veterans of World War I," in Paul Longmore and Laurie Umansky, eds., *The New Disability History: American Perspectives* (New York: New York University Press, 2000).

34. Quoted in Steven Hall, "Amputees Find Employers Want Only Super-Men," *Washington Daily News,* October 2, 1947.

35. Louise Maxwell Baker, *Out on a Limb* (New York: McGraw-Hill, 1946), 37.

36. See, for example, Serge Guibault, *How New York Stole the Idea of Modern Art* (Chicago: University of Chicago Press, 1983), or Robert Haddow's discussion of the circulation of American objects during the Cold War in *Pavilions of Plenty: Exhibiting American Culture Abroad in the 1950s* (Washington, DC: Smithsonian Institution Press, 1997).

37. For an interesting discussion of pinup girls as domestic politics, see Robert B. Westbrook, "'I Want a Girl, Just Like the Girl, That Married Harry James': Amercian Women and the Problem of Political Obligation in World War Two," *American Quarterly* 42 (December 1990): 587–614.

38. See Barbara Ehrenreich, *The Hearts of Men: American Dreams and the Flight from Commitment* (Garden City, NY: Anchor Books, 1983). See also Angel Kwolek-Folland, "Gender, Self, and Work in the Life Insurance Industry, 1880–1930," in Ava Baron, ed., *Work Engendered: Toward a New History of American Labor* (Ithaca: Cornell University Press, 1991). For historical background about the image of the white-collar corporate Organization Man, see C. Wright Mills, *White Collar* (New York: Oxford University Press, 1951); and William H. Whyte, *The Organization Man* (New York: Simon and Schuster, 1954).

39. See Ellen Herman, *The Romance of American Psychology: Political Culture in the Age of Experts* (Berkeley: University of California Press, 1994); and David Riesman, Nathan Glazer, and Reuel Denney, *The Lonely Crowd: A Study of the Changing American Character* (Garden City, NY: Doubleday, 1953 [1950]).

40. Anderson and Sollars, *Manual of Above-Knee Prosthesis*, 20.

41. New York University College of Engineering Research Division, *The Function and Psychological Suitability of an Experimental Hydraulic Prosthesis for Above-the-Knee Amputees*, 21–22.

42. See, for example, Eric T. Dean, *Shook Over Hell: Post-Traumatic Stress, Vietnam, and the Civil War* (Cambridge: Harvard University Press, 1997).

43. See Elspeth Brown, "The Prosthetics of Management: Motion Study, Photography, and the Industrialized Body in World War I America," in this volume. See also Rabinbach, *The Human Motor*, esp. 280–88; and Michael Adas, *Machines as the Measure of Men: Science, Technology, and Ideologies of Western Dominance* (Ithaca: Cornell University Press, 1989).

44. Henry Dreyfuss, *Designing for People* (New York: Simon and Schuster, 1955), 160.

45. All information about Dreyfuss Associates accounts taken from chronologies in his "Brown Books" microfiche, Henry Dreyfuss Papers, Henry Dreyfuss Memorial Study Center, Cooper-Hewitt National Museum of Design, New York, New York.

46. See Stephen Mihm, "'A Limb Which Shall Be Presentable in Polite Society': Prosthetic Technologies in the Nineteenth Century," in this volume.

47. A. A. Marks annual merchandise catalogue (New York, 1908), 226. From the collection of Katherine Ott.

48. Dreyfuss, *Designing for People*, 29.

49. For more about disruptions of gender normativity (and their consequences) in the late 1940s and early 1950s, see, for example, Richard Corber, *In the Name of National Security: Hitchcock, Homophobia, and the Political Construction*

of Gender in Postwar America (Durham: Duke University Press, 1993); and Alan Nadel, *Containment Culture: American Narratives, Postmodernism, and the Atomic Age* (Durham: Duke University Press, 1995), esp. 117–54.

50. See "Playboy's Penthouse Apartment" (1956), reprinted in Joel Sanders, ed., *Stud: Architectures of Masculinity* (New York: Princeton Architectural Press, 1995), 54–65.

2

Re-Arming the Disabled Veteran

*Artificially Rebuilding State and Society in
World War One Germany*

Heather R. Perry

WHILE THE BATTLEFIELDS of the First World War left unprecedented numbers of German soldiers dead, the intensity of the conflict fostered medical innovations that enabled a far greater percentage of severely injured men to survive. Over the course of the war, doctors gained enough experience with amputation surgery and antiseptic procedures to save lives that would have been lost to gangrene or infectious disease in previous wars. Nonetheless, the alarming rate at which soldiers lost arms or legs in battle forced German medicine to take stock of its existing rehabilitation programs and prosthetic devices. German doctors interpreted it as their patriotic duty to heal and repair the broken bodies of war, and orthopedists and engineers worked together toward this end. Along the way they revolutionized artificial limb technology and invented modern German orthopedics.

The crippled veterans whom they sought to assist faced a difficult transition to civilian life. They returned to a new German Republic fraught with social violence and political turmoil. Though publicly lauded during the war, many soon felt cast aside by the fatherland they had so bravely defended. Previous studies of this "front generation" have tended to focus on either government pension and demobilization programs[1] or the postwar politics of veterans.[2] In an effort to understand the "outsider" position of Germany's veterans, these studies argue that German veterans were dissatisfied with their war pensions, or felt forgotten in the larger postwar crisis of Weimar Germany, or simply rebelled against an unwanted liberal government in the violent manner they had "learned" during the war. None of these histories, however, have considered the consequences of the government's attempted reintegration of crippled soldiers. This is particularly surprising, given that it was the conspicuous and unresolved dislocation of the returning disabled soldiers that fundamentally stamped Weimar culture. From the paintings of Otto Dix and George Grosz to the pacifist literature of Erich Maria Remarque to the uniform-clad beggar on the streets and cinema screens of Berlin, the ubiquitous presence of the broken soldier was one that all Germans ultimately confronted.

This essay examines how German orthopedists attempted to solve this crisis—a crisis that not only threatened the existing welfare and social insurance system, but also left the country with a desperate postwar labor shortage. In an effort to both legitimize their field in the eyes of the state and reconstruct men disabled in battle, German orthopedists painstakingly developed new rehabilitation programs and innovative prosthetic devices for disabled veterans. By returning the disabled veterans to the workforce, orthopedists hoped to alleviate the financial pressure on the national insurance system and thereby win the favor of the government. In doing so, they produced scores of artificial arms, revolutionizing prosthetic design in Germany. Along the way, however, they lost sight of their patients' needs, focusing instead on the reproduction of prewar class boundaries and the stabilization of wartime society.

GERMANY BEFORE THE WAR: SOCIETY, WELFARE, AND ORTHOPEDICS IN THE EMPIRE

Wilhelmine Germany was a highly stratified society where interclass mobility was extremely rare. The bourgeoisie strictly guarded the educational and structural gateways to the middle class, and blocked members of the working class from gaining access to the universities, civil bureaucracy, and military. Moreover, in Prussia a three-tiered voting system further weighted the votes of the wealthy and privileged, ensuring that the nobility and bourgeoisie maintained control of German politics.

The prewar German national insurance system was an intricate web of administrative laws and regulations primarily designed to preserve the existing social order, not to administer any kind of compensatory justice. In order to defuse an increasingly restless working class in the 1880s, the German Chancellor Otto von Bismarck passed a series of legislative acts creating a national insurance program. This system calculated benefits on the basis of wages lost, not medical condition. In practice, this meant that two workers could experience the same injury—the loss of a hand, for example—yet receive substantially different pensions. The goal of the insurance system was to maintain the worker's socioeconomic status, ensuring that he would neither rise above nor fall below his present level.

Insurance officials strictly guarded the public coffers and eyed every claim with skepticism. Because they suspected many applicants of angling for a "free ride" from the government, insurance officials intentionally calculated medical benefits just high enough to keep the injured or ill from starving, but low enough to encourage them to get back to work quickly, if possible. The ideology informing this system was one that viewed Germany's workers as children who would unscrupulously try to exploit the state's welfare if not inspected closely.[3]

The German military's medical disability program, though administratively and legally separate from the national insurance laws, reflected a similar set of principles. Military officials administered disability pensions in order to keep a soldier (or his surviving family) within an accustomed socioeconomic level, not to compensate for the loss of a particular body part. The amount calculated for a disability pension was therefore tied to a soldier's rank and not his injury. Just as under the national insurance system, the exact same injury could result in widely different pension sums for soldiers of differing ranks. In his study of German war victims, Robert Whalen notes that disabled sergeant-majors received pensions nearly twice those of privates, *for the exact same injury*. Those whose disabilities were classified as minor received even less. Additional funds helped those officers whose pensions did not meet what was considered an appropriate officer-level wage.[4] Through its pension program, the military too reinforced its own internal social order.

Insurance officials and military courts were not the sole evaluators of disability claims, however. German doctors played an important role in determining the actual extent to which a man was permanently disabled. Doctors sent a medical evaluation of the physical injury combined with an estimate of the patient's "lost movements," education, and social position to the insurance committee. This report helped dictate the type and amount of benefits. In more ways than one, Germany's doctors determined the disabled veteran's future.[5]

The First World War both complicated and strained this system. Between 1914 and 1918 some 13.2 million men shuffled through the German armed forces. They came from all social segments of the German population, though the majority of them originated from rural regions of the empire.[6] In civilian life these men had been farmers, industrial workers, teachers, craftsmen, and professional soldiers, but the overwhelming majority of the recruits came from the working classes.[7] Roughly 2 million died. Approximately 4.3 million were injured, of whom 67,000 lost a limb.[8] The prospect of eventually pensioning off even a fraction of this number was a staggering thought for the military administration. Moreover, while many of the volunteers and draftees had been inducted as low ranking foot-soldiers, some of these men had claims to a much higher social status in civilian life. To return a highly skilled artisan home with a private's pension would not just compromise the existing social order of Wilhelmine Germany. Existing tensions between the classes would erupt, breaking down the temporary *Burgfrieden* (social peace) established on the political home front.

Realizing the potential strain the mass of war-injured posed to the existing system, in 1915 the German government made clear its policy toward soldiers disabled by the war: the Imperial War Office would assume responsibility for and oversee the immediate physical care of wounded soldiers. Rehabilitation and retraining, however, would fall to private organizations and the individual German states. In short, the military authorities wished only to treat those soldiers *who could be returned to active service*. Once a soldier was declared *dienstunfähig* (unfit for duty), he was discharged; in a neat bureaucratic maneuver, he no longer fell under the medical jurisdiction of the military.[9] In 1917 the German government further limited the future role of the military in the welfare of disabled soldiers, declaring, "The military authority must accord every possible support to the upbuilding and the intensive growth of the civilian cripple care work because, after demobilization, the further social care of our war cripples will fall entirely on these civilian agencies."[10] Modern trench warfare was draining the German army of both material *and* human resources. Ultimately, the military had to choose to support those men who could continue the war effort and cut its losses on those who could not. The burden of caring for Germany's war-wounded was thus shifted to volunteer civilian groups and private medicine.

Until the First World War the demand for orthopedics had been relatively small in Germany. Crippled care (*Krüppelfürsorge*) had been limited to the care of either congenitally disabled children or accident victims. Privately run convalescent homes supported by religious charity groups or working-class fraternal aid societies handled the majority of these cases, but a few doctors took on wealthier patients who could afford private care. Before 1914, few universities had established orthopedic clinics; the field was simply too young. Moreover, orthopedics was not covered in the states' medical boards (*Staatsexamen*) and was therefore a specialty that existed without official examination.[11] Few doctors felt the need to familiarize themselves with such a marginal field. Indeed, the first textbook for orthopedics was published only a few short months before the war. When the fighting broke out, few German doctors had the skills needed for dealing with the disabled.

Published in 1914 by Dr. Fritz Lange, *Lehrbuch der Orthopädie* was the first comprehensive teaching and training guide for orthopedists. This prewar medical textbook listed only two models of artificial arms: the "Sunday arm" (*Sonntagsarm*) and the "work claw" (*Arbeitsklau*). A Sunday arm was a cosmetic prosthesis typically carved from a lightweight wood and modeled after a natural, human arm. These were so named because most amputees wore them on Sundays and holidays for public or special occasions. Incapable of movement, they served only to hide the disability. By contrast, a work claw consisted of a metal hook or clamp fixed to the end of a leather casing. This "sleeve" was then slipped over the stump and strapped around the wearer's body. Its appearance was crude, mechanical, and foreign; it did, however, enable the wearer to firmly hold or carry an object. Its practical applications compensated for its aesthetic failings. A few wealthy Germans purchased advanced models from companies in the United States, the most popular being the so-called Carnes arm. At the time, this was the state-of-the-art in artificial arms, replicating as closely as possible the appearance of the human hand. Otherwise, though, there was neither the technology nor the demand for more advanced prostheses in Germany prior to the war.

THE ORTHOPEDIC RESPONSE TO WAR

When German forces marched into Belgium in August 1914, the military high command predicted a short war; an easy victory would bring everyone home by Christmas. The medical community was less sanguine, and as the first trainloads of heavy casualties arrived back in the homeland, they began to panic. The empire had neither a centralized disability pension office for the war-injured nor an empire-wide organizational apparatus to oversee and standardize care for the wounded. Traditionally the role of the state in the German welfare system had been rather limited. Rather than supporting national social or welfare services, the government had chosen instead to let this work fall to volunteer organizations, religious charities, fraternal aid societies, trade unions, or the individual German states (*Länder*). In 1914 the German empress requested that all private homes for the crippled, the elderly, and the orphaned open their doors to the nation's war-injured.[12] But this could have been little more than a show for the public, as these institutions could accommodate only a small fraction of the injured. To say that German medicine was overwhelmed by the war is to put it mildly.

Nonetheless the nation's orthopedists responded quickly. Many volunteered to work in field hospitals. They called conventions and gathered in research symposia.[13] Expert orthopedists edited field manuals for frontline doctors and published civilian guides for the care of the disabled at home. They developed on-site measures to mitigate previously deadly bullet fracture wounds and perfected stable methods of transport so that travel no longer posed a danger to the severely wounded. Not least of these wartime accomplishments was the technological revolution in artificial limbs. Orthopedics became indispensable in the treating of the war-wounded and orthopedists themselves—formerly at the margins of medicine—became unquestioned experts in the care and rehabilitation of the disabled.

In 1915 Dr. Konrad Biesalski published a short pamphlet for the war-disabled and their families, *Caring for War Cripples: A Word of Explanation to Both Comfort and Warn*.[14] As the director of the Oskar-Helene Home for the Treatment and Education of Disabled Children in Berlin and founding member of both the German Association for Crippled Care (*Deutsche Vereinigung für Krüppelfürsorge*) and the German Orthopedic Society (*Deutsche orthopädische Gesellschaft*), Biesalski was a recognized expert in the orthopedic care of crippled children.[15] He was an obvious choice to draft the guide for both the rehabilitation of the disabled soldier and the reeducation of the general public. By publishing this pamphlet, orthopedists hoped to allay the economic fears of the war-crippled and their families by showing how modern technology and physical reeducation could enable the disabled to return to their civilian line of work. Through medical explanations, a wide variety of diagrams and photographs, and several case studies, Biesalski "proved" that any disabled soldier could be successfully rehabilitated and returned to work. At the same time, he counseled the rest of the nation on the proper ways of handling the disabled and discouraged them from seeing cripples as helpless. In his opinion, successful rehabilitation depended on both the physical reeducation of the war-injured and the psychological re-education of the entire lay public.[16]

Biesalski considered it a "proven fact" that any disabled man could recover and be returned to his profession.[17] In his opinion, the biggest obstacle to recovery was not the injury itself, but the veteran's lack of will to fully recover and return to work. Too often, he noted, the disabled became convinced they could not resume their pre-accident lives and allowed themselves to become dependent on the charity of others. He argued that these men freely chose to remain disabled in order to continue collecting their pensions. This willful refusal to return to work was symptomatic of what he termed "pension psychosis," a phenomenon he believed to be widespread among Germany's disabled veterans.[18] Moreover, he added, many unenlightened members of society tended to reinforce this behavior by stereotyping the war-crippled as incapable of further productive work, as well. In criticizing those around the disabled, he wrote,

> The sentimental type says, "How can one be so unfeeling as to expect the poor man—who has lost his hand for the fatherland and has endured so much pain—to work again, especially when it is clear that a one-handed man is not able to work anymore." However, socially healthy human reason responds: "The cripple should earn his bread for himself and his dependents completely on his own, so that he does not . . . fall into misery and poor relief—for us, the hero of this war is too good for that—instead he should be an upstanding, economically independent member of our society, just as before."[19]

Biesalski argued that the will to work must be reawakened in every disabled veteran and that it was incumbent on those surrounding him to support this. Without constant reinforcement and positive publicity, the veteran would fall irreversibly victim to this "pension psychosis," remaining forever "delusional and uncooperative."[20]

Reading through the pamphlet designed to "comfort" disabled veterans, one is struck by the lack of empathy for the disabled veteran. By reducing the process of rehabilitation to a matter of will, Biesalski shifted responsibility onto the patient. In Biesalski's view, the disabled veteran who did not resume his work was easily labeled lazy, uncooperative, and will-less. Moreover, this redefinition of "disability" itself as a conditional state easily overcome radically recast the disabled veteran's public image from crippled war hero to stubborn slacker.

As if to underline the indisputable ease and certainty of rehabilitation, Biesalski further warned that the disabled veteran should not expect the German state to financially support him simply because he had lost an arm or leg. This practice was outdated, belonging to a past when it had not been possible to replace lost limbs or fully restore disabled men. According to Biesalski, instead of being a burden to the state, the disabled veteran ought to say to himself,

> Yes! I don't need to remain a useless cripple, I may once again eat my own bread with my family and I will be the same man that I was before, even up to the little injury [*kleinen Schaden*] that I want to accept— for the sake of the fatherland—as a sign of honor.[21]

The language that Biesalski used to describe disabled veterans and the counseling he prescribed for them tended to cast the disabled veteran as a childlike and self-centered individual who needed to be persuaded, even pushed, to work again. It was up to those people around him—family and friends, but especially the medical community—to practice a kind of vigilance against his desire to exploit the welfare state. On the one hand, Biesalski's paternalistic manner mirrored the larger, prewar middle-class attitudes toward the working classes; on the other hand, it was no doubt influenced by his ten years of professional experience with treating disabled children, not adults. However, Biesalski was not alone in holding these ideas. His pamphlet merely reflected prevailing opinions in orthopedic circles calling for the disabled to return to work as quickly as possible—not only for their own personal well-being, but more important, for the well-being of the entire German nation.

In 1916 the German Orthopedic Society and the German Association for Crippled Care held successive special conferences to discuss the future treatment of disabled soldiers. In addition to orthopedists and surgeons, attendees included representatives of heavy industry, insurance officials, private cripple homes, the German empress, and the Austro-Hungarian archduke.[22] For three days those present discussed medical strategies to heal and restore the rapidly increasing number of crippled war veterans. When Biesalski opened the conference by reminding the attendees of the importance of "awakening the will to work" in wounded soldiers, he was quickly supported.[23] Dr. Schultzen of Berlin agreed, adding that "of the utmost importance is social reinforcement. Prevention of the pension psychosis epidemic must be practiced. Healing and treatment is simply a pre-stage to the ability to work. Therefore job retraining should begin earlier and, under the supervision of doctors, be led with strict discipline."[24] The district administrator for Düsseldorf noted, "The goal of all medical care must be to make the wounded fit again to work in productive labor. . . . The will to work will not be supported through little manual skills or theory, but instead through practical job training. This is also the best manner for overcoming the pension fear."[25] Dr. Riedinger of Würzburg added that older men returned more quickly and with less resistance to their work than younger ones, because younger disabled veterans "hoped to better their social stations."[26] Dr. H. Gocht, professor of orthopedics at the University of Berlin, was even more explicit in his comments. In discussing the fundamental goals of prosthesis design, Gocht argued that the disabled placed overwhelming importance on the artificial limb's capacity to hide the disfigurement. He argued, rather, that

> the restoration of function, that is, the ability to work again and the ability to accomplish something, was of the greatest importance. And not simply with regard to the limbs of the severely injured and his will to work, but also for the general public, for the entire nation, and for the state.[27]

Discussion of rehabilitation centered on the outfitting and retraining of soldiers in order to return them to their professional work.

Orthopedists also obsessed about extinguishing so-called pension psychosis among the disabled. Assuming a dual role, as guardians of both the state *and* the disabled, German orthopedists treated Germany's war-amputees as opportunistic and interpreted it as their duty to send these men back to work. In this respect, orthopedists' philosophy simply fell in step with the longer tradition of German welfare. That the goal of welfare should be to preserve social status was the dominant principle of social insurance. Orthopedists, however, allowed this ideology to dictate more than rehabilitation goals; it also guided the design of specific limbs.

As war casualties mounted and the number of amputees appearing in Germany's hospitals continued to increase, orthopedists recognized the inadequacy of their current resources and the urgent need to update them. The choice of prostheses available to disabled soldiers was far too limited. If the new orthopedics was to return the thousands of Germany's disabled to the workforce, amputees would need more than the wooden Sunday arm and the simple work claw. Furthermore, the delivery of those available arms remained consistently behind order; many soon argued that designs should be Taylorized to allow for quick, factory production. In response, orthopedists and engineers created new artificial arms, highly specialized and divided along class lines. At first these designs concentrated on arms for general occupational fields, such as those for agricultural workers, for workers in light or heavy industry, and for *Kopfarbeiter*, those men whose professions relied more on mental "work." Gradually, however, doctors realized that developing job-specific arms created more efficient workers and concentrated on the manufacture of trade-specific prostheses, too. These new work arms were considered to be the only ones appropriate for Germany's war-disabled. Orthopedists no longer recommended Sunday arms for use as anything other than "supplementary arms."

Indeed, the First World War—and the total economic mobilization of society that accompanied it—made cosmetic arms largely obsolete. According to Biesalski and others, Sunday arms should not be assigned to Germany's war-disabled because they were "useless" in the workplace. Intended primarily as a cosmetic piece, an artificial arm of this type was capable of little more than masking the disability. In recalling the prewar Sunday arm, Lange described it as having a "hand which due to the inexpedient movement of the outer three fingers was practically useless—even for simply holding or carrying an object."[28] In his pamphlet Biesalski argued,

> An artificial arm with a hand is, as all laypeople must be told, essentially useful for nothing more than to hide the disfigurement. That is, it should be worn during strolls and used for simple movements: eating, holding a piece of paper, while writing and reading, etc. For any kind of *important function*, it has little value.[29]

Apparently, the German government also supported this opinion. From his post at the military hospital in Offenbach, Dr. Rebentisch reported a decree from the Medical Department of the Ministry of War that had recently "definitively ruled the unsuitableness of the purely decorative arm, which was to only cover the sustained loss."[30]

Of course, the construction of a natural-looking arm that was capable of work remained beyond current technology. In discussing artificial arms and hands for war-disabled, the military surgeon O. Witzel remarked, "The human hand—whether it be performing high culture or serving the wage-laborer—remains at present irreplaceable. It is especially impossible to fulfill demands that a prosthesis take into consideration both appearance and work ability."[31] This fundamental approach to arm design did not change over the course of the war. Dr. Theodor Mietens remarked two years later,

> In the question of the artificial arm it appears more and more self-evident that a universal appliance, as suitable in all ways as the natural human hand is, can neither be developed, nor does it need be. And the decorative arm and the work arm do not permit themselves to be combined in one and the same tool.[32]

Orthopedists could not combine their vision of a practical, useful arm with that of a cosmetic one and so opted to dispense with hiding the disability.

In designing substitutes for lost body parts—and replacing their functional capacity—orthopedists turned to the theories and practices of *Arbeitswissenschaft*, or the science of work. In the mid-nineteenth century, the human body was conceptualized as an animate machine that could be finely tuned and trained. Human engineers concentrated on harmonizing the physical movements of the human body with the increasing mechanization of work under industrial capitalism. By streamlining the corporeal activity of a worker, German scientists of work aimed to eliminate wasted motion and thereby increase worker productivity.[33] German orthopedists adhered to a similar set of principles while developing artificial limbs, analyzing the various occupations in minute detail and listing the motions absolutely necessary to their performance. By reducing each job to a series of movements, doctors determined which particular functions a worker had "lost" along with his arm and created a corresponding "work arm" capable of performing them. In short, form followed function in German prosthetic design.

Of course, the development of a single prosthesis capable of replacing all the movements of the human hand remained beyond their reach. Despite ever-new developments in prosthetic arms, Dr. Peter Janssen contended that no single perfect work arm yet existed. Explaining why, he argued, "this is because of the demands we must place on an artificial arm, which are completely different, depending on whether it has to do with the *Kopfarbeiter*, the industrial worker, or the agricultural worker."[34] In addition, noted Janssen, because of the crucial importance of job-specific working prostheses, his hospital conducted job counseling before dispensing arms in order to ensure that the disabled patient was completely "clear" with regard to his future profession.[35] By crafting job-specific prostheses and returning disabled workers to their former professions, orthopedists thus helped maintain the stability of the social structure.

Reporting on his experiences with disabled soldiers in Nürnberg, Dr. Adolf Silberstein emphasized the new demands placed on orthopedic rehabilitation as a result of the war. Before the war, he reminded his colleagues, no one truly expected a disabled man to return to a self-sustaining lifestyle and professional career through the aid of a prosthesis. To be sure, he acknowledged instances of the occasional attentive doctor who painstakingly crafted an individualized prosthetic for a disabled patient and then patiently trained him in the use thereof, but these cases were extremely rare. Even rarer, he continued, were those disabled individuals who could then use their prostheses comfortably and assuredly. He characterized such successful patients as demonstrations, mere witnesses to advances and technological possibilities in orthopedics. No one had seriously expected the disabled patient to earn a full-time living with the device. Furthermore, those men who had demonstrated work capacity with the artificial limb had been employed in orthopedic workshops. That is, they remained in the rehabilitation hospital. None had been subject to job competition on an open market.[36]

The war created new conditions, however, and doctors needed to create more than a capable prosthesis. Disabled soldiers needed to be able to perform to the same capacity, endurance level, and skill that their able-bodied competitors could. For this, new guidelines in the design of artificial limbs would have to be followed.[37] Modernizing prosthetic design would eliminate the need for the individual attention of doctors by creating more standardized but practical arms. The high-pressure atmosphere of war made it crucial to restore the disabled quickly and return them to work as soon as possible where they could resume being "productive members of human society."[38]

Silberstein recommended the Siemens-Schuckart arm for both industrial and agricultural workers. This prosthesis consisted of a leather harness strapped around the wearer with a metal rod extending from the shoulder area. Running parallel to the wearer's body, the "arm" had a metal joint at the end into which any number of specially designed working "hands" could be inserted and securely fastened. These "hands" ranged in form and shape from simple tools (e.g., a hammer), to brushes or cutlery with elongated handles, to specially crafted inserts designed to fit perfectly with corresponding industrial machinery. Figures 2.1 and 2.2 illustrate many of the "hands" available with the arm. Essentially, this prosthetic working arm was a tool holder.

According to Silberstein, each amputee was given a set of inserts to match his profession and was then considered equipped for work. In addition, the attachment joint was so constructed that it allowed the insertion of those ordinary, everyday tools used by skilled workers, but also conformed to a standard hand attachment size. This meant that any hand attachments produced by other manufacturers could be used with the Siemens arm. In the artificial arm industry, hand attachments became both standardized and interchangeable, much like the soldier-workers who eventually received them. Just as the principles of *Arbeitswissenschaft* denied the individual identities of workers in their quest for efficiency, the principles informing artificial limb design denied the identities of their wearers. Figures 2.3 and 2.4 show disabled soldiers in various professions at work with the arm.

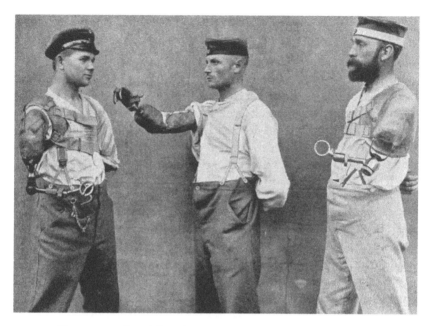

FIG. 2.1. Three examples of "hands." From Karl Nieny, "Die Behandlung und Ausrüstung der Amputierten im Marinelazarett Hamburg," *Zeitschrift für orthopädische Chirurgie* 37 (1917): 313.

Silberstein considered the Siemens arm revolutionary when compared to other arms—not merely in its outward form, but in the fundamental principles of its design. Other arms, he claimed, made the mistake of adhering to the form of the human hand. Instead, he argued, one must think of the prosthesis for the worker (but not the *Kopfarbeiter*) as nothing but a machine. Once the functions and demands of a prosthesis had been determined, the device itself needed to be built by an engineer, not a doctor.[39] Only the Siemens arm could fulfill these conditions. "It is the first artificial arm that has been constructed exclusively as a work tool. The uncompromising implementation of this idea—to create a machine and not an 'arm' [sic]—led logically to the considerable divergence from all previous systems."[40] In Silberstein's opinion, this was the first useful arm designed for Germany's workers. In addition to the abundant supply of interchangeable inserts, advantages of the arm were that it could be worn by either left- or right-arm amputees and that it did not include a leather stump-case requiring personalized fittings. Essentially the Siemens-Schuckart could be attached to practically any disabled body.

These arms could bring together nearly any disabled body with a range of standard industrial tools, from a simple carpenter's plane to a piece of heavy machinery. Many of these prosthetic "hands" physically fastened the disabled man to his work station. With the prosthesis attached to the amputee on one end and to machinery on the other, the disabled man's body gradually blended into his work. The quest for efficiency blurred the boundary between man and machine. In these cases the identity of the wearer was not so much denied as blatantly subjugated to that of his working equipment. The worker became nothing more than a living appendage or *human prosthesis* to his machine. A

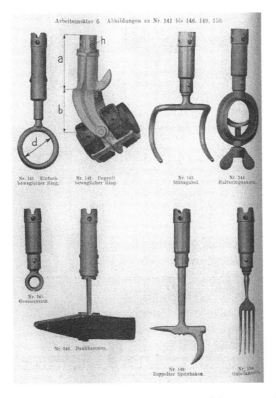

FIG. 2.2. Arm tools. From Adolf Silberstein, "Bein- und Armersatz im Kgl. Orthopädischen Reservelazarett zu Nürnberg," *Zeitschrift für orthopädische Chirurgie* 37 (1917): 376–77.

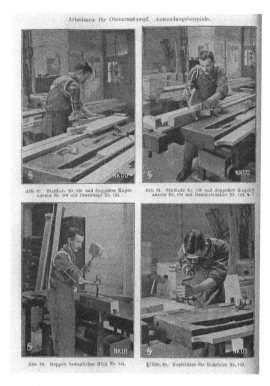

FIG. 2.3. Men at work. From Adolf Silberstein, "Bein- und Armersatz im Kgl. Orthopädischen Reservekazarett zu Nürnberg," *Zeitschrift für orthopädische Chirurgie* 37 (1917): 378–79.

closer look at the photos in figures 2.3 and 2.4 illustrates this point more clearly.

Fastening the prosthesis to industrial machinery may have drastically increased worker efficiency in some cases. It could also prove hazardous. Dr. F. Sauerbruch in Zurich noted two fundamental problems with an arm of this kind. First, the constant replacement and exchange of the inserts required both considerable time and the use of one healthy hand. The good hand loosened the joint, removed the old tool, exchanged it for the new tool, secured it in the joint, and tightened the closure. The constant attendance of the good hand to the artificial one meant a considerable loss of time, according to Sauerbruch. In his opinion, an arm of this kind was particularly useless to the double-amputee, who would not be able to open and close the joint. The need to quickly maneuver the arm is even more critical when the worker is attached to motorized machinery. Sauerbruch reported having observed the upper-arm stump of a disabled worker ripped from his body when the prosthesis he was wearing became caught up in factory machinery.[41]

In addition to standardization of design, production of prostheses in an inexpensive and timely manner became increasingly important as the war continued. In describing the perfect artificial limb, Dr. Mietens from Munich argued that it must without question meet the following demands: "have a good display of strength, freedom of movement, a simple construction, the use of which is easily learned, be easy to repair, and last, but not least, be cheap in price."[42] Given the inexhaustible material demands of the war that Germany faced, this was perhaps a somewhat tall order; however, it was one with which other doctors

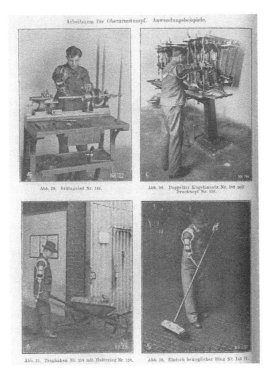

FIG. 2.4. Men at work. From Adolf Silberstein, "Bein- und Armersatz im Kgl. Orthopädischen Reservekazarett zu Nürnberg," *Zeitschrift für orthopädische Chirurgie* 37 (1917): 380–81.

agreed. Biesalski too supported the idea of factory-made arms, Taylorized for easy construction and repair. He argued that

> Only then can prosthesis construction become so inexpensive that truly every disabled man could acquire that prosthesis which is absolutely suitable for him, just like the wide dissemination of the automobile, the bicycle, the electric light, etc. was first possible when the standard parts became factory-made, available cheaply and everywhere.[43]

The push for standardization of arms was also due to the heavy demand placed on existing resources. As the war progressed, German prosthetic manufacturing companies could not keep up with the ever-increasing orders for artificial limbs. At the naval hospital in Hamburg, delivery of artificial arms was so far behind demand that the doctors there developed their own models of artificial limbs. In explaining this, Dr. Karl Nieny cited the factory's inability to keep up with demand as well as the pernicious effects of forcing amputees to wait for prostheses, noting that "there is no opportunity to keep them adequately busy and therefore they are losing quickly and in great quantity their desire to return to work, one which is most often impossible to reinstill."[44]

The prosthetic arm that he and his colleagues devised could be mass-produced in Hamburg. Local production drastically reduced the waiting period, provided substantial savings, and facilitated quick repairs. The hospital had spent considerable time and energy on the original design and manufacturing. However, in an effort to spare others such loss, he wanted to share their results. Now they were able to outfit their men with a new arm much faster, decreasing the waiting period and potential threat it posed to rehabilitation.

According to Nieny, the primary principle of development had been to "create an instrument designed to replace the human arm in as many functional ways as possible, and most importantly in the performance of productive work."[45] Specifically, the doctors concentrated on reproducing holding and grasping motions so the arms could act as clamps holding tool handles and nails and steadying machinery (see fig. 2.5).[46] As in most recovery hospitals during the war, an adjacent workshop training room had been set up to help men learn and practice the use of their arms. Nieny noted that in Hamburg they could outfit and train the men in the following professions: locksmithing, black-

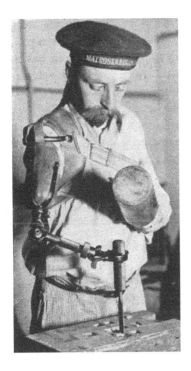

FIG. 2.5. Close-up of man at work. From Karl Nieny, "Die Behandlung und Ausrüstung der Amputierten im Marinelazarett Hamburg," *Zeitschrift für orthopädische Chirurgie* 37 (1917): 328.

smithing, plumbing, cabinet making, lathe turning, and other wood-working trades, and as tailors, shoemakers, and harness makers.[47] He regretted, however, that the majority of recovering workers showed little interest in excelling in these exercises, preferring rather to relearn their penmanship and apply for positions at the government's postal or train administrations. Continued counseling, he was sure, would bring these men into line. He did note that disabled men from the "educated professions" or those who had previously been independent businessmen showed far more enthusiasm for their prewar work. In the final analysis, however, he emphasized that "given the important meaning of rehabilitation for the national economy [*Volkswirtschaft*], there is no such thing as expending too much work or effort" and urged his fellow orthopedists to renew efforts at rehabilitation, despite the resistance of those who did not want to return to their prewar occupations.[48]

Not all of Germany's amputees, however, required the equivalent of an industrial tool holder in order to resume their old professions. The disabled *Kopfarbeiter*—or mental worker (literally head worker)—was categorized and treated differently than the injured manual laborer. In the main, these amputees had been civil servants, teachers, bookkeepers, or office workers. Whereas doctors methodically sought to distill the movements necessary for carrying out the work of the blacksmith or the woodworker, it was not necessary to rationalize the movements of the *Kopfarbeiter*. He worked with his head, *not* his hands. The "teacher's arm" or the "civil servant's arm" was neither created nor even proposed. The work of the *Kopfarbeiter* was considered substantially different from that of the industrial or agricultural worker, demanding less physical strength or manual dexterity. Therefore, whereas work arms were assigned to laborers and skilled workers, orthopedists deemed cosmetic or simple artificial arms sufficient to meet the needs of the *Kopfarbeiter*. The physical work required in these professions often consisted simply of holding papers, carrying light objects, or perhaps writing; orthopedists were far less preoccupied with the physical reconstruction of these men. What this amounted to in practice is that disabled *Kopfarbeiter* often received the "useless" but more natural-looking arms denied to other disabled veterans.

Many orthopedists ruled the Carnes arm—or one of similar construction—to be the ideal prosthesis for *Kopfarbeiter*. Both Nieny and Silberstein recommended it for those in the "intellectual professions."[49] In his lengthy analysis of the Carnes arm, Dr. Rudolf Ritter von Aberle noted its many advantages. The numerous levers and intricate gears enabled the wearer to perform more detail-oriented movements that were beyond the scope of tool-like work prostheses. These activities included tying a necktie, picking up coins from a flat surface, riding a bicycle, and taking banknotes out of a wallet (see fig. 2.6). This was apparently the kind of manual dexterity more appropriate for the *Kopfarbeiter*. According to von Aberle, an arm as delicate and finely crafted as the Carnes arm could not withstand the heavy labor of the field and factory. Furthermore, its high price and costly repairs should reserve this arm for those patients in intellectual professions.[50] In short, the Carnes arm was a middle-class arm.

In a brief discussion of the types of artificial arms available for Germany's disabled, Dr. P. Guradze of Wiesbaden also defined the Carnes arm as strictly for *Kopfarbeiter* and intellectuals.[51] This assessment of the Carnes arm was not limited to orthopedic circles: engineers, too, argued that such a mechanically sophisticated arm was impractical for many of

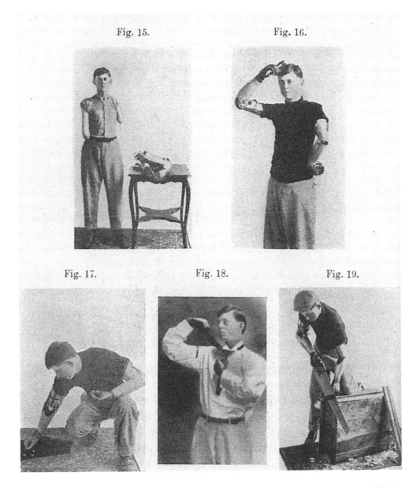

Fig. 15.   Fig. 16.

Fig. 17.   Fig. 18.   Fig. 19.

FIG. 2.6. "White-collar" arm picking up coins, tying necktie. From Rudolf Ritter von Aberle, "Künstliche Gliedmassen für Kriegsverwundete," *Zeitschrift für orthopädische Chirurgie* 35 (1916): 598.

Germany's disabled. In their evaluation of the Carnes arm, the engineers Arthur Ehrenfest-Egger and Siegfried Neutra could not recommend the prosthesis for the majority of arm amputees due to its high maintenance costs. Instead, they noted, the arm was far more useful and valuable for the "invalid intellectuals, especially for those in well-to-do circumstances."[52]

As the war continued, the development of artificial arms became increasingly patriotic. Orthopedists sought to remove German doctors and patients from their dependency on foreign nations. Dr. Max Cohn, a disabled orthopedist in Berlin, wore a Carnes arm himself. But after demonstrating the arm's usefulness in opening an umbrella and holding a pen, he conceded that "It is desirable that leading circles succeed in realizing that one should take pains to build this prosthesis here domestically in order to prevent a foreign firm—perhaps even an enemy one—from economically exploiting the thing after the war."[53] Biesalski argued that German factories could design and manufacture an arm similar to the Carnes arm as well as the Americans and at lower costs. Moreover, he noted, "it can hardly lie within the taste of the German soldier to accept an artificial arm as a replacement for one lost, when the prosthesis possibly stems from the same source as the grenade which brought him down."[54]

The entrance of the United States into the war brought an even more urgent push to develop German alternatives to the Carnes arm. In May 1917, Fritz Lange introduced a new prosthesis that was to replace the American arm. In his opinion, the Carnes arm was too heavy, complicated, and expensive. Most amputees, he argued, did not actually wear the arm. Instead, after just a few months of wear, they tended to go armless rather than use the device. He pointed out that of the 356 arms distributed in the Rhineland, already 310 had been discarded. On the other hand, his Lange hand was simple, sturdy, and inexpensive. Weighing in at just two hundred grams, it was a full three hundred grams lighter than the Carnes arm and "despite its light weight even more hearty than the heretofore produced wooden hands."[55] As if that were not enough to recommend his arm, Lange concluded triumphantly, "Therefore we now have every reason to rejoice that a German doctor has found the way to at least partly return to our amputees what the war has taken away from them."[56]

CONCLUSION

In reinventing and legitimizing their field, German orthopedists generated volumes of essays, medical reports, and how-to procedures during the First World War. Medical journals specializing in surgery, cripple care, and orthopedics brimmed with discussions of how to return Germany's war veterans to productive work. In 1915 Fritz Lange and J. Trumpp published a pocket-sized volume entitled *War Orthopedics*. Named for the emergent specialty that it described, the manual was a guide for medical officers with no official training in the field.[57] In 1917 the *Journal for Orthopedic Surgery* (*Zeitschrift für orthopädische Chirurgie*) published a special 828-page volume devoted to the development and construction of artificial limbs, including over 750 pictures, diagrams, and sketches.[58] In an expanded version of the *Lehrbuch der Orthopädie* published in 1922, Fritz Lange cited the new field of war orthopedics, the progress in prosthetic science, and the revolution in orthopedics as justifications for the new edition.[59] He also noted the existence of sixty-five newly founded institutes in Germany conducting research in the new orthopedics and the establishment of a state medical exam for orthopedics. Thanks to their contributions, orthopedists had won significant official recognition from the German state.

The wartime goals of German orthopedists expanded far beyond the simple rehabilitation of the nation's disabled soldiers. To orthopedists, the wounded veteran represented the larger German nation, one who was crippled in battle and needed to be economically and physically rebuilt. Since they mapped their concerns about German society onto the body of the German soldier, the physical reconstruction of the disabled veteran became tantamount to the rebuilding of the nation itself. In the *weltanschauung* of orthopedists, the rehabilitation of the German soldier's body became crucially linked with the reconstruction of the German social order. Orthopedists sought to manage the postwar relocation of Germany's veterans, sending them back to prewar professions and standards of living. This effort to stabilize an empire caught in the political and economic upheaval of war resulted in the physical reproduction of class boundaries. Since a disabled soldier's artificial arms were tailored to meet his professional needs, prostheses themselves became markers of class identity. The work prostheses firmly bound the worker to his profession, and by extension, to his class: a veteran with a specially crafted arm or set of working hands could not easily change jobs. This job inflexibility would have catastrophic implications during the inflationary period and unemployment crisis of the Weimar Republic.[60] In this respect, orthopedists physically reproduced prewar identities on Germany's veterans, as class status was now inscribed upon the body.

NOTES

The research for this essay was supported by an exchange fellowship between Indiana University and the Christian-Albrechts-Universität zu Kiel (Germany). From October 1997 through July 1999 I profited from the overwhelming intellectual and material generosity of my fellow researchers at the Zentrum für interdisziplinäre Frauenforschung (ZiF) at the CAU. This study (and my stay in Kiel) could not have been completed successfully without their support.

1. See, e.g., Robert Weldon Whalen, *Bitter Wounds: German Victims of the Great War, 1914–1939* (Ithaca: Cornell University Press, 1984). Also Richard Bessel, *Germany after the First World War* (Oxford: Oxford University Press, 1993).

2. Here, for example, see James M. Diehl, *Paramilitary Politics in Weimar Germany* (Bloomington: Indiana University Press, 1977).

3. For a brief but relevant description of both the German welfare tradition and the military pension laws, see Whalen's appropriate chapter thereon. He offers a concise, clear and readable discussion of the subject. Whalen, *Bitter Wounds*, 83–93.

4. Whalen, *Bitter Wounds*, 88–89.

5. Whalen, *Bitter Wounds*, 59–60.

6. Bessel, *Germany after the First World War*, 10.

7. See Whalen, *Bitter Wounds*, 41 for a brief discussion of class composition among casualties.

8. Yet even Whalen points out that in the confusion of war the wounds of some 604,533 (84 percent of Germany's total wounded) remained unclassified. Whalen, *Bitter Wounds*, 40, 55–56. Bessel cites a figure of 2.7 million permanently disabled men, but does not distinguish between amputees and other forms of disability. Bessel, *Germany after the First World War*, 275.

9. Garrard Harris, *The Redemption of the Disabled* (New York: D. Appleton, 1919).

10. As quoted in Douglas McMurtrie's analysis of the response to war cripple care in Germany, *Evolution of National Systems of Vocational Rehabilitation Reeducation for Disabled Soldiers and Sailors* (Washington, DC: Government Printing Office, 1918), 138.

11. Fritz Lange and J. Trumpp, *Taschenbuch des Feldarztes*, part 3, *Kriegs-Orthopädie* (Munich: J. F. Lehmann's Verlag, 1915).

12. Konrad Biesalski, *Kriegskrüppelfürsorge: Ein Aufklärungswort zum Troste und zur Mahnung* (Leipzig: Leopold Voss Verlag, 1915), 25.

13. Of these, the more significant were the Ausserordentliche Tagung der Deutschen Vereinigung für Krüppelfürsorge, held 7 February 1916 in Berlin, and the Ausserordentliche Tagung der Deutschen Orthopädischen Gesellschaft, held immediately thereafter, 8–9 February 1916. Reports from

these and other "exceptional conferences" held during the war can be found in the journals *Zeitschrift für orthopädische Chirurgie* and *Zeitschrift für Krüppelfürsorge*.

14. Biesalski, *Kriegskrüppelfürsorge*.

15. Biesalski founded the DVK in 1908 with Eduard Dietrich. The founding of the DOG followed shortly thereafter. See H. Eckhardt "Die Entwicklung der Krüppelfürsorge in Deutschland," *Zeitschrift für Krüppelfürsorge* 23 (1930): 394 for a description of the founding and development of cripple care shortly before the war.

16. By August 1916 over 140,000 copies of the pamphlet had sold. It was translated and published in Hungarian; and (unrealized) plans were made for translating the work into Polish and Slovenian. For a more detailed discussion of the brochure, see Klaus-Dieter Thomann, "Die medizinische und soziale Fürsorge für die Kriegsversehrten," in *Die Medizin und der Erste Weltkrieg*, ed. Wolfgang U. Eckart and Christoph Gradmann (Pfaffenweiler: Centaurus-Verlagsgesellschaft, 1996).

17. Biesalski, *Kriegskrüppelfürsorge*, 15.

18. Biesalski, *Kriegskrüppelfürsorge*, 18.

19. Biesalski, *Kriegskrüppelfürsorge*, 13–14.

20. Biesalski, *Kriegskrüppelfürsorge*, 18.

21. Biesalski, *Kriegskrüppelfürsorge*, 17.

22. See note 13 for more information about this conference.

23. Konrad Biesalski, in "Bericht über die ausserordentliche Tagung der Deutschen Vereinigung für Krüppelfürsorge," *Zentralblatt für chirurgische und mechanische Orthopädie* 10 (1916): 74–88, 75 (hereafter cited as "Bericht DVK").

24. Schultzen, in "Bericht DVK," 75–76.

25. Horion, in "Bericht DVK," 77.

26. Riedinger, in "Bericht DVK," 77.

27. Gocht, in "Bericht der ausserordentlichen Tagung der Deutschen Orthopädischen Gesellschaft," *Zeitschrift für orthopädische Chirurgie* 37 (1916): 209–671, 215 (hereafter cited as "Bericht DOG").

28. Fritz Lange, ed., *Lehrbuch der Orthopädie*. 2d ed. (Jena: Verlag von Gustav Fischer, 1922), 553.

29. Biesalski, *Kriegskrüppelfürsorge*, 12.

30. Rebentisch, "Erfahrungen bei der Beschaffung von Kunstgliedern für Kriegsbeschädigte," *Zeitschrift für orthopädische Chirurgie* 37 (1917): 334–50, 337.

31. O. Witzel, "Die Aufgaben und Wege für den Hand- und Armersatz der Kriegsbeschädigten," *Münchener medizinische Wochenschrift* 44 (1915): 1491–92, 1491.

32. Theodor Mietens, "Ein willkürlich beweglicher Arbeitsarm," *Feldärztliche Beilage zur Münchener medizinische Wochenschrift* 3 (1917): 100–103, 101.

33. In Germany scientists emphasized the social utility of their discoveries, specifically the creation of more efficient workers, the reduction of fatigue (the debilitating *mal de siècle*), and higher industrial productivity. Two good sources for further reading on this subject include Matthew Hale, *Human Science and Social Order: Hugo Munsterberg and the Origins of Applied Psychology* (Philadelphia: Temple University Press, 1980); and Anson Rabinbach, *The Human Motor: Energy, Fatigue, and the Origins of Modernity* (New York: Basic Books, 1990), 179–205.

34. Peter Janssen, "Was muss der Lazarettarzt von der Prothese wissen?" *Feldärztliche Beilage zur Münchener medizinische Wochenschrift* 12 (1917): 398–401, 400.

35. Janssen, "Was muss der Lazarettarzt wissen?" 400.

36. Adolf Silberstein, "Bein- und Armersatz im Kgl. Orthopädischen Reservelazarett zu Nürnberg," *Zeitschrift für orthopädische Chirurgie* 37 (1917): 350–84, 361.

37. Silberstein, "Bein- und Armersatz," 364.

38. Silberstein, "Bein- und Armersatz," 362.

39. Silberstein, "Bein- und Armersatz," 363–4.

40. Silberstein, "Bein– und Armersatz," 382.

41. F. Sauerbruch, "Willkürlich bewegbare Arbeitsklaün," *Münchener medizinische Wochenschrift* 10 (1918): 257–58, 257.

42. Mietens, "Ein willkürlich beweglicher Arbeitsarm," 101.

43. Konrad Biesalski, "Über Prothesen bei Amputationen des Armes insbesondere des Oberarmes," *Münchener medizinische Wochenschrift* 44 (1915): 1492–96, 1496.

44. Karl Nieny, "Die Behandlung und Ausrüstung der Amputierten im Marinelazarett Hamburg," *Zeitschrift für orthopädische Chirurgie* 37 (1917): 302–33, 325.

45. Nieny, "Die Behandlung und Ausrüstung," 318.

46. Nieny, "Die Behandlung und Ausrüstung," 318–19.

47. Nieny, "Die Behandlung und Ausrüstung," 328–29.

48. Nieny, "Die Behandlung und Ausrüstung," 330–31.

49. Nieny, "Die Behandlung und Ausrüstung," 327; Silberstein, "Bein- und Armersatz," 365.

50. von Aberle, "Künstliche Gliedmassen für Kriegsverwundete" *Zeitschrift für orthopädische Chirurgie* 35 (1916): 584–610, 601.

51. P. Guradze, "Über Amputationsstumpf und Prothesen," *Zeitschrift für orthopädische Chirurgie* 37 (1917): 83–93, 93.

52. Arthur Ehrenfest-Egger and Siegfried Neutra, "Die Carnesarmprothese," Mitteilung des Vereins "Die Technik für die Kriegsinvaliden" (1915), no. 2, as noted in *Zeitschrift für orthopädische Chirurgie* 38 (1918): 695.

53. Max Cohn in "Bericht DOG," 264.

54. Biesalski, "Über Prothesen bei Amputationen," 1494.

55. Fritz Lange, "Eine neü Kunst- und Arbeitshand," *Feldärtzliche Beilage zur Münchener medizinische Wochenschrift* 20 (1917): 661–664, 662.

56. Lange, "Eine neue Kunst- und Arbeitshand," 664.

57. Lange and Trumpp, *Taschenbuch des Feldarztes,* part 3, *Kriegs-Orthopädie,* iii–iv.

58. "Gesammelte Arbeiten über die Prothesenbau," *Zeitschrift für orthopädische Chirurgie* 37 (1917).

59. Lange, *Lehrbuch der Orthopädie.*

60. See Bessel, *Germany after the First World War,* esp. 277, for further discussion of the reemployment and unemployment problems facing disabled and healthy veterans alike.

3

From Cotton to Silicone

Breast Prosthesis before 1950

Kirsten E. Gardner

IN 1904 LAURA WOLFE, a single woman who worked as a saleslady in downtown Columbus, Ohio, filed a patent for an "artificial breast pad."[1] After earning her patent two years later, she described the product as "durable and efficient and simple and comparatively inexpensive to make."[2] Like many inventors seeking patents for breast forms, she relied on basic and accessible products to create the forms. By combining a clever design with uncomplicated production, Wolfe and other women filing patents in the early 1900s earned a niche in the male-dominated fields of retail sales, manufacture, and business. Moreover, in filing for a patent application, inventors articulated their designs, intent, and purpose and rendered a detailed record of the material culture of these early artificial parts.[3]

Many of the first patents for breast forms, filed as early as 1873, identified the aesthetic value of their product. Beginning in 1919 some applicants distinguished a medical application for the form. By then, surgeons performed a radical mastectomy as standard treatment for breast cancer and increasing numbers of women survived a breast cancer diagnosis.[4] An expanding market emerged for women who wanted to disguise the results of this extensive surgery by wearing breast forms. As one inventor explained, a surgical bust form offered a "convenient and comfortable substitute for the bust of a woman, which has been removed by surgical operation, and which will relieve the flattened appearance caused by the operation and will reproduce the exact shape of the amputated part."[5]

Historically inventors have conflated the aesthetic and medical application of the breast form. In midcentury, however, as refined and synthetic materials became part of breast form production, inventors' designs reflected a heightened sensitivity to the needs of post-mastectomy patients. Moreover, patent production shifted to factories, overseas locations, and corporate ownership. Tracing breast prosthesis patents from the late nineteenth century to the mid-twentieth illuminates the functions of this form as both a fashion accessory and a therapeutic surgical device. The history records inventors', and moreover common laypersons', knowledge of breast cancer treatment, the medical implications of radical surgery, and a woman's sensitivity to the amputated breast. References to surgical scars from the radical mastectomy, indentations that resulted in the chest and shoulder, and the disfigurement that accompanied this operation speak to the inventors' familiarity with breast cancer treatment. The record in the patent further employs language and visual representation of different shapes and forms of the breast and suggests how value was attached to the various characteristics of a replacement breast. Finally, all inventors of breast forms, whether their products were designed for cosmetic or medical purpose, stressed the importance of natural appearance in an artificial form and recognized a profitable market as they sought proprietary claims on their designs.

In spite of the specificity apparent in the breast prosthetic market by midcentury, both aesthetic and medical breast forms relied on similar popular conceptions of femaleness, womanhood, and "wholeness." Comparing early patents for breast forms offers a lens through which to compare images of the female body, particularly the breast, and efforts to augment and imitate it. This essay explores the design, construction, and material culture of external breast prostheses designed before 1950.

EARLY BREAST FORMS

In 1874 the U.S. Patent Office issued its first patent for a breast prosthesis to Frederick Cox.[6] This "breast pad" introduced the basic components of the first breast prostheses—a fabric casing filled with an artificial material meant to serve as a substitute for human breast tissue. The first "breast pad" design relied on a cotton "cushion" as casing and "inflatable india-rubber breast pads" as fill material. It served a cosmetic func-

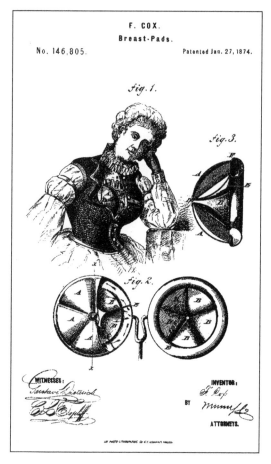

FIG. 3.1. "Breast Pad" by Frederick Cox. U.S. Patent 146,805 (27 January 1874).

tion and created the illusion of larger breasts. Most early prostheses were based on this "casing model" and varied according to their shape, choice of fill material, and adaptations for comfort or ventilation. Using cheap and accessible supplies, designers often made casings of cotton, and fill material ranged from cotton to feathers, sponge, rubber, or hair.

In figure 3.1 the model's appearance, including her refined clothing, hair design, and corset-imposed shape, point to Cox's assumption that his part be associated with upper-class customers concerned with contemporary notions of female fashion and standards of beauty.

For Cox, air-filled rubber offered a substitute for the breast that could be worn over the existing breast, appear real, and maintain a level of comfort and ventilation for the wearer. His reliance on inflatable rubber as fill material came under attack by future inventors, however. Patents filed post-1874 that relied on a solid fill material argued that inflatable models might puncture, burst, or prove less durable than solid fill. As Wolfe explained in her initial patent application in 1904, her design improved the artificial breast by ensuring the breast would maintain its shape when punctured. Replacing the inflatable model with a solid model, she promised her design would be "less liable to incur

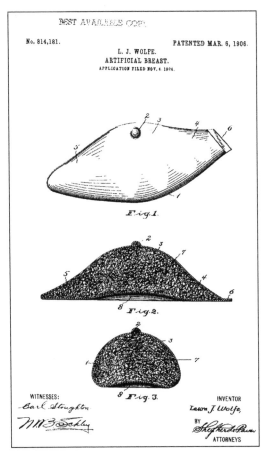

FIG. 3.2. "Artificial Breast" by Laura Wolfe. U.S. Patent 184,182 (6 March 1906).

humiliation upon the wearer than similar devices now known to the trade."[7]

Wolfe further articulated the three major concerns for artificial breast wearers: comfort, appearance, and product quality. She recommended a form made of rubber casing and stuffed with a soft fill material such as down or silk floss. In addition, she noted that the rubber casing could be dyed to match skin tone and lend a more realistic appearance. While this could be construed as an early awareness of racial diversity, no other evidence suggests that this was her intent. Although she articulated her concern for matching a woman's skin tone in her 1904 patent application, this concern seemed to disappear from later patents. In recent decades it has resurfaced as breast prosthetic companies expand their product line to include a range of skin tones, introduced specifically for African American women who needed breast prostheses.

Although Wolfe identified the aesthetic nature of her form, she introduced a second innovation that became a critical component of good medical breast prostheses. Insistent that larger breast size would look natural only if additional fill material were inserted near the edges of the breast form, Wolfe introduced extra pieces of fabric in her design. Depicted in her patent drawing (fig. 3.2) as parts 4 and 5, the "extension" promised to lend the appearance of additional tissue surrounding the breast. Wolfe also added small, flat, rectangular sections of material, depicted in part 6, to the side of each breast form to enhance its realistic appearance. "It will be understood that when the female chest and bust increases in size it is not only the breast or gland which grows larger, but the fatty portions upon the outer side thereof also increase."[8] This material flap would ultimately be imitated in surgical forms to help fill the indentations that resulted from the Halsted mastectomy.

MASTECTOMY AND PROSTHESES

The radical mastectomy, frequently referred to as a Halsted mastectomy after William S. Halsted popularized this type of operation in America in 1894, included the surgical removal of the breast, lymph nodes, pectoral muscles, and all surrounding tissue that might be cancerous.[9] The operation could be even more extensive depending on the surgeon. As one physician described it,

This operation consists in the removal of the mammary gland with a considerable amount of skin. The thorough dissection of the axilla. Removal of the sternal portion of the pectoralis major muscle. Division of the pectoralis minor, and occasional removal of this muscle. If necessary, exploration of the infra-clavicular and supra-clavicular spaces. This operation requires perfection of technique; operative skill; experienced judgement. It is comprehensive, thorough, far-reaching.[10]

As medical practitioners standardized breast cancer treatment in the form of the radical mastectomy throughout most of the twentieth century, breast prostheses manufacturers articulated a medical application for artificial breasts.

Laura Mailleue promised in her patent application, "Surgical Bust Substitute," a "perfect restoration of the original figure."[11] Mailleue earned this patent in 1922. She shared Wolfe's concerns about comfort, realistic appearance, and durability, but also articulated the medical usefulness of this part. She explicitly identified the surgical results of mastectomy and the prosthetic nature of the artificial breast.

Mailleue explained that her design would restore "the natural appearance of the figure" after surgical removal of the breast. Without mentioning cancer or mastectomy, she alluded to the surgical removal of the breast throughout her application and stressed the design's import in re-creating a woman's "natural appearance." As she explained, "a perfect restoration of the original figure is obtained and the elastic holding bands are flattened over the sides and back and shoulder so that they can not be noticed underneath the clothing." Mailleue also clarified that a firm material, in this case, whalebone, lent structure to an artificial breast in the absence of a natural breast.

Employing descriptive rhetoric, Mailleue relied on vocabulary often associated with images of femininity to describe the material culture of her part. She suggested a "dainty" casing material. In addition, she encouraged designers to improve the appearance of the form. "The edge may be finished with a border of lace if desired, thus giving an attractive appearance to the device." Finally, her reference to manufacturers as artists and her inclusion of advice for individual adaptations to the part suggest that production was often assumed by those trained in the craft of sewing and operating business in a very small-scale manner. She articulated that her design was meant to serve as a prototype that would enable "others skilled in the art" to employ her ideas.

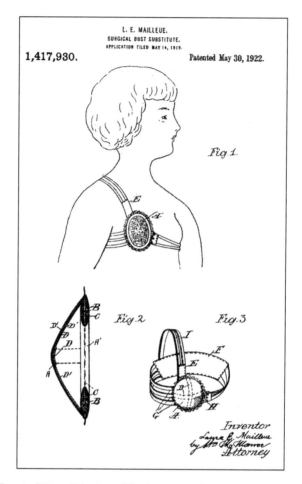

FIG. 3.3. "Surgical Bust Substitute" by Laura Mailleue. U.S. Patent 1,417,930
(20 May 1922).

Mailleue's drawing was a striking part of her application. The
childlike appearance of the model, the small size for the breast pad, and
the deliberate attention paid to the frill surrounding the prosthesis triv-
ialized the mastectomy. It ignored the biological female form and the
manipulative effects of surgery, and presented the prosthesis as an un-
derwear garment meant to be attractive. She depicted a young girl's
body, thereby ignoring the reality of cancer diagnosis, most often occurring in midlife. Finally, she included a drawing that seemed inap-

propriate, but may also have reflected an uninformed attempt to depict a woman recently treated for breast cancer.

Like many patents for artificial breasts, this patent also included directions for wearing the false breast. Mailleue suggested that the form be permanently attached to a belt that could be worn around the chest, with two narrow elastic bands attached to serve as shoulder straps, connecting the top of the breast form to the back of the belt. This arrangement ensured that the artificial breast would remain in place and provide comfort for the wearer. This device could be adjusted to accommodate either a right or left breast form.

The drawing and description of this prosthesis illustrate how artificial medical parts reflected notions of gender. Mailleue's attention to the physical appearance of the device and her choice of adjectives to describe the part both suggest a concern that consumers perceive this product as "feminine." She devoted considerably more attention to the cosmetic nature of the breast prosthesis than its practical function, foreshadowing similar emphases in the breast prosthetic marketing in the second half of the century.[12]

Although Wolfe's "Artificial Breast" and Mailleue's "Surgical Bust Substitute" had distinct functions, each shared common characteristics. In fact, the detailed classification system created by the U.S. Patent Office did not distinguish breast forms for beauty purposes and prostheses meant to replace an amputated breast. The patent office classified both Wolfe's and Mailleue's patents under the category "prosthesis" within the subclass of "breast prosthesis."

As the patent classification system suggested and Wolfe and Mailleue's patents attest, breast enhancement products or "falsies" and prosthetic breasts closely resembled each other. Both attempted to replicate the characteristics of a human breast and match its natural weight, size, texture, color, and form. In fact, with a few exceptions, many of the patented breast forms—with minor adjustments—could serve either purpose.[13]

In 1937 Blanche Wiggers, a widow who lived in downtown Baltimore and worked as a clerk for the Maryland and Pennsylvania Railroad Company, earned a patent for her "Breast Adapter."[14] Within several pages that described the various attributes of this part, Wiggers explained that it would "have arrangements for giving a filled-in structure for the breast portion of the body after surgical incidents." Specifically, Wiggers argued that current breast forms did not replace the "bodily injuries that have resulted in the removal of the breast, muscles and flesh of the human body in the vicinity of the chest."[15] Wiggers recognized the extensive nature of radical mastectomy and demonstrated familiarity with medical terminology and breast cancer. She explained that a mastectomy led to "severe depression" throughout the breast, chest, and shoulder region. Her design filled all these areas. She introduced the idea of creating a fill for the hollow area above the breast and extending to the shoulder.

> The muscle structure that leads to the breast follows across the pectoral plane of the body towards the deltoidal interconnections, and its removal brings about a severe depression extending from the lower base line of the breast, upwardly and apexed towards the shoulder juncture.[16]

Wiggers's artificial breast was made of a "special nonabsorbent spongy rubber." This material gave the form resiliency in every direction. In addition to offering a natural appearance, sponge rubber reduced the number of "embarrassing displacements" that might occur with other, more slippery materials. She pierced the material for better ventilation. Wiggers also included a small hump in the sponge rubber to give the appearance of a nipple.

Although Wiggers's description indicates a familiarity with the radical mastectomy, her drawing reflects her reliance on the model of false breasts meant to augment existing breasts. First, although she employs frills above the breast to offset the unnatural spherical shape of the false breast, she does not indicate how these frills could be used to fill the gaps under the arms and often in front of the shoulders. Second, as figures 1 and 3 in Figure 3.4 indicate, her design offered little support for wearing an artificial part and securing it in place, especially in the absence of an existing breast. Finally, figure 2 devotes considerable attention to accommodating the existing breast, a concern that post-mastectomy consumers would not have.

While surgeries varied depending on the surgeon, the type of cancer, and the extent of the cancer's growth at the time of the operation, most women undergoing a mastectomy lost much more than a breast. Wiggers's patent was one of the first to discuss extensive loss of flesh, muscles, and breast tissue and she was aware that the surgery caused indentations in the chest and shoulder. "The conventional breast form

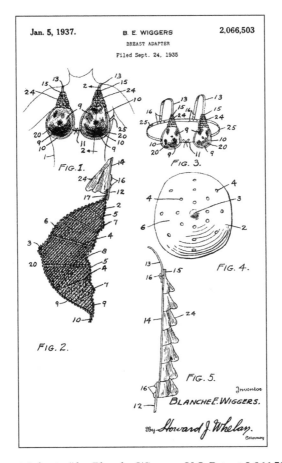

FIG. 3.4. "Breast Adapter" by Blanche Wiggers. U.S. Patent 2,066,503 (5 January 1937).

does not provide for the physical depression above the breast caused by the removal of the muscular structure and thus leaves a noticeable dent in the clothes at this portion of the body."[17] Wiggers included a "depression insert" in her design, similar to Mailleue's tongue appendage. Depicted as parts 15 and 24 in the patent, the fill offered a soft and gradual fill between the breast and the upper chest. In addition to filling space, this prosthesis was designed to ensure adequate ventilation, thereby preventing heat pockets that might cause a woman to sweat excessively.

In 1949 two women filed a patent for a "Restoration Surgical Breast" that was designed to "take the place of a breast that has been removed, as by surgery."[18] Instead of basing the model for an artificial breast on an imagined perfect breast, Mildred Wright and Dora Gates proposed a design that would allow the manufacturer to imitate the size and shape of the existing breast. The inventors devoted considerable attention to post-mastectomy needs, identifying common problems with skin irritation and tenderness after surgery. Recognizing the needs of the wearer, they used inexpensive material that could be easily washed with soap and water. Women could safely wear the artificial breast while swimming. Finally, it was designed to stay in place when the arm was moved or raised.

Wright and Gates expressed familiarity with mastectomy. For instance, they recognized the different results of surgery on each woman's body and therefore promised that the "artificial breast is individually designed to fit the scar tissues."[19] Instead of designing a post-mastectomy bra to accommodate the breast form, the inventors assured that it could be worn in any standard brassiere. Finally, the inventors of the restoration breast identified the psychological implications of breast cancer treatment. They wrote, "By means of the present invention . . . a woman's body will have a natural appearance so that the woman can live a normal life without being self-conscious as a result of the loss of a breast." Figure 1 of the patent design (fig. 3.5) represented "a front elevation view showing a woman with one of her breasts removed, as from a mastectomy." Although many women faced scars more severe than that depicted in figure 1, this patent demonstrated concern with the effects of mastectomy. Figure 2 reflects a familiarity with the need to create a holding mechanism in the absence of a breast. Figure 3 offers a realistic depiction of a chest wall after a breast amputation, and figure 6 reflects the fact that the surgery left a concave gap in the chest wall.

WEARING A PROSTHESIS

Popular women's magazines devoted articles to cancer as early as 1913, offering a detailed discussion of the early symptoms of breast cancer and encouraging women to consult a doctor immediately if they noticed any indications of cancer.[20] Throughout the early decades of the

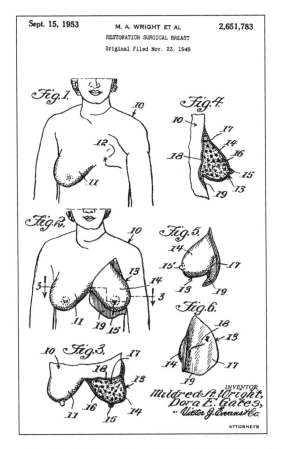

FIG. 3.5. "Restoration Surgical Breast" by Mildred A. Wright and Dora A. Gates. U.S. Patent 2,651,783 (23 November 1949).

twentieth century, magazines such as *Ladies' Home Journal, Good Housekeeping*, and *Scientific America* spread the message of early detection regularly, and presented surgery as a cure for this dreaded disease. Popular medical wisdom suggested that cancers discovered in their first stages could be excised by surgery, before the growth had metastasized. Despite the continual emphasis on surgery as a cure, few journalists discussed the details of mastectomy, effects of treatment, and postoperative care before midcentury.

Marion Flexner's 1947 autobiographical story "Cancer—I've Had It" reflected a shift in the popular discussion of breast prostheses.

Flexner recounted her breast cancer diagnosis and subsequent mastectomy. She explained,

> One of my first problems was to get a false breast, which I knew I would have to wear as soon as I put my clothes on. I called a local department store and ordered one over the telephone. It came—a small, pincushionlike affair to be shoved into the empty side of my old brassiere.[21]

Flexner explained that the "falsie" did not fit and did not resemble a human breast. She then visited a "surgical *corsetiere*" and bought a false breast made of sponge rubber. This form served its purpose, resembled a breast, and restored Flexner's confidence.

Patent applications filed in midcentury articulated the rapidly changing production and standards of breast prostheses. The distinctions between breast forms for aesthetic augmentation and forms intended to replace an amputated breast reflected different types of production and distinct customer bases. Many inventors clarified the purpose of their forms as surgical. Abe Silverman said his invention "relates to the surgical breast pads which are adapted to be used and worn by women who have a breast amputated due to cancer, tumor, or for other causes." Indicating his familiarity with the radical mastectomy, he promised that his surgical form "fills in the void caused by the removal of the cancerous tissue which is customarily removed in such surgical operations." Employing a combination of foam rubber particles held together with rubber cement, Silverman envisioned his breast pad as an improved and realistic replacement form for women surgically treated for breast cancer.[22]

Throughout the 1950s popular women's magazines also described the medical dimensions of breast cancer treatment more starkly. Moreover, articles reminded readers that a prosthesis could hide the results of mastectomy. As one journalist noted, "No one outside the immediate family need know she has had the operation—just as she does not know that many women whose names are household words have undergone the experience."[23] As the article entitled "After Breast Surgery" indicated, entire articles focused on caring for one's health after a mastectomy, suggested the importance attached to this artificial part, and offered advice about purchasing one. The public discussion of prosthetic breasts also indicated the expanding product line available by midcentury. "The device may be made of plain rubber, foam rubber, liquid-filled plastic, or air-filled plastic. It should match the remaining breast as closely as possible, at the sides, front, and top."[24]

In addition to providing information about the material culture of the breast prosthesis and advice about buying the product, magazine articles discussed the psychological impact of losing a breast and the healing powers of a prosthetic form. One woman revealed her discomfort with the prosthesis:

> The hardest lesson for me was how to cope with fear. For months *after* the mastectomy I lived in a new kind of terror. I had lost part of myself for which there could be no compensation—an integral part of my femininity. I hid away in my room, feeling like a criminal every time I put on my new foam-rubber breast. It seemed a sort of deception I was perpetuating on the general public because it allowed me to pretend to be a whole woman.

Comparing herself to people who had lost limbs, this woman continued, "I would have preferred losing an arm or leg—something that could be discussed publicly without flinching—anything unconnected with sex."[25] While this reaction stressed the initial discomfort with the breast form, eventually the author learned to appreciate the artificial breast and attributed her returning sense of "normalcy" to it.

In a 1957 article, "I'm Glad I Had My Breast Removed," the author discussed her reticence to ask her doctor about her post-mastectomy concerns. Finally, her doctor introduced the discussion and encouraged the woman to wear a proper prosthesis after surgery. "Wearing an artificial breast . . . will give you the confidence and the pleasure of knowing you look perfectly natural to others." Relieved, the author described her first fitting for a breast prosthesis:

> A nurse came and took my measurements, and by the time I was ready to leave the hospital my new brassieres were ready and waiting for me. The form was exactly like my other breast in size and shape, built to replace even the underarm fullness that was taken away. Its soft, pliable composition makes it feel natural against my body.[26]

CONCLUSION

Patents offer a wealth of evidence about the material culture of this artificial part, including descriptions of the materials used to create the part, arguments about its intent and purpose, and explanations of how each design improved on or contributed to previously patented prostheses. Typical patent applications included a description of the invention, a drawing of the product, a list of its objectives, and references to preceding patents of a similar product. Surgical trade journals offered similar information about the part, but also discussed concerns such as price, supply company, and availability.

Because of the homemade nature of early breast prostheses and their limited durability, few survive today. Historians interested in the material culture of these parts can use patent applications to better understand the material of the parts, their purpose, and applicability for post-mastectomy care. Moreover, this history suggests the evolution of breast cancer care today and indicates a burgeoning market that has its roots in earlier inventions.

The history of breast prostheses is also tied to the history of breast surgery and breast cancer treatment. Until the 1970s, Halsted's extensive surgical treatment for breast cancer, and moreover his logic that breast cancer was a local disease, dominated medical practice.[27] Women faced extensive surgical scars ranging from indentations in the chest and shoulder region to recurring lymphedema. Early breast prosthesis designs included innovative methods to hide the effects of radical surgery. Designs included new ways to fill indentations, secure the artificial breast in place, and lessen the skin irritation caused by surgery. Other concerns were met with the creation of appendages that enhanced the realistic nature of the part, including false nipples and "tongues." Finally, inventors tried to create a part that a woman could wear confidently and comfortably.

NOTES

1. Columbus City Directory. I have not been able to locate specific references that confirm who bought and sold these products in the early 1900s, only circumstantial evidence such as Wolfe's career in sales and her patented invention for a breast form. In Cincinnati a famous artificial parts manufacturer,

William Autenrieth, included in the city directory that Mrs. Autenrieth was "in attendance for ladies," perhaps supplying breast forms. See the Williams Cincinnati City Directory (1901), 127.

2. "Artificial Breast" by Laura Wolfe. U.S. Patent 184,182 (6 March 1906).

3. For an insightful examination of changing representations of the breast throughout history, see Marilyn Yalom, *A History of the Breast* (New York: Ballantine, 1997), esp. chap. 6, "The Commercialized Breast: From Corsets to Cyber-Sex."

4. Late-eighteenth-century and early-nineteenth-century statistics lacked scientific rigor. Moreover, statistical comparisons were often based on different criteria, including various definitions of recurrence and metastasis.

5. "Surgical Bust Substitute" by Laura Mailleue. U.S. Patent 1,417,930 (30 May 1922).

6. "Breast Pad" by Frederick Cox. U.S. Patent 146,805 (27 January 1874).

7. "Artificial Breast" by Laura Wolfe (1906). Wolfe filed the patent in 1904; it was awarded in 1906.

8. Ibid. Wolfe explained that the artificial breast would accommodate the existing breast in the space represented by part 8 in figures 2 and 3. The space is depicted as very small, perhaps reflecting Wolfe's perception that this be used on unusually small breasts.

9. William S. Halsted, "The Results of Operations for the Cure of Cancer of the Breast Performed at the Johns Hopkins Hospital from June 1889 to January 1894," *Johns Hopkins Hospital Report 4* (1894): 297–350.

10. William Francis Campbell, "The Early Recognition of Carcinoma Mammae," *Transactions of the Associated Physicians of Long Island* 1 (June 1898): 124–32.

11. "Surgical Bust Substitute" by Laura Mailleue (1922).

12. Ibid. I would argue that Mailleue also used this drawing to distinguish her product from a breast form meant to merely enhance breast sizes. The small size of the replacement breast distinguishes it from "artificial" breasts meant to be worn on top of natural breasts, such as the designs by Cox and Wolfe.

13. The U.S. Patent Office grants a patent when an inventor proves that he or she has created a "new and useful process, machine, manufacture, or composition of matter" (see Title 35 of U.S. Code 101). On June 30, 1999, the U.S. Patent Office listed 178 patents under the classification code 623/7. Much of this evidence comes from United States patent applications.

14. See *Polk's Baltimore City Directory, 1936* (Baltimore: R. L. Polk, 1936). Wiggers also had a phone.

15. "Breast Adapter" by Blanche Wiggers. U.S. Patent 2,066,503 (5 January 1937).

16. Ibid.

17. Ibid.

18. "Restoration Surgical Breast," by Mildred A. Wright and Dora E. Gates. U.S. Patent 2,651,783 (23 November 1949).

19. Ibid.

20. Samuel Hopkins Adams, "What Can You Do about Cancer?" *Ladies' Home Journal*, May 1913.

21. Marion W. Flexner, "Cancer—I've Had It," *Ladies' Home Journal* 64 (May 1947): 57+.

22. "Surgical Breast Pad," by Abe Silverman. U.S. Patent 2,482,297 (20 September, 1949)

23. Maxine Davis, "After Breast Surgery," *Good Housekeeping* 139 (September 1954): 28.

24. Ibid.

25. Genevieve Zeiss, "A New Life after Breast Cancer," *Ladies' Home Journal* 74 (October 1957): 52–53.

26. Charlotte George, "I'm Glad I Had My Breast Removed," *Today's Health* 35 (August 1957): 50–51.

27. I. Craig Henderson, "Paradigmatic Shifts in the Management of Breast Cancer," *New England Journal of Medicine* 332, no. 14 (1995): 951–52; Barron H. Lerner, "Fighting the War on Breast Cancer: Debates over Early Detection, 1945 to the Present," *Annals of Internal Medicine* 129 (1998): 74–78.

4

"How a One-Legged Rebel Lives"

Confederate Veterans and Artificial Limbs in Virginia

Jennifer Davis McDaid

ON 3 JUNE 1861, a cannonball tore eighteen-year-old James E. Hanger's left leg off at the knee during a skirmish with Union troops at Philippi, the first battle of the Civil War. A student at Washington College in Lexington, he had returned home at the outset of the war and joined Confederate troops on the battlefield. Grievously wounded two days later, Hanger was taken prisoner and had his leg amputated by an Ohio surgeon. After being exchanged for a Union prisoner, the wounded veteran returned home to Augusta County, where he joined the Staunton Home Guard and applied unsuccessfully for a job with the War Department. He later worked as a jeweler and a teacher before achieving success as a manufacturer and inventor of artificial limbs.

Years later, Hanger's niece remembered that a cannonball was prominently displayed in the family parlor. It seemed to the child to be "as large as a man's head—in reality—it was about the size of a grapefruit." By then a prosperous businessman with a prizewinning patented limb design, Hanger claimed that the six-pound cannonball had taken his leg, making him the war's first amputee. It was a dubious honor. Few veterans needed such a weighty souvenir to remind them of the bloody conflict. The twenty-six major battles and over four hundred smaller skirmishes fought on Virginia soil had left their mark in burned homes, empty barns, and limp sleeves.[1]

While the end of the war brought peace for some, many disabled veterans of the Confederacy struggled to regain physical mobility and economic stability. Using disability applications and other sources, this

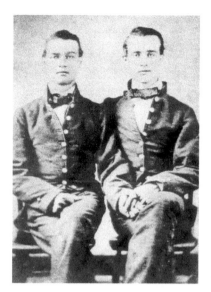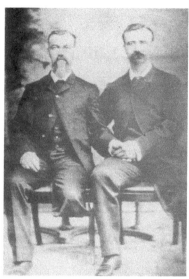

FIG. 4.1. The Walker brothers of Mecklenburg County, North Carolina, before and after the war. Both enlisted in the Thirteenth Regiment and each had his left leg amputated. Dr. H. J. Walker (seated on the left in both photographs) lost his leg during the retreat from Gettysburg. His brother L. J. lost his at Fredericksburg. Reproduced by permission of the Library of Virginia.

essay documents the sometimes poignant attempts of war amputees in Virginia to survive and thrive in the postbellum years. Not all proved able to turn their misfortune into an asset as Hanger did; indeed, most found themselves in a struggle to survive comparable to the war itself.

Traveling from Mechanicsville to Richmond during the war, Fannie Gaines Tinsley recoiled at the sight of dead and wounded soldiers "strewed on every side" of the road. "I had to keep my eyes shut all the way," she recalled in 1902, "to keep from seeing the most horrible sights." Throughout the South, the war's cost had been immense, leaving 260,000 Confederate soldiers dead and at least as many wounded.[2] The war routinely broke bodies in ways that doctors could not mend. Writing from "the stinking hole of Cold Harbor," the New York surgeon Daniel M. Holt bitterly related the extent of his medical duties during and after the bloody battle: "dressing stinking maggoty wounds and taking off the mangled tagends of what was once arms, legs, &c." Amputations, Holt and his fellow surgeons believed, were "the very *worst* part of the business." Nonetheless, the procedure prevented infection and gangrene, and was often the only way to save the life of soldiers who ended up in one of the short-staffed and unsanitary field hospitals.[3]

Surgeons for the North and South together performed approximately sixty thousand amputations during the course of the war. The operation took only minutes in practiced hands. It was best performed by a surgeon and three assistants: one to administer chloroform, one to compress the main artery, and one to support the limb. For circular amputations, the physician cut through muscle and bone and brought skin over the resulting stump, then sewed it shut. For a flap amputation, the surgeon trimmed skin and tissue into a crescent shape, then protected the severed bone with the flaps. A patient's chances of survival depended in large part on the location of the wound; the closer it was to the body, the more likely the occurrence of severe blood loss and secondary infection.[4]

Although many soldiers pragmatically accepted amputation as a lifesaving procedure, the experience was nevertheless traumatic. Surgery manuals recommended that the operation be performed as soon as possible after the injury, "while the patient had his sensibilities depressed by the shock." Even then, complications could occur. Writing home to his brother, Walter, from a Lynchburg hospital in August 1864, the soldier Milton A. Clark reported that after his leg was amputated, a stitch broke, allowing an artery to bleed. A surgeon stopped the flow with his thumb, then tore out the faulty stitches and sewed up the stump again. A few days later, another stitch failed, and Clark had to be taken to surgery. By "sawing off a piece of the bone and cutting up higher in the flesh," the doctor was able to secure the artery again. It was "almost equal to a second amputation," Clark grimly reflected. Despite this, he maintained that the operation was safer than nursing a shattered limb, telling his brother that in the end an injured man would "suffer a great deal less if he had his leg amputated, at least that is my experience." A doctor writing for *United States Service Magazine* in 1864 agreed. "Life is better than limb," he argued, especially when complications, like the hemorrhaging experienced by Clark, waited "at every turn, like harpies to seize their victims, and shout back in derision, too late!"[5]

After the war, the demand for artificial limbs in the former Confederacy was overwhelming. Some amputees couldn't wear a prosthesis because of insufficient padding on their stumps. But for those who could, filling an empty sleeve or trouser leg with a functional, lightweight, artificial limb became an imperative. "I am one of the unfortunate disabled soldiers of the late Confederate army," wrote Samuel F. Abraham in a shaky hand to the newly created Virginia Board of Commissioners on Artificial Limbs in 1867. A Buckingham County native, Abraham had lost his "most usefull member" on 2 June 1864 at the Battle of Cold Harbor, when a minie ball shattered the bones in his right arm. The soft-lead bullets lost their shape on impact, shattered several inches of bone, and carried skin and clothing into the torn flesh. The Confederate surgeon J. Julian Chisolm bemoaned the ammunition's destructive efficiency. "In steady hands," he explained, "frightful wounds are produced by the minie ball, which require all the resources of surgery to manage successfully."[6]

While Samuel Abraham wrestled with his pen left-handed, other veterans depended on neighbors, friends, and relatives to make their requests. Edward Acree requested an artificial eye for his brother, Alexander, who had served in the Fifth Virginia Cavalry. "It is probably more necessary that he should have an eye," he explained, "than it is for most soldiers to have arms," since the prosthetic orb would protect a painfully exposed portion of Acree's brain, and "there are very few who will be most benefitted except in looks by artificial arms." Despite this desperate plea, the state didn't supply glass eyes until 1876. By then, Acree was working as a clerk in his brother's Halifax County dry goods store, using his one good eye. The other may have been covered with a patch; if business was good, the brothers may have scraped together enough money to purchase a replacement.[7]

Acree's belief that artificial limbs were of little practical use was a common one. Many veterans considered prosthetic arms and legs noisy, uncomfortable, and cumbersome. In a letter to the auditor, Rockbridge County resident Henry D. Bishop explained that he had received two Hanger-manufactured legs during the war, but could not wear them regularly because army surgeons had left too much bone near the surface of his stump. Other men lamented that their prostheses wore out or broke under the wear and tear of daily use. Otto J. Whitlock, of Louisa County, had constant trouble with artificial legs after losing his own at Chancellorsville. The one he received in the summer of 1872 lasted only through the winter and "broke down as a worthless thing" the following spring. After trying both the Hanger and Bly legs (both of which he judged "instruments of severe torture"), Whitlock resorted to wearing a wooden peg leg. His injuries *were* severe: he lost his left leg below the knee, took two minie balls in the right, and was also afflicted with crippling rheumatism. Whitlock found his job as a teacher to be physically difficult and poorly paid; with a wife and six children to support, he was anxious to receive both a new, wearable leg and a Confederate pension. Limbs issued by the state had a five-year warranty, so Whitlock's leg was repaired, not replaced; he did receive pension payments from the state until 1917, when he died from liver cancer. His widow, Virginia, applied for and received a pension the following year.[8]

Some veterans expressed doubts as to whether their new limbs would stand up under heavy use. William H. Tolley wondered whether his would be sturdy enough for his increasingly hefty frame. "I weigh now about 200 lbs," he wrote from Augusta County, "and wish you would make the irons very strong." Sidney Turner, who lost his leg below the knee at Gettysburg, was equally concerned. "I have had a great deal of walking and traveling about to do here in this rough part of the country," he explained from Fincastle, in Botetourt County. "My business was such for a good while, that I had to be all the time on my feet to Attend to it, and my leg has Worne out and Broken down." Turner had been a teacher, but found the work increasingly difficult. With no family and in poor health after the onset of "disease of the lungs," he traveled to Richmond in April 1885, entered the Soldiers' Home, and died that August.[9]

Overwhelmed with the demand for artificial limbs, the state failed to keep pace. Already ailing, Sidney Turner had applied for benefits in the spring of 1882, explaining that "whether I get the money or not, I would like to know Soon as Possible as I wish to make arrangements with some one about getting a Leg." His check for sixty dollars was finally mailed out in February 1886, over six months after his death and nearly four years after he had initially requested help. George B. Keezell, Rockingham County's senator, sent the payment back to Richmond the following month, adding a note to the auditor that, since Turner was dead, he should bestow his money on "some other *Rockingham* man." By 1894, more than six thousand veterans, either amputees or those otherwise disabled, received limbs or commutation (financial payments for disability) from the Virginia government. In addition, over three thousand men entered the R. E. Lee Camp Confederate Soldiers' Home in Richmond after it was established in 1885.[10]

In response to the overwhelming number of war amputees, the Virginia General Assembly passed more than twenty laws designed to provide artificial limbs to those Confederate veterans in need of them between 1867 and 1894. In 1866 Francis H. Pierpont, a Unionist whom President Andrew Johnson recognized as governor in 1865, urged the assembly to supply relief to maimed soldiers. Pierpont pragmatically argued that veterans with artificial limbs would be able to work and, as a result, would not depend on the state for their support. A group of Richmond physicians echoed this call for action on behalf of "this unfortunate class of men." Faced with large numbers of injured and unemployable veterans, other southern states, including North Carolina, South Carolina, and Georgia, enacted similar legislation.[11]

Even during the war, the shortage of artificial limbs was painfully apparent. Meeting in Richmond in 1864, surgeons, clergymen, and concerned citizens had formed the Association for the Relief of Maimed Soldiers. Designed to supply prostheses free of charge to "all officers, soldiers, and seamen" injured fighting for the South, the association appealed to "benevolent and patriotic Confederate citizens" for financial support. Membership dues were ten dollars; among those who joined was Robert E. Lee, who admired the work of the association in assisting "the brave defenders of our Country" and donated five-hundred dollars in September 1864. Unfortunately, artificial limbs remained in short supply: only four companies in the state regularly manufactured limbs; two more made them only occasionally.[12]

By the association's estimates, more than ten-thousand southern men had already lost arms and legs in battle. Maimed soldiers became a common sight. On Christmas Day 1863, the diarist Mary Chesnut noted that, among her after-dinner visitors, many were "without arms, without legs." "We have all kinds now," a guest commented dryly, "but a blind one." Faced with "the sight of empty sleeves, and of men hobbling on wooden pegs, or swinging on the galling crutch," the association ambitiously planned to raise funds to purchase limbs and to encourage their manufacture. But while prostheses had the potential to increase mobility, the group warned potential wearers that "the best is but a poor substitute for the natural member." In January 1864 the association invited southern limb manufacturers to submit samples of their work and propose production schedules. Artificial legs, the directors reminded them, should be "light, strong, and durable, as labor is the lot of the majority of those who wear them."[13]

In February 1864 James E. Hanger wrote to the association from his factory in Staunton, promising that an artificial leg was on its way to Richmond for inspection. "It is not as neatly finished as we desired," he warned, "the painting being deficient in appearance only on account of the difficulty of getting proper material." Hanger promised to produce ten to fifteen legs a month, and proposed a price of $200 for above-the-knee models, $150 for below-the-knee styles. Constructed of "light and tough" wood and enclosed in rawhide, the legs (Hanger boasted) were more durable than other artificial limbs and weighed only four pounds, fourteen ounces. Not everyone agreed with Hanger's assessment. One surgeon reported to the association that he had yet to see an "efficient specimen" of Hanger's leg; instead, he reported to Richmond that he had seen soldiers throw "their [Hanger] leg aside and return to the *peg* leg." William A. Carrington, the association's corresponding secretary and a surgeon, was "much disconcerted" by this news and requested that Hanger provide him with references immediately.[14]

Hanger and Brother, meanwhile, had other troubles and was falling behind in production. "Our factory is at present at a perfect stand still," he explained in June 1864, "the hands being ordered to the fields by Gen Imboden how [long] he will keep them we do not know." In September, Hanger's contract with his shoemaker expired, and when the man demanded a pay increase, Hanger refused and wrote to the association in Richmond, hoping instead to hire a free black to do the work. "We are very much in need of workmen at this time," he admitted. "Your orders are accumulating somewhat." Military operations in the valley and a shortage of seasoned timber forced him to halt production repeatedly; nevertheless, in October 1864 he requested a pay raise himself, since the cost of materials had increased and his brother had recently enlisted in the army, leaving him alone to handle the business. In December he twice requested an exemption for "the heavy *tax* imposed on manufacturers," since he had "not made enough to pay for *Grub*, much less the various other expenses" of running the factory.[15]

Hanger failed to win Carrington's wholehearted support for his endeavors. In January 1865, after he inspected a Hanger limb worn by an Alabama private, Carrington fired off an angry letter to A. M. Fauntleroy, the doctor in Staunton responsible for inspecting Hanger's work:

[The leg] is rude in workmanship inefficient and *very* inferior to the specimens he deposited with the Association. The color is unsightly, the toes are not fastened by hinges as the specimen was, but by wooden pegs which will soon be worn off. The braces to the knee are too straight and not curved to the convexities of the knee—the sole leather thigh box made of leather much too rough and too rough entirely—The color of the specimen was near flesh color—I am dissatisfied with the leg and hope you will not pass any more such, as they are a discredit to the Association and will soon be of little use to the men.

Undeterred, Hanger sent a new five-pound model for Carrington's review in February 1865. Perhaps with the association's recent objections in mind, Hanger explained that "the men sometimes prefer [legs] without any painting whatever." "They are durable," he assured the surgeon, "but do not look so well."[16]

At least two Virginia companies—Wells and Brother in Charlottesville (located near a hospital) and Hanger and Brother in Staunton—eventually contracted with the Confederacy to fabricate artificial limbs. Because the directors of the association failed to find an efficient arm prosthesis with "both the semblance and the grasping power of the original," many upper-body amputees had to make do with a limp sleeve—despite the fact that considerably more men lost arms (or parts of arms) than legs. Most postwar patents for prosthetics thus consisted largely of artificial legs, crutches, and wheelchairs.[17]

Benefits for wounded veterans went beyond physical rehabilitation. On 4 March 1864, Virginia legislators passed an act providing for the education of disabled soldiers. Men "of suitable character and capacity" who could no longer pay tuition became eligible to attend classes at the University of Virginia in Charlottesville and board at the school free of charge. The rector's report of December 1865 is telling: of the school's fifty-five students, twenty-one were disabled veterans paying no tuition. Another twelve paying students had lost an arm, leg, or foot. Most studied law or medicine, traveling from as far away as Mississippi, South Carolina, and Texas to enroll. While education proved useful to some injured veterans, who found posts as clerks or teachers, most of the disabled found schooling an impractical alternative.[18]

Efforts to extend benefits to servicemen continued after the war. On 29 January 1867, the General Assembly created the Board of Commissioners on Artificial Limbs (consisting of the governor, the auditor of public accounts, and a physician) to oversee the purchase of $20,000 worth of artificial limbs. In order to get a limb from the board, veterans had to fill out disability applications with information on the command in which they served; when, where, and how they were wounded; and their medical history. Newspapers across the commonwealth published notices encouraging disabled veterans to apply, while railroads and steamboats furnished the men free transportation to Richmond, where the limbs were distributed. Once in the capital, each veteran could schedule an appointment with a state-appointed doctor, who (for a fee of two dollars a leg) checked the quality of limbs and made the final fit.[19]

Navigating the bureaucracy of state government proved frustrating for most veterans. James M. McCoy, an Alleghany County native, wrote directly to James E. Hanger in April 1874 to explain why his disability application was incomplete:

> In regard to my certificate about my leg I did not get it the reason was I went to the county seat but before I could get there our butifull county court had adjourned it only last[ed] about two hours. The judge told me to write to you and inform you of my bad luck and to say to you that he would give me a certificate next court. So if you can take this as an application it will be all right.

Even when veterans completed their applications, money often ran out before all of those entitled to benefits received their share. McCoy, who lost his left leg in an 1864 skirmish at Mount Madison in Augusta County, finally received his artificial limb ten years later. His problems, however, had only begun. In 1877 he complained to the auditor that the long-awaited Hanger limb was "worn out and worthless," and noted that he had replaced the tattered foot and ankle joint himself "at considerable expense." As a depot agent for the railroad in Allegheny County, McCoy depended on the mobility the limb provided. In June 1884, he contacted the auditor again, after his approved application had been passed over for lack of state funds. "At last the Legislature they passed a bill appropriating So Much Money for Crippled Confederates," he wrote with relief. "Has it all been taken yet and How will I proceed to Get my part," he inquired anxiously "I am one of the unfortunate ones." More than two decades after his crippling injury, the state provided McCoy with a sixty-dollar commutation.[20]

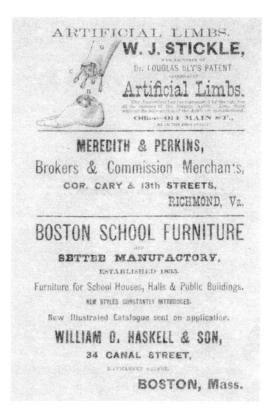

FIG. 4.2. Manufacturer William J. Stickle sold patent legs from an office on Main Street in Richmond, and advertised for patients in the city directory. He promised to provide a natural (or flexible) ankle—a feature much in demand among veterans who wore their legs long hours and often worked on their feet. Reproduced by permission of the Library of Virginia.

By 1870 at least one manufacturer of artificial limbs had opened for business in Richmond itself. William J. Stickle made and sold Dr. Douglas Bly's "celebrated artificial legs" at a shop on Main Street, just down the hill from the Capitol. As Bly's local representative, Stickle distributed this revolutionary "anatomical leg . . . with all the motions of the Natural Ankle," collected payments from the state government, and forwarded the profits to the home office in Rochester, New York. Edward F. Lockett, a teacher who had lost a leg at Chancellorsville, wrote to the auditor's office from Amelia County in 1867, recommending

Bly's leg with its specially designed ankle. William B. Wise, a Norfolk veteran who lost a foot, echoed his enthusiasm. On the other hand, Ausbert G. L. VanLear, an Augusta County physician who also lost his leg at Chancellorsville, complained bitterly about the durability of his Bly leg. "After I wore it about two years," he wrote in 1872, "it broke intirely in two."[21]

James E. Hanger was Bly's prime Virginia competitor. Writing to the governor on his behalf in 1867, Staunton mayor Nicholas K. Trout maintained that Hanger, who was both "a *home* manufacturer and maimed," should, like the northerner Bly, receive a state government commission. Some veterans, like W. J. M. Yount of Allegheny County, were anxious to try the Hanger leg for its promised snug fit; others undoubtedly signed up specifically to have a southern-made leg. With the commonwealth as a client, Hanger moved his business from Augusta County to Richmond, locating his workshop on Main Street near the competition. He boasted, with no small amount of sectional pride, that medical associations had recommended his patented legs as preferable "to the best Northern limbs."[22]

As the board distributed limbs, it encountered problems. In 1872, after numerous complaints from veterans, the General Assembly amended the law providing artificial limbs to allow veterans to return unusable legs. In 1884 the assembly stipulated that the state would offer a reimbursement if veterans returned the unwanted limbs in good condition with a certificate from their county clerk confirming that they could not use them. So many men took advantage of the offer that the auditor fretted over the several hundred returned artificial arms and legs stored in Richmond. Because the rejected limbs were rapidly "going to destruction from natural decay," the auditor reissued them to other veterans capable of wearing them.[23]

Artificial limbs served both practical and cosmetic purposes. With a wooden leg, a veteran could stand, walk, and work. Advertisements, like those for the Hanger factory, often featured "before and after" pictures of veterans transformed by the purchase of a prosthesis.[24] For a 1911 promotion, W. N. House, a double amputee (with one leg missing from above the knee and the other from just above the ankle) was photographed sitting in a chair clad in only a shirt. Thanks to Hanger's "Orthopedic Appliances," he stands tall in the next picture, wearing a suit and holding a natty bowler. In 1902 House (a telegraph operator on the Baltimore and Ohio Railroad) wrote to Hanger praising the durability

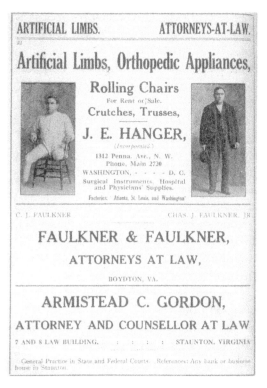

FIG. 4.3. James E. Hanger moved his business from Richmond to Washington, D.C., where he manufactured and sold artificial legs, rolling chairs, crutches, and surgical supplies. This 1911 advertisement featured W. N. House, a double amputee and Hanger customer who worked on the Baltimore and Ohio Railroad. Reproduced by permission of the Library of Virginia.

and comfort of his artificial limbs. Hanger himself claimed that his limbs hid all signs of injury and guaranteed them to be comfortable, well-fitting, and "thoroughly tested," with a patent socket that promised "no chafing, no jarring, no cords, no springs"—in short, "the best and cheapest artificial leg." Every year, Hanger changed his copy in city directories to reflect the number of years he had himself worn a prosthesis, realizing that he was his own best advertisement: "Forty-six years experience wearing, studying and manufacturing artificial limbs," he trumpeted in 1907.[25] Clearly, the design of Hanger's prostheses had improved by this time.

While Adelaide Smith, a Union nurse, claimed that one of her patients received a government-issue leg that fit so well "he could jump off a moving car," most amputees struggled to adjust to their physical limitations. Many hoped that, like Smith's mending charges, they could walk on an artificial leg with only a slight limp, or use a "neatly gloved" artificial hand so well that no one would notice their infirmity. In an effort to produce more lifelike prostheses, manufacturers used India rubber for hands and feet, and covered wooden legs with parchment paper, then painted and varnished them "to resemble the complexion of the natural skin." Most Virginia veterans, however, were interested in substance more than style, looking to artificial limbs as a practical means to regain mobility and return to work. [26]

After the war, a missing limb served as a badge of bravery and sacrifice. "All women," nurse Louisa May Alcott assured a patient, "thought a wound the best decoration a brave soldier could wear." Some amputees faced their situation with bravery: "I had rather have my leg blown off by a rebel shell," one philosophized in 1864, "than crushed by a locomotive, or bitten off by a crocodile." Others were understandably despondent. An absent limb was a nagging reminder of the struggle for survival in an age when physical work was a large part of many men's lives. Nurse Arabella Wilson recognized that "to go through life deprived of the cunning of the right hand or the exceeding service of the foot or the eye, is, no doubt, a great calamity." Returning home without arms and legs, veterans found longed-for reunions with loved ones difficult and jobs nearly impossible to find.[27]

Virginia's financial woes after the war only exacerbated their troubles, and many questioned the state auditor's judgment. Writing from Massies Mill in Nelson County, W. A. B. McComb complained in 1882 that his neighbor James W. Bolton, "a very poor man" who had received thirty dollars (instead of the full sixty dollars he was entitled to) in 1879, had been shortchanged. McComb had heard rumors in the county that some veterans had received sixty dollars "for having lost part of one finger," while others "who had their hands so maimed that they can not grip any thing except with one or two fingers" received the same amount. McComb assured the auditor that he would prepare the necessary paperwork for Bolton if funds were forthcoming. McComb expressed skepticism that the state would distribute the funds equitably, and ended his letter in frustrated resignation: "I suppose these things will not pertain to your duties."[28]

Preston Bledsoe summed up the feelings of many of his fellow veterans when he wrote in his disability application that "I no that my helth was ruind by being in the war." In 1862 he had enlisted as a private in the Twenty-first Battalion Virginia Infantry, along with five other Bledsoes. Stricken with measles and weakened from exposure, Bledsoe had lost the sight in one eye by the time he returned home to Scott County in 1865. Lamenting that he was of "no use" to himself, he petitioned the auditor for funds in 1882, since he was depending on his friends for support and they were "verry poore." Two years later, someone wrote the auditor for him, since he was by then totally blind and suffering from lung disease. Bledsoe finally received sixty dollars in 1886. Other returning soldiers expressed similar sentiments. Buckingham County native Samuel F. Abraham, who lost his right arm at Cold Harbor, was discharged from the Fifty-sixth Virginia Infantry in 1864. The Medical Examining Board declared him permanently disabled and recommended that he return to farming, since they knew "of no duty he could well perform" for the Confederacy. Despite his fear that he could not benefit from an artificial arm, Abraham applied for and received one in 1867. He later returned it unused. In 1888 he successfully applied for a Confederate pension of thirty dollars a year.[29]

Disabled veterans often found themselves unable to reconstruct their former lives. After William B. Moody's arm was amputated in 1861, he enrolled in the Medical College of Virginia, but withdrew for lack of funds to pay tuition. In 1867 Thomas E. Sims wrote to the auditor pleading his nephew's case. Moody's property, held largely in slaves, had been lost as a result of the war. Left with no financial resources, Moody abandoned his education and took a job as a clerk in a Richmond tobacco factory. Other veterans, like E. L. Bennett, of Loudoun County, had scraped together the money to purchase artificial limbs themselves but were unable to use them. Bennett hoped that his new leg would fit better than his old one, which "like the majority of Yankee inventions proved to be a 'humbug.'"[30]

Many veterans found they could not return to their prewar occupations. Henry Clay Fergusson, formerly a painter, applied for a position with the capitol police in 1874. A member of the First Virginia Cavalry, Fergusson lost his left arm in Pickett's Charge at Gettysburg, was captured two days later and imprisoned, and was discharged as disabled in 1864. His police application ungranted, he labored as a finisher and painter in the city of Richmond until 1879, when he finally obtained a position as a watchman at city hall. Unable to use an artificial arm, Fergusson received a payment of sixty dollars from the state. When he died in 1893, Fergusson was eulogized as a "gallant member" of the First Virginia and a valuable "attaché of the City Hall." Nevertheless, his death left his widow and children in a precarious financial state. To support the family, three of his five children went to work for their uncle, J. W. Fergusson, as printers and bookbinders. His widow, Margaret, received a pension in 1928 at the age of seventy-seven.[31]

Other families found themselves in equally desperate circumstances. After the war, Thomas E. Drinkard had been employed as a city tax collector in Petersburg and as a capitol policeman before losing his job as an engineer at the Capitol building in 1887. With only one arm, he had been unable to find more work and was on the verge of losing his farm. With the money he had received from the state in 1873 long since spent, Drinkard urged the governor to prod the legislature into relieving impoverished veterans. "Please do what you can," he wrote. "*I am very much in need.*" William P. Purcell, an unemployed clerk, decided to write the governor only after unsuccessfully searching for a job for two months; with "winter near at hand" and his wife, Sarah, crippled by rheumatism worsened by her work as a nurse during the war, Purcell was desperate for any "light employment" to support his family. James Lawson Kemper, who served as Virginia's governor from 1874 to 1878, was himself battle-scarred: leading his brigade at Gettysburg on 3 July 1863, he was struck by a minie ball, which lodged near the base of his spine. He was hampered for the rest of his life by limited locomotion and constant pain. Having an ex-Confederate brigadier general as the commonwealth's chief executive evidently prompted his fellow veterans to action. S. J. Hurst, who lost a limb in the "late struggle for Independence," wrote to the governor (whom he knew was "a friend of the Boys in Grey") with a suggestion. "If the members of the Legislature could place themselves in my condition for a few moments," he argued, "immediate action would be taken for the benefit of those who fell defending the Honor of Va."[32]

Some disabled veterans had better luck. John S. Robson took full advantage of nearly all the benefits the state of Virginia had to offer Confederate veterans. A corporal in the Fifty-second Virginia Infantry,

Robson returned home to Woodville, in Rappahannock County, after the surrender at Appomattox, with a bullet-shattered leg, which was soon amputated. He applied for a Hanger limb in 1871, a commutation in 1882, admission to the Confederate Soldiers' Home in 1887, and a pension in 1888. He received all but admission to the Soldiers' Home. Robson studied medicine briefly and, despite his physical limitations, kept a boardinghouse along the Chesapeake and Ohio Railroad line and worked as a bookseller, barkeep, and bottled water merchant, finally settling down and earning a meager living as a constable in Rappahannock and Culpepper Counties. "I have been no idler," he explained, "even though I am a cripple."[33]

Robson also penned a memoir, *How a One-Legged Rebel Lives*. "I have an object in writing," he admitted in the preface, "and that object is the money I expect to obtain from its sale." His "little pamphlet" speaks plainly about his disability and the financial difficulties that resulted from it. Robson maintained that the loss of a limb and its replacement by "a bogus representative . . . made out of good strong oak" marked him as "unable to do battle, in the strife of the world, with strong and more fortunate" able-bodied veterans. "One thing is sure," he reflected. "I find this world a pretty hard place to flourish when you have no money, and only one leg to make it with." *How a One-Legged Rebel Lives*, published in 1876 and reprinted in 1898, was his last chance to be economically self-sufficient:

> Could I find employment in any way, I assure my readers I would not resort to authorship, but in these days of depression, when so many young and willing persons, sound of mind and whole in limb, are out of employment and can find nothing to do, my chances are hopeless indeed. For hard and laborious work, I am physically unfit and few would be willing to pay me reasonable wages.[34]

Although determined not to be a burden on relatives, Robson lived with family members until his death, spending the last forty years of his life in the home of his younger brother, William, a Rappahannock County farmer also wounded in the war. When John Robson died in 1920 at the age of seventy-five, the state paid his funeral expenses. Suffering from the lingering consequences of a wartime head wound, rheumatism, and heart trouble, his brother applied for a pension that same year.[35]

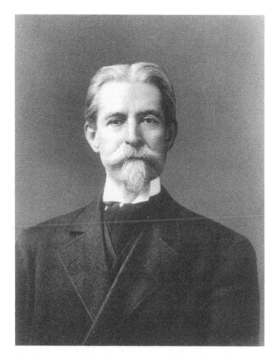

FIG. 4.4. The only known surviving portrait of the Confederate veteran, inventor, and manufacturer James E. Hanger. "From the efforts of a one-legged man with a crudely designed substitute for the leg lost in the War," he boasted, "the concern which bears my name has grown into the world's foremost manufacturer of artificial limbs." Courtesy of the Hanger Orthopedic Group Collection, Bethesda, Maryland.

James E. Hanger had considerably more success in turning his disability to commercial profit. Around 1890 he moved from Richmond to Washington, D.C., where he established a second branch of his limb manufacturing business; by 1911 he had opened factories in Atlanta and St. Louis. His reasonably priced legs were popular, promised "perfect comfort," and won awards at the 1881 Cotton Exposition and the 1907 Jamestown Ter-Centennial Exposition. In 1873 Hanger married twenty-year-old Nora McCarthy (a graduate of Hollins Institute) in Richmond. Of their twelve children, eight survived, and by 1900, nineteen-year-old Hugh was a "leg maker" in the Hanger factory. Other children joined the family business and collaborated with their father on a variety of patented inventions (including limbs, wheelchairs, and beds) designed to assist the disabled. Confederate (and later Union) veterans wore Hanger limbs; so did English and French soldiers injured in World War I. Founded in war, the business profited from its casualties. When Hanger died in 1919, at age seventy-six, he left behind a thriving company that still survives today. [36]

Unlike Hanger, most Virginia veterans fought a grueling battle against poverty once they returned home. Joseph M. Hodge, of Warm Springs, struggled with spelling to write the auditor in June 1884. He summed up the obstacles that disabled veterans faced in postwar Virginia: "i was a soalder and amde to doo the duty that was required of me," he explained, "now i am not able to work i recking I will hafto be sold out and sent to the pore house Just for the lack of a few Dollars." With a family of ten to support, Hodge feared the worst. W. H. Carter, of Abingdon, likewise wrote to Richmond in desperation. Unable to wear his artificial leg, he gave it to a veteran who could use it and was also in dire straits. "Our Cripple Soldiers is Starving & many of them [are] in the poor house," he cried. "I for one am a one legged man all most on Starvation." Like many of their fellow veterans, Carter found the postwar battle for economic survival and physical mobility nearly as difficult as the war itself.[37]

NOTES

The author would like to thank Conley L. Edwards III, Virginia's state archivist, for his research advice, thoughtful reading, and good cheer; archivist Robert Young Clay, who kindly searched the 1900 District of Columbia census at the National Archives; and the rest of the Library of Virginia's Archival Research Services staff. Confederate disability applications are available online at the Library of Virginia's Web site www.lva.lib.va.us.

1. Orderly Book, Churchville Cavalry (1861), Museum of the Confederacy, Richmond; Mark Mayo Boatner III, *The Civil War Dictionary* (New York: Vintage Civil War Library, 1991), 651; James M. McPherson, *Battle Cry of Freedom: The Civil War Era* (New York: Oxford University Press, 1988), 299–300; "Record of Services," written by James E. Hanger for his daughter Alice Hanger Cook's application for the United Daughters of the Confederacy, March 1914; "Hanger History," 28 January 1954; undated notes for an address by McCarthy Hanger to the West Virginia Academy of Science; and "Biography of J. E. Hanger," *Philippi Republican*, 3 April 1941, all in the Hanger Orthopedic Group Collec-

tion, Bethesda, MD; Compiled Service Records of Confederate Soldiers Who Served in Organizations from the State of Virginia (National Archives microfilm), 23 Virginia Infantry; U.S. Census, State of Virginia, Augusta County, Population Schedules (National Archives microfilm), 1850, 1860, 1870, 1880; District of Columbia census, 1900; *J.-E. Hanger et Fils, Membres Artificiels* (Paris, n.d.), Hanger Orthopedic Group Collection. History of Churchville (Churchville, VA: Women's Club, 1932), 33; Sara B. Bearss, *The Story of Virginia: An American Experience* (Richmond: Virginia Historical Society, 1995), 38–39.

2. "War Experiences of Mrs. S. G. Tinsley," Works Progress Administration, Virginia Historical Inventory, Hanover County, Library of Virginia (LVA); William J. Cooper Jr. and Thomas E. Terrill, *The American South: A History*, 2d ed. (New York: McGraw-Hill, 1996), 363–64.

3. James M. Greiner et al., *A Surgeon's Civil War: The Letters and Diary of Daniel M. Holt, M.D.* (Kent, OH: Kent State University Press, 1994), 203–04; Milton A. Clark to his brother, Walter, 28 November 1864, Milton A. Clark Letters, Confederate Miscellany Ib #20 (folder 19), Special Collections Department, Robert W. Woodruff Library, Emory University.

4. Laurann Figg and Jane Farrell-Beck, "Amputation in the Civil War: Physical and Social Dimensions," *Journal of the History of Medicine and Allied Sciences* 48 (October 1993): 454, 457–58; Mary C. Gillett, *The Army Medical Department, 1818–1865* (Washington, DC: Center of Military History, 1987), 285–86.

5. J. Julian Chisolm, *A Manual of Military Surgery for the Use of Surgeons in the Confederate States Army* (1864; reprint, Dayton, OH: Morningside, 1983), 360; Milton A. Clark Letters, Emory University; "Military Surgery, Ancient and Modern," *United States Service Magazine* 1 (1864): 132–33.

6. Samuel F. Abraham to the Board of Commissioners on Artificial Limbs, 17 March 1867, Auditor of Public Accounts (entry 112), LVA; Compiled Confederate Service Record, 56 Virginia Infantry; Confederate Disability Application, Buckingham County, Act of 1886–87, LVA; Chisolm quoted in Figg and Farrell-Beck, "Amputation in the Civil War," 455.

7. E. F. Acree to Board of Commissioners on Artificial Limbs, 15 March 1867; Compiled Confederate Service Record, 5 Virginia Cavalry; King and Queen County, Virginia, census, 1870, 1880; Act of the Assembly, 29 March 1877.

8. Henry D. Bishop, Confederate Disability Application file, Rockbridge County, Act of 1882, LVA; Compiled Confederate Service Record, 60 Virginia Infantry; Otto J. Whitlock, Confederate Disability Application file, Louisa County, Act of 1884, 1886–87; Compiled Confederate Service Record, 44 Virginia Infantry; Goochland County census, 1870, 1880; Confederate Pension Application, Goochland County, Act of 1888, LVA; Virginia A. Whitlock, Confederate Widow's Pension, Richmond City, Act of 1918.

9. William H. Tolley, Confederate Disability Application file, Augusta County, Act of 1884; Rockbridge County, Virginia, census, 1870; "An Act, for the

Relief of William H. Tolley," approved 27 February 1886; Sidney Turner, Confederate Disability Application, Rockingham County, Act of 1884; Compiled Confederate Service Record, 21 Virginia Infantry; R. E. Lee Camp Confederate Soldiers' Home, Application for Admission, and Register of Residents, 1:25–25a, LVA.

10. Sidney Turner, Confederate Disability Application file, Rockingham County, Act of 1884; R. B. Rosenburg, *Living Monuments: Confederate Soldiers' Homes in the New South* (Chapel Hill: University of North Carolina Press, 1993), appendix.

11. Michael B. Chesson, *Richmond after the War* (Richmond: Virginia State Library, 1981), 88; *Senate Journal*, 4 December 1866; Ansley Herring Wegner, "Phantom Pain: Civil War Amputation and North Carolina's Maimed Veterans," *North Carolina Historical Review* 75 (July 1998): 277–96; Patrick J. McCawley, *Artificial Limbs for Confederate Soldiers* (Columbia: South Carolina Department of Archives and History, Public Programs Division, 1992).

12. *Brief Review of the Plan and Operations of the Association for the Relief of Maimed Soldiers* (Richmond, 1865); R. E. Lee to Dr. J. B. McCaw, 8 March 1864; R. E. Lee to Rev. Charles Minnegerode, 9 March 1864; and Treasurer's Account, 4 November 1864, all in the Association for the Relief of Maimed Soldiers Records (ARMS), Record Group 109 (chap. 6, file no. 463, Confederate Archives), National Archives and Records Administration.

13. C. Vann Woodward, ed., *Mary Chesnut's Civil War* (New Haven: Yale University Press, 1981), 515. *Brief Review*, 6; letters soliciting samples of artificial limbs, 26 January 1864, 8 February 1864, 26 February 1864, ARMS.

14. James E. Hanger to William A. Carrington, 16 January 1864, 16 February 1864; Carrington to Hanger, 28 January 1864, ARMS.

15. Hanger to Carrington, 3 June 1864, 7 September 1864, 29 October 1864, 4 December 1864, 22 December 1864; Report of the Corresponding Secretary, 10 October 1864, ARMS.

16. Carrington to A. M. Fauntleroy, 5 January 1865; Fauntleroy to Carrington, 10 January 1865; Hanger to Corresponding Secretary [Carrington], 15 February 1865, ARMS.

17. *Brief Review*, 2, 6, 10.

18. Berkeley Minor and James F. Minor, *Legislative History of the University of Virginia* (Charlottesville: University of Virginia, 1928), 34–35; Douglas Southall Freeman, *A Calendar of Confederate Papers* (1908; reprint, New York: Kraus Reprint Company, 1969), 193; *Report to the Rector and Visitors of the University of Virginia to the General Assembly, December 1865* (Charlottesville: University of Virginia Press, 1865), 18.

19. Act of Assembly, 29 January 1867.

20. James M. McCoy to Board of Commissioners on Artificial Limbs, 22 April 1874; Confederate Disability Application file, Allegheny County, Act of

1884; Compiled Confederate Service Record, 2 Virginia Cavalry; Allegheny County, Virginia, census, 1870.

21. Richmond City, Virginia, census, 1870; *Dudley's Richmond City Directory*, 1870; power of attorney agreement between Bly and Stickles, 8 May 1861, Board of Commissioners on Artificial Limbs (entry 112, box 265); letters to Board of Commissioners on Artificial Limbs, Edward F. Lockett (11 February 1867), William B. Wise (12 March 1867), and Ausbert G. L. VanLear (30 May 1872, 28 January 1873).

22. N. K. Trout to Governor Pierpont, January 1867, Office of the Governor, Letters Received, LVA; *Chataigne's Business Directory and Gazetteer*, 1884–1885, 1888–1889; W. J. M. Yount to Board of Commissioners on Artificial Limbs, 24 January 1873.

23. Acts of Assembly, 25 March 1872, 1 December 1884.

24. *Virginia Business Directory and Gazetteer*, 1911, LVA.

25. *Chataigne's Virginia Business Directory and Gazetteer*, 1911; *Hanger Substitute Limbs, Nature's Rivals: A Complete Illustrated Treatise* (Washington, DC, n.d.), 104, Hanger Orthopedic Group Collection; *Boyd's Directory of the District of Columbia*, 1907.

26. Adelaide W. Smith, *Reminiscences of an Army Nurse during the Civil War* (New York: Greaves, 1911), 129, 189; "On Marks' Artificial Limbs," *Journal of the Franklin Institute* 127 (May 1889): 329, 333.

27. Quoted in Figg and Farrell-Beck, "Amputations in the Civil War," 469 (Louisa May Alcott), 471–72 (soldier), 470 (Arabella Wilson).

28. W. A. B. McComb to Board of Commissioners on Artificial Limbs, 29 March 1882.

29. Preston Bledsoe, Confederate Disability Application files, Scott County, Act of 1882, 1884; Compiled Confederate Service Record, 21 Battalion Virginia Infantry; doctor's receipt, Samuel F. Abraham, 12 March 1867, Board of Commissioners on Artificial Limbs; see also note 8.

30. Thomas E. Sims to Board of Commissioners on Artificial Limbs, 8 February 1867; Richmond City, Virginia, census, 1870; E. L. Bennett to Board of Commissioners on Artificial Limbs, 13 February 1867.

31. Shelby Foote, *The Civil War: A Narrative* (New York: Random House, 1958–74), 2:564, 569; Henry C. Fergusson to Governor James L. Kemper, 20 January 1874, Office of the Governor, Letters Received; Richmond city directories, 1869–1894; Richmond City, Virginia, census, 1880, 1900; BVS Deaths, Richmond City, 26 January 1893; Confederate Disability Application file, Richmond City, Act of 1884; Confederate Widow's Pension Application, Richmond City, Act of 1924; obituary in *Richmond Dispatch*, 27 January 1893.

32. Thomas E. Drinkard, Confederate Disability Application, King George County, Act of 1884; Dinwiddie County, Virginia, census, 1870; BVS Marriages, Petersburg, 29 November 1865; BVS Births, Petersburg, 13 November 1867;

Commutation for Disabled Soldiers, Register, 1876–1880, LVA; Petersburg city directories, 1866, 1868–1871; Richmond city directories, 1874–1885; William P. Purcell to Governor James L. Kemper, 21 September 1874, Office of the Governor, Letters Received; Richmond City, Virginia, census, 1870; Jack Welsh, *Medical Histories of Confederate Generals* (Kent, OH: Kent State University Press, 1995), 125–26; S. J. Hurst to Governor James L. Kemper, 14 December 1874, Office of the Governor, Letters Received.

33. Confederate Disability Application file, Augusta County, Act of 1884; R. E. Lee Camp Confederate Soldiers' Home, Application for Admission (rejected), 5 February 1887; Confederate Pension Application, Culpeper County, 21 May 1888; John S. Robson, *How a One-Legged Rebel Lives* (Richmond: W. H. Wade and Company, 1876), v, 7, 112–18; *How a One-Legged Rebel Lives* (Durham, NC: Educator Company, 1898); Virginia census, 1850 (Madison County), 1860 (Rappahannock County), 1870 (Augusta and Rappahannock Counties), 1880 (Rappahannock County), 1910 (Culpepper County), and 1920 (Culpepper County).

34. Robson, *How a One-Legged Rebel Lives* (1876), iii–v, 115.

35. Confederate Pensions, Journals and Registers, 1918–1919/1920–1921: 29, for the funeral expenses of John S. Robson, and 1921–1922/1922–1923: 26, for the funeral expenses of William T. Robson; Confederate Pensioners, Funeral Expense Roll Book, 1914–1920; Confederate Pension Application, William T. Robson, Culpeper County, Act of 1920.

36. Richmond city directories, 1870–1888; *Chataigne's Virginia Business Directory and Gazetteer*, 1871–1872, 1877–1878, 1884-1885, 1888–1889, 1890–1891, 1893–1894, 1911; Boyd's *Directory of the District of Columbia*, 1902, 1904–1908; BVS Marriage Register, Richmond City, 21 October 1873; Hollins Institute, Certificates of Distinction for Nora McCarthy, 1867–1868, Hanger Orthopedic Group Collection; Augusta County, Virginia, census, 1880; District of Columbia census, 1900; *Annual Report of the Commissioner of Patents*, 1872, 1874, 1904, 1907–1908, 1910, 1913, 1915, 1917–1918; obituary, *Staunton Morning Leader*, 17 June 1919; death notice, *Washington Post*, 16 June 1919; *Hanger Substitute Limbs, Nature's Rivals*, 5–11, Hanger Orthopedic Group Collection. Hanger's success story is similar to that of the northern manufacturer B. Frank Palmer, who lost his leg at age ten. Lisa Herschbach, "Prosthetic Reconstructions: Making the Industry, Re-Making the Body, Modeling the Nation." Online: http://www.nyam.org/library/history/hist99_1.html (17 December 1998).

37. Joseph M. Hodge to Board of Commissioners on Artificial Limbs, 9 June 1884; Bath County, Virginia, census, 1870, 1880; W. H. Carter to Board of Commissioners on Artificial Limbs, n.d.

BIBLIOGRAPHY

Manuscript Sources

Emory University, Atlanta, Georgia
  Milton A. Clark Letters

Hanger Orthopedic Group Collection, Bethesda, Maryland

Library of Virginia, Richmond, Virginia
  Board of Commissioners on Artificial Limbs Records
  Bureau of Vital Statistics Births, Deaths, and Marriages
  Confederate Disability Applications
  Confederate Pension Records
  Office of the Governor, Letters Received
  R. E. Lee Camp Confederate Soldiers' Home Records
  Senate Journal
  Works Progress Administration, Virginia Historical Inventory

Museum of the Confederacy, Richmond, Virginia
  Orderly Book, Churchville Cavalry

National Archives and Records Administration, Washington, D.C.
  Association for the Relief of Maimed Soldiers Records
  Compiled Service Records of Confederate Soldiers Who Served in Organi-
      zations from the State of Virginia (microfilm)
  U.S. Census, Population Schedules, District of Columbia, 1900
      (microfilm)
  U. S. Census, Population Schedules, Virginia, 1850, 1860, 1870, 1880, 1900,
      1910, 1920 (microfilm)

Official Records

Annual Report of the Commissioner of Patents, 1872–1918
Report of the Western Lunatic Asylum, 1884, 1886–1887
*Report to the Rector and Visitors of the University of Virginia to the General Assembly,
    December 1865*. Charlottesville: University of Virginia Press, 1865.
Virginia Acts of Assembly, 1867–1894

Directories

Boyd's Directory of the District of Columbia, 1902–1908
Chataigne's Business Directory and Gazetteer, 1884–1885, 1888–1889

Petersburg city directories, 1866–1871
Richmond city directories, 1869–1894
Virginia Business Directory and Gazetteer, 1871–1911

Contemporary Printed Sources

Brief Review of the Plan and Operations of the Association for the Relief of Maimed Soldiers. Richmond, 1865.
Chisolm, J. Julian. *A Manual of Military Surgery for the Use of Surgeons in the Confederate States Army*. 1864. Reprint, Dayton, OH: Morningside, 1983.
"Military Surgery, Ancient and Modern." *United States Service Magazine* 1 (1864): 125–34.
"On Marks' Artificial Limbs." *Journal of the Franklin Institute* 127 (May 1889): 329–36.

Newspapers

Richmond Times-Dispatch
Staunton Morning Leader
Washington Post

Published Letters and Memoirs

Greiner, James M., et al. *A Surgeon's Civil War: The Letters and Diary of Daniel M. Holt, M.D.* Kent, OH: Kent State University Press, 1994.
Robson, John S. *How a One-Legged Rebel Lives*. Richmond: W. H. Wade and Company, 1876.
———. *How a One-Legged Rebel Lives*. Durham, NC: Educator Company, 1898.
Smith, Adelaide. *Reminiscences of an Army Nurse during the Civil War*. New York: Greaves, 1911.
Woodward, C. Vann. *Mary Chesnut's Civil War*. New Haven: Yale University Press, 1981.

Secondary Sources

Bearss, Sara B. The Story of Virginia: An American Experience. Richmond: Virginia Historical Society, 1995.
Boatner, Mark. *The Civil War Dictionary*. New York: Vintage Civil War Library, 1991.
Chesson, Michael. *Richmond after the War*. Richmond: Virginia State Library, 1981.

Cooper, William J., Jr., and Thomas E. Terrill. *The American South: A History*. 2d ed. New York: McGraw-Hill, 1996.

Figg, Laurann, and Jane Farrell-Beck. "Amputation in the Civil War: Physical and Social Dimensions." *Journal of the History of Medicine and Allied Sciences* 48 (October 1993): 454–75.

Foote, Shelby. *The Civil War: A Narrative*. 3 vols. New York: Random House, 1958–74.

Freeman, Douglas Southall. *A Calendar of Confederate Papers*. 1908. Reprint, New York: Kraus Reprint Company, 1969.

Gillett, Mary C. *The Army Medical Department, 1818–1865*. Washington, DC: Center of Military History, 1987.

Herschbach, Lisa. "Prosthetic Reconstructions: Making the Industry, Re-Making the Body, Modeling the Nation." Online: http://www.nyam.org .library/history/hist99_1.html. 17 December 1998.

History of Churchville. Churchville, VA: Women's Club, 1932.

McCawley, Patrick J. Artificial Limbs for Confederate Soldiers. Columbia: South Carolina Department of Archives and History, Public Programs Division, 1992.

McDaid, Jennifer Davis. "With Lame Legs and No Money: Virginia's Disabled Confederate Veterans." *Virginia Cavalcade* 47 (winter 1998): 14–25

McPherson, James M. *Battle Cry of Freedom: The Civil War Era*. New York: Oxford University Press, 1988.

Minor, Berkeley, and James F. Minor. *Legislative History of the University of Virginia*. Charlottesville: University of Virginia, 1928.

Rosenburg, R. B. *Living Monuments: Confederate Soldiers' Homes in the New South*. Chapel Hill: University of North Carolina Press, 1993.

Wegner, Ansley Herring. "Phantom Pain: Civil War Amputation and North Carolina's Maimed Veterans." *North Carolina Historical Review* 75 (July 1998): 277–96.

Welsh, Jack. *Medical Histories of Confederate Generals*. Kent, OH: Kent State University Press, 1995.

PART II

DESIGN

5

Hard Wear and Soft Tissue

Craft and Commerce in Artificial Eyes

Katherine Ott

IN 1881, FORTY-THREE-YEAR-OLD Jacob Groff was using an uncooperative ox to haul logs through the countryside of Elkhart County, Indiana. Groff cracked his whip at the unruly animal and the whiplash struck him in the eye. The injury blinded him at once and he felt so sickened he nearly vomited. Groff's neighbor, John Mann, a nineteen-year-old farmer, began his day as usual, long before dawn, groping around in the dark for his boots. On this particular day, as he stooped over, Mann jammed his eye against the spool holder on the sewing machine.[1]

Although both of these men regained their vision, at least in the short term, their experiences were typical of people living in the nineteenth and early twentieth centuries. Blunt trauma from blows to the head and face and foreign body penetration were constant hazards. Janitors lost vision while breaking coal for furnaces; stonecutters lost eyes to rock splinters and iron chips flying off the edges of chisels and hammers; farmers found everything from wheat chaff to tree branches and the hooves of a recalcitrant horse thrust into their eyes. Gun cap shrapnel, cinders from the family fireplace, errant insects, and factory work also posed dangers.[2] In the American South and on the prairie frontier of the nineteenth century, a winning strategy in wrestling fights involved biting and eye gouging. Such injuries usually resulted in inflammation (commonly called ophthalmia), infection, and vision loss (called amblyopia). Before the 1920s, protective eyewear was virtually unknown, except for the occasional carriage, and later, railroad goggles.[3] There were only a handful of medicaments: various collyria or

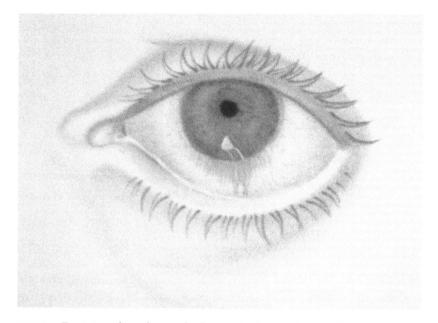

FIG. 5.1. Eye injury from foreign body penetration, such as cinders, wood chips, or this millet husk lodged in the cornea, frequently led to vision loss in the nineteenth century. From Julius Sichel, *Iconographie ophthalmologique* (Paris: J. Bailliere, 1852).

eyewashes, atropine, after 1884 cocaine and its anesthetic cousins such as holcaine and nucaine; chloral hydrate was a common sedative.[4] Consequently, corneal and retinal injury and deep eye lesions wreaked havoc. Partial and total loss of vision was a fact of life.

By the early 1800s, sight itself had assumed a new status in the hierarchy of the senses.[5] In Western culture until recent times, all the senses carried equal weight and interest for poets, philosophers, priests, and laypeople. Touch, smell, hearing, taste, and sight contributed to understanding the everyday world of affairs. During the Renaissance, scholars and thinkers began to elevate the sense of sight above other senses. Visual metaphors abounded. In science and medicine, illustrations, drawings, and demonstrations achieved new prestige. By the nineteenth century, the sense of sight was firmly at the top of the hierarchy of the senses. Its dominance was assured by graphic reproduction techniques, such as engraving, lithography, and photography, which made possible the mass production and dissemination of images. People actively engaged with the world added visual discrimination to their portmanteau of important life skills. Scientists plunged into the study of optics, centered on the function of the human eye. The "regime of vision," as Jonathan Crary has characterized these events, with its kaleidoscopes, stereoscopes, kymographs, compound microscopes, zoetropes, prisms, and ophthalmoscopes, provided the cultural context for understanding expectations about artificial eyes.

Injury often resulted in an eye so damaged that physicians believed removal of the eyeball to be the best course of action. For most of the nineteenth century, physicians were of the opinion that, although the injured eye may seem to have recovered fully, eventually the eye would deteriorate and, even more importantly, in the process, the pathology would spread to the other, healthy eye. Known as sympathetic ophthalmia, the process might take from a few hours to many years, but physicians in the late nineteenth century believed it to be inevitable.[6] So doctors practiced preventive surgery based on the opinion that it was better to remove the jeopardized eye at the time of injury.

This practice was not merely due to the doctor's desire to collect larger fees for surgery and its attendant procedures. Minute particles embedded somewhere in the eye (in the retina, conjunctiva, choroid, or elsewhere) were hard to locate, even with the aid of the ophthalmoscope (invented in 1851), and consequently went undetected. In one reported case, a man wounded at the battle of Chancellorsville during the Civil War had no problem for fourteen years and then developed severe neuralgia, or pain, and sympathetic ophthalmia. His eye was enucleated and inside was found a piece of bone.[7]

Enucleation entailed the surgical removal of the entire globe. It became a popular operation in the 1860s and 1870s.[8] Until then, the procedure was very messy, bloody, and dangerous. Before the 1860s, the instruments were crude and mortality was high. The eye was literally pulled out with pliers or scooped with a spoon. Surgeons avoided enucleation as much as possible, leaving patients to die with malignancies that slowly overtook their faces, rather than inflict death from the consequences of enucleation. In the 1840s, as the anatomy of the eye was more accurately described, surgeons figured out a way to cut the four rectus muscles that gave movement to the eyeball, making removal an easier and more practical procedure.[9] Not surprisingly, the new technique advanced rapidly in industrial areas of Europe, where eye

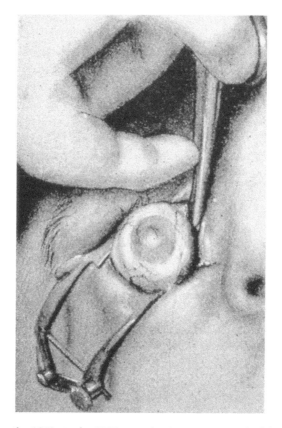

FIG. 5.2. From the 1860s to the 1920s enucleation, or removal of the eyeball, was a common treatment for eye injuries. Physicians removed the injured or inflamed globe in hopes of preventing sympathetic ophthalmia, a condition in which impairment spread from the damaged eye to the healthy one. From Charles May, *Manual of the Diseases of the Eye* (New York: William Wood, 1924).

injuries were a major problem. There is also evidence that physicians used a patient's class background as a criterion for whether to perform enucleation or not. A Richmond physician recommended immediate enucleation for working-class patients but a wait-and-see strategy for members of the "educated class," whom he believed were capable of better vigilance about troublesome symptoms.[10] Conversely, another physician suggested that poor people might be better served by leaving the "shrunken and disfigured globe" rather than performing enucleation, because the procedure would entail the expense of an artificial eye.[11]

The popularity of enucleation brought demand for a different design in prostheses. Over the centuries, a variety of designs, materials, and techniques were employed in artificial eye making. Underlying all attempts at artificial eyes was the search for a "good fit," Since the definition of a "good fit" depended on the availability of materials as well as the interplay of cultural aesthetics and medical practices, the design of artificial eyes has varied across time and place. In one community, an eye patch served well enough, but in another era, a painted metal eye tied around the head was the best solution.

All materials selected to make the eye have limitations of one sort or another. Weight mattered because of the relative fragility of the orbit. Most materials were too heavy and distorted the face, made the lower lid droop, or caused headaches and distress to other, surrounding areas. Substances that were light enough quickly irritated the orbit and so were inadequate. Celluloid, for instance, was tried shortly after its invention in the late 1800s, but it became rough after a little use. It irritated the membrane and emitted an offensive odor. Other substances, glass included, tended to spontaneously implode, break, or become scratched and rough over time. Hollow globes of glass or other substances were often so large, the surgeon found it necessary to trim the eye socket.[12] Since makers had no means to lessen the size of the artificial implant, physicians altered the body to accommodate the technology.

Ambroise Paré, a brilliant and ingenious French physician, was one of the first people to make a usable artificial eye and describe it in print. In 1579 he fabricated a metal plate covered with chamois and painted the eye, lid, and lashes on to it. Since it was worn over the lid, Paré called it an ekblepharon. The prosthesis attached to a cord or thin iron bar that wrapped around the head to keep it in place.[13] Paré's foray into ocular prostheses was part of his ongoing interest in artificial replacement parts for the human body. No doubt influenced by his tenure as a battle surgeon, he also designed hands and legs.

Beginning in the 1700s, makers turned to glass as the material of choice. Venice, as the center of glassblowing, dominated the market for most of the eighteenth century and strictly guarded the secrets of eye making. But by the late 1700s, eye makers began to appear in other countries, France and Germany in particular.

In the early 1800s in France, eyes were most often made of enamel (silicon, potash, and minium or lead and tin), seldom of ordinary glass. Since enamel was fragile and corroded over time, ocularists tried many other substances, such as lead, aluminum, ivory, bone, caoutchouc, vulcanite, and hollowed out marbles. None of these substances was as satisfactory as enamel. In France, several expert eye makers began writing about and training students in the craft. French ocularists widely adopted glass and dispensed with painted or leather-wrapped metal plates. Hazard-Mirault wrote an important book on eye making in 1818, in which he recommended glass and explained the ocular fabrication process.[14] The first successful enamel glass prosthesis was probably made by the Boissonneau family of Paris, about 1822. Paris dominated the artificial eye market for fifty years. The Boissonneau eye received first place at the 1855 Paris Exposition, where artificial eyes, in general, were a sensation.[15] The eyes intrigued people because, as one observer wrote, they "restore the patient's peace of mind and his proper place amongst his fellow creatures."[16]

The social and symbolic rather than the medical value of artificial eyes played an increasingly important role in the design of eyes as the nineteenth century progressed. Bourgeois customers placed a premium on appearance and decorum, which meant that an empty socket or a crudely fashioned globe became an indication of lower socioeconomic standing. The Boissonneaux made distinctions among their clientele by requiring potential customers to first fill out a questionnaire, to ensure that they could pay.[17]

Whether or not mid-nineteenth-century enamel eyes could pass unnoticed in our own time is of little importance. Certainly the majority of persons wearing artificial eyes today go unnoticed. But in the nineteenth century, people embraced different aesthetic standards. Bodily difference was taken for granted—everyone had scars, bad teeth, a unique gait, or some other mark of physical diversity. How the individual presented his or her own diversity in public indicated both their social and economic background and their aspirations. A farmer, expecting no deviation in his lifetime's labor, might carve an eye from a piece of wood or quartz to use for special occasions and wear a patch the rest of the time. He need only please himself, his family, and his cows. But young persons with big ideas and any of the thousands of newly apprenticed lawyers and doctors responded to other social pressures. They were cognizant of prejudice against the wearing of crudely made eyes. As one critic observed, such eyes gave the face an "uncertain and wild" appearance, or "imparted to the face a repulsive aspect."[18] These sentiments addressed bourgeois conventions of propriety and gentility and appreciation of others who behaved accordingly. One's artificial eye may not have passed for a natural one, but the gesture of wearing one, as well-made as possible, was what middle-class members and aspirants approved of and found significant. As a New York City eye doctor wrote in his 1829 newspaper ad to persuade clients to purchase his artificial eyes, "Nothing is more offensive to look upon than a sightless closed eye, and the loss . . . renders the patient unfit to mingle in society."[19]

Meanwhile, French dominance of artificial eye making was short-lived. The French used lead glass, which was adequate, but German makers found a way to improve the aesthetic results by substituting soda glass, which was noticeably lighter in weight. Manufacturing gradually shifted to Germany, especially Wiesbaden, which became one of the commercial centers of eye making. In the 1870s and 1880s, Germany was in the midst of an intense period of industrial and economic change. German researchers and scientists developed techniques and systems in chemistry, synthetics, and electricity-based industry. Glass eye making was part of that blossoming of science, engineering, and industry. German oculists started using cryolite (also called creolite) glass in the 1870s. Its advantage was that it was easier to work and it finished to a more lifelike, opalescent shine.

Once the medical necessity for more and better artificial eyes combined with the oculists' craft experience in working the object in glass, a new design emerged. Before the new design, descriptively dubbed the "reform" eye or Snellen eye, artificial eyes were thin curved shells of glass. Since a shell-style eye needed a stump to support it, it was useless in the post-enucleated, empty socket. The edges cut into the surrounding tissue, causing fluids to build up behind it. With nothing to rest against, the shell was woefully inadequate. Wearers needed a prosthesis that could be worn not only behind the eyelid but within the eye, since the socket was emptied. The "reform" or Snellen eye was thus a great boon to both the surgeon and oculist.

The new design, which is still the basis of most artificial eyes in use today, called for the shell to be expanded to fill more of the socket. It looked and felt better. The shell was fattened by the addition of another wall with a hollow space in the middle. Instead of a thin plate, the arti-

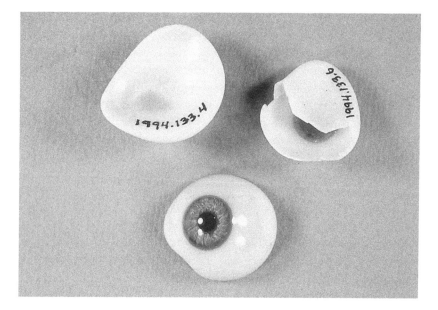

FIG. 5.3. These glass eyes illustrate aspects of design. The back view, on the left, shows the curve of the shell. The broken eye on the right provides a glimpse of the expanded internal space characteristic of the reform or Snellen eye. The middle eye shows the notch indicating which socket the eye fit. Courtesy of the National Museum of American History, Smithsonian Institution.

ficial eye became a hollow pillow. The design was named for Hermann Snellen, a well-respected and internationally known ophthalmologist from the Netherlands (among other things, Snellen created the familiar eye charts still used to measure vision). Snellen did not actually invent the design; rather, he challenged the Müller-Uri family of glassblowers in Wiesbaden to come up with a design to better meet the needs of physicians and patients. Snellen's patented reform eye was introduced in the 1890s and quickly became the preferred design throughout Europe and the United States.

Patients and ocularists preferred the Snellen design because it reduced the sunken appearance of the orbit and socket area of the face. It also eliminated the need for operations to introduce implants of sponge, gelatin, or globes of glass, metal, or other substances, for the purpose of forming a better supporting stump for the superimposed artificial eye. Late in the nineteenth century, a few ophthalmic surgeons turned their attention to procedures for implanting support spheres that would give a better outcome to placement of the artificial eye. The most popular technique of this sort was Mules's operation, in which a glass sphere was inserted into Tenon's capsule, after evisceration of the globe. The sphere functioned as an artificial vitreous, the semifluid material between the retina and the lens of the eye. Mules introduced his technique in 1885 and the buried implants soon became a common accompaniment to the reform eye. Until World War II, Mules implants dominated this procedure. Many surgeons preferred to eviscerate the globe and implant a Mules sphere, instead of performing the more severe enucleation of the entire orbit.[20]

German ocularists ruled the eye-making market primarily because of their ability to control glass exports and their superior raw materials. The soda glass from German factories was well suited to eye making. Sand from the Black Forest region had a low iron oxide content, which meant the glass made with it resisted corrosion from human tears. Alkaline secretions from the lachrymal duct more easily dissolved and damaged the lead glass commonly available in France, England, and the United States. Consequently, eye makers depended on German makers to supply the glass tubes needed for blowing artificial eyes.

To make a glass eye, the ocularist began with a hollow tube of glass. The ocularist examined the socket and shaped the eye as he or she blew it. The tube was heated at one end, a bulb blown, and the piece gradually pulled off from the rest of the tube. The iris color resulted from applications of pigmented glass rods. The maker heated the bulb and rod and used the pigment stick like a crayon, to lay on color around the slightly flattened face of the globe.[21]

The dependence of ocularists in the United States on German glass became intolerable in 1933. During the mobilization of German industry for war, the Nazis forbade exportation of many products and raw materials, including glass. Among the Allies, glass shortages became acute, as supplies of artificial eyes and glass tubing disappeared. Although the need for eye tubing was critical, consumers comprised a small niche market. As had happened during World War I, when supplies dwindled, glass manufacturers did not find it cost-effective to put their scarce resources into research for perfecting glass eye tubing. It was left to army medical officers to search for alternatives.

Where and by whom the first successful acrylic eye was made is a subject surrounded in dispute and confusion. Plastic eyes first began to

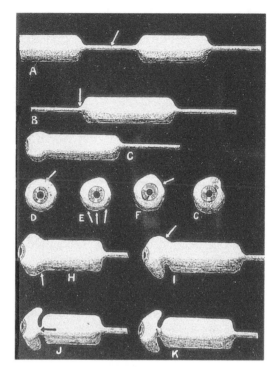

FIG. 5.4. In fabricating a glass eye, the maker begins with a hollow glass tube. The tube is heated and stretched, a bulb blown at the tip, and the eye piece broken off; finally, the maker sucks the air out of the bulb to collapse it. From J. H. Prince, Ocular Prosthesis (Baltimore: Williams and Wilkins, 1946).

appear in the late 1930s, and news of their existence spread by word of mouth.[22] Three army dentists, Milton Wirtz, Stanley Erpf, and Victor Dietz, have been credited with producing the first acrylic eye in 1943. What they actually did was adapt existing materials and techniques to create a system for mass production of acrylic eyes. The three men had been experimenting with acrylic eyes in their own labs and were dispatched together to Valley Forge, Pennsylvania.[23] Since they were dentists, they turned to common denture-making processes, instruments, and substances. They achieved success with acrilan, also known as methyl methacrylate, the thermoplastic from which dentures were made. Acrilan was easy to mold and harden, although the process took a few days. Plastic dentures had evolved from the rubber ones popularly used in the late 1800s. An international trust controlled the rubber market of the time and set prices exorbitantly high, so dentists searched for alternative materials. They first used celluloid with good results (and tried other materials similar to the ocularists' list of substitutes) and then switched to methyl methacrylate in the 1930s, once it became commercially available.[24] Acrylic plastic came into its own during World War II, when war researchers studied its potential use in aerodynamics, automobiles, and other applications (Plexiglas was another important acrylic plastic, introduced in 1936, as was Lucite, in 1939). By then, methyl methacrylate was readily available, its chemistry was well known, and a cadre of dentists existed who were experienced in working with it.

To make an acrylic eye, the ocularist began by taking an impression of the patient's socket for use as a pattern in shaping the artificial eye.[25] This was done by injecting the socket with alginate. Once the alginate set, it was removed and the positive cast was used to form a plaster cast. The other method of creating a pattern of the socket was to put a wafer of pliable wax over a ball bearing and sculpt it freehand, while observing the contours of the socket. A gauge was used to measure the size of the area, the measurement imposed on the wax, the iris spot marked, and the wax trial piece tested on the patient.[26]

When the plaster cast was finished the ocularist filled it with dental wax and used the resulting trial prosthesis to adjust the fit within the patient's socket and position the iris. The corrected wax prosthesis was then embedded in a halved dental stone mold. When the mold was set and the wax removed, the mold was filled with the methyl methacrylate and heat cured, under several hundred to several thousand pounds of pressure. Since acrylic is porous, it needed to be fused under great pressure to make the eye dense. The greater the density, the less chance of infection. The sclera, pupil, and iris were made separately and then fused. The tiny iris was shaped like a button, with a tab with which to grasp it, for placement. Thin strands of colored rayon thread embedded on the scleral piece gave the illusion of veins. The ocularist painted each iris by hand, to match the companion eye. After the parts were fused in place, the ocularist laminated the entire eye with a wrapper of clear acrylic.[27] The eye was further adjusted by lathe grinding and then polished. Although each eye was custom made, the use of molds and

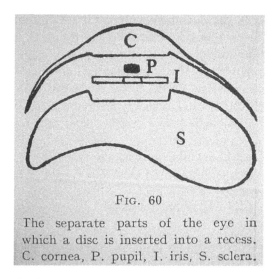

FIG. 60

The separate parts of the eye in which a disc is inserted into a recess. C. cornea, P. pupil, I. iris, S. sclera.

FIG. 5.5. The individual parts of the acrylic eye, introduced in the 1940s. From J. H. Prince, *Recent Advances in Ocular Prosthesis* (Baltimore: Williams and Wilkins, 1950).

multiple dies, iris color guides, and stock sclera streamlined production and ensured that the product had consistent quality.[28]

The use of stock eyes for mass distribution began in the nineteenth century. Medical supply houses, such as George Tiemann and Company, offered artificial eyes for sale to physicians and "oculists" through the mail.[29] The purchaser supplied a sketch and some basic measurements, including left or right eye, and received an appropriate, if approximate, prosthesis by return post. The mail-order clerk might send one eye or select several from the company supplies, requesting the buyer to select the most congenial one and return the rest. Failing a mail-order eye, residents of rural and remote areas relied on a chance encounter with one of the itinerant peddlers who traveled the back roads, fixing pots, sharpening edge tools, selling combs and spectacles, and fitting eyes. In cities, jewelers, opticians, and eye doctors dispensed artificial eyes. American Optical Company was a leader in supplying stock eyes for several decades. The trade in stock eyes declined in the 1960s, perhaps as a result of the efforts of ocularists, who successfully made the case that eyes should be custom made and fitted. Display boxes and table-top storage cabinets used in dispensing artificial glass eyes occasionally turn up in opticians' back rooms and doctors' closets, as curiosities of a bygone era.

Walter Spohn learned the technique of acrylic eye making in the army during World War II.[30] Spohn's career as an ocularist was typical of many twentieth-century practitioners who loved their work, experimented with their craft, and questioned the structure of the profession. Spohn was working in a Paterson, New Jersey, bakery when he was drafted into the army in 1941 and his life abruptly changed course. He found himself stationed in Texas, glad to be out of the bakery, knowing he wanted a more challenging job, and hopeful that he could find a kind of work in which he could apply his deep-rooted spiritual beliefs (Spohn had earlier considered becoming a Christian missionary). He took a dental technician course and learned about denture materials and articulation of teeth. He met a dentist who was taking eye socket impressions using the wax and ball method for making acrylic eyes. Afterwards, Spohn joined the plastic eye clinic at Fort Sam Houston and eventually ended up at the Veteran's Hospital in San Francisco, where he was chief of the Plastic Eye and Restorations Clinic from 1948 until his retirement in 1971.

Spohn never made glass eyes. His work with acrylics led him, as it did many other ocularists, to tinker with and adjust the process (in 1949, for example, he worked out a method to shorten fabrication time to one day). But unlike most ocularists, Spohn made more than eyes. He also fabricated facial prostheses, or restorations, in collaboration with plastic surgeons and prosthodontists (specialists in mouth and oral cavity repair medicine). Spohn experimented with new plastics such as silastic and silicone and was a consultant in anaplastology at Stanford University's Department of Surgery for ten years after he retired from the Veterans Administration. And unlike most other ocularists, Spohn did not learn his craft as an apprentice in a family business, but in a career track in the army. At the Veterans Administration and at Stanford, Spohn trained students who had no family legacy or inherited interest in eye making, but only a strong vocational drive. Consequently, his understanding and broader experience of the profession led him in a unique direction.

If Walter Spohn exemplified one branch of eye making, the New Jersey ocularist Earle C. Schreiber Jr. represented the other: Schreiber learned his craft as a teenager from his father and mother. Earle Sr.

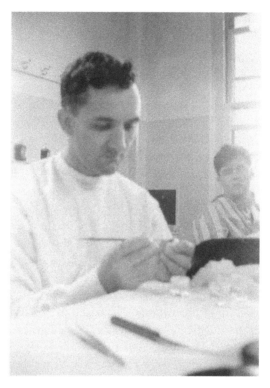

FIG. 5.6. Unlike many twentieth-century ocularists, who learned the craft as part of the family business, Walter Spohn, shown here finishing an eye in the 1940s, learned to make acrylic eyes in the army. Courtesy of the National Museum of American History, Smithsonian Institution.

worked for many years for the prestigious Mager and Gougelmann business, after he married the daughter of partner George Mager. In 1931, following George Mager's death, all the Mager relatives departed the firm. The economic crisis of the Depression was deepening and the Gougelmann clan reduced staff by dismissing all the Magers. Four years later, Earle Sr. died, leaving a young wife and seventeen-year-old son. Young Earle dropped out of high school and with the blessing of his mother, Laura Mager Schreiber, went off to San Francisco to apprentice with his father's friend, Gottlieb Danz. After six months of training, he and his mother began practicing together in Newark. In the 1940s Schreiber met Fritz Müller and Otto Greiner and periodically studied with them in Chicago to perfect his craft. During World War II, when American nativists denounced Japanese and German Americans as untrustworthy and potential spies, some ocularists came under suspicion, perhaps because of their ties to and dependency on imported glass manufacturers. At any rate, citing his participation in the German-American Vocational League, FBI agents arrested Otto Greiner at his Chicago office. Greiner was indicted by a grand jury in Newark, New Jersey, and Schreiber testified on his behalf (Schreiber had been present during the arrest as well). Greiner was eventually acquitted of all charges.[31]

The ocularist profession has two main and sometimes competing branches: the American Society of Ocularists, organized in 1958, and the American Anaplastology Association, founded in 1980. The makers of artificial eyes call themselves ocularists. Ocularists rarely make restorations of the eye socket or other parts of the face; they concentrate on making eyes. Historically, the craft of eye making has been exceedingly insular and closed to outsiders. For most of the nineteenth and twentieth centuries, artificial eyes were made of glass. Since glassblowing required specialized knowledge and skill, methods of eye making were closely guarded. Eye making was often a family business, with the craft knowledge passing from generation to generation and rarely to outsiders. Members of competing ocularist families often intermarried, but like Capulets and Montagues, they fiercely guarded their professional capital.

To some extent, the insularity of the ocularist profession was a natural consequence of the nature of the work culture. Many of the great U.S. eye makers were German immigrants, or had ties to other stellar European makers: Gottlieb Danz (father and sons), Fritz Jardon, and Arno and Otto Greiner, to name a few. Peter Gougelmann, founder of perhaps the most respected and long-lived ocularist family in the United States, immigrated from Switzerland to New York City. Gougelmann spent several years working with Auguste Boissonneau in Paris, before opening his shop in New York City in 1851.[32]

Family ties ran deep and loyalty in times of stress further solidified the insularity of the craft. By the mid-twentieth century, the dispersed yet conjoined nature of the profession gave rise to distrust, secrecy, and jealousy. Skilled craftwork, such as eye making, has been fraught with internal pressures throughout modern history. In the Middle Ages, artisans formed guilds to protect their labor skills, oversee training, regulate prices and competition, and control markets in paper making, glassblowing, shoemaking, metalworking, barbering, and numerous other trades. Eye making has retained its craft, artisanal characteristics far longer than most other kinds of work. Like earlier artisans, ocularists worked for themselves and set their own hours and rates (once their apprenticeship was completed), owned their tools, and formed trade organizations based upon specialized knowledge accumulated over generations.[33]

In the 1940s and 1950s, leading members of the ocularist community got together and decided to institutionalize their profession, end the internecine battles, and increase recognition and prestige by forging stronger ties with the American Academy of Ophthalmology and Otolaryngology. The stated goals of the new group, named the American Society of Ocularists, was to solidify the base of ocularists, share knowledge more openly, and raise professional standards.[34]

The new society immediately faced challenges from ophthalmologists, who fit eyes but did not actually fabricate them. The ocularists were wary of the eye-fitting ophthalmologists and feared that with large numbers of ophthalmologists the society would become sidetracked by issues not related to their needs. The ocularists and ophthalmologists solved the problem by creating two groups, a larger one for everyone (American Academy of Ophthalmic Prosthetics) while maintaining the smaller one only for the ocularists (the American Society of Ocularists, or ASO). The two groups existed peacefully and with shared membership for a few years, but by 1965 most of the ophthalmologists had moved into other areas, such as the then new and enticing field of contact lenses. Only the American Society of Ocularists remained. The ASO closely monitored its membership requirements and rigorously reviewed all applicants. In the early 1970s the society instituted a formal educational program under which all new ocularists were required to follow a five-year training program and pass examinations administered by an ASO board of examiners. The curriculum was developed and supervised by ASO members. Admission to the program—and by consequence, to the profession—was controlled by the ASO.[35]

Inevitably, ASO ocularists experienced pressures to change, coming both from within the profession and from changes in American society. Throughout the 1960s and 1970s, more and more eye makers collaborated with plastic surgeons to create facial prostheses for cancer patients and patients who had suffered automobile and workplace injuries. Nowhere was this work more intense than in veterans' hospitals, where medical practitioners constantly sought new techniques to aid the wounded soldiers returning from Vietnam. The high-velocity weapons used in Vietnam, such as the M-16 rifle and other missiles, damaged more tissue and resulted in larger sockets needing repair. Subcutaneous implants, bone grafts, and skin augmentation methods improved with the sheer number of soldiers injured.

Elsewhere, microsurgery, antibiotics, steroids, and other drugs, new reconstruction materials, and new operating room and diagnostic technologies contributed to changes in the medical profession and its ancillary fields, such as prosthetics. Following World War II, interest in ocular implants revived. Ophthalmologists had generally sewn a Mules sphere or a variation of it into the empty socket. But beginning in the 1950s, new designs, using tantalum, stainless steel mesh, clips, pegs, magnets, acrylic, Teflon, silicone, silastic, and other plastics appeared.[36]

Despite the changes disrupting the medical profession in the 1960s and 1970s, the American Society of Ocularists remained small and tightly knit. In 1980 there were 225 members at various stages of expertise, such as trainee, associate, and honorary. But tensions over their continued insularity and monopoly over eye making erupted in 1980 and led to formation of a rival organization, the American Anaplastology Association.[37]

Not surprisingly, Walter Spohn helped lead the exodus into anaplastology. In fact, Spohn has been credited with the neologism, combining the important aspects of the work into the single word, anaplastology. Spohn was a respected and active member of the ASO who gave papers at annual meetings, served on the board of directors for many years, and served as its secretary and the chair of several committees. But over the years, Spohn became increasingly frustrated in trying to get his students into (as well as interested in) the ASO. He came to believe that "Nepotism is prevalent in great numbers within the Society," and that a new professional group was needed.[38]

The new group was formed partly in opposition to the ASO, and partly to meet the expanded professional interests of some ocularists. By 1980 there existed a significant number of eye makers who had learned their craft through military and government training or university programs, such as the ones Walter Spohn directed at the Veterans Administration and then at Stanford University (Foothill College).

These oculars differed from the family dynasty oculars in several ways.

Since members of the upstart group were usually the first generation of makers in their families, they tended to have less loyalty and commitment to ocularist traditions. They also usually fabricated more than ocular prostheses and included cranial implants, ears, noses, and other facial restorations in their work. This meant that they worked closely with a greater variety of medical specialists as well as spent time in operating rooms and clinics. In addition, anaplastologists more often had university degrees or class credits than did family-trained ocularists. The expertise of each group was equally solid; their conceptions of the field and their professional interests were frequently at odds. Nevertheless, the two groups continue to share members and maintain overlapping interests.

The artificial eye, in aesthetics and technology, is a product of the mechanical age. It tries to imitate or mimic our organs and muscles. It replicates the literal appearance of the eye but does not produce vision.

Part of the renewed interest in implants after World War II had been the desire to improve mechanical motility of the eye. Designers wanted to make the artificial eye move as though it were the real thing. Since most of the manufacturing and materials problems were resolved, physicians and oculars turned their attention to achieving optimum motility of the replacement eye. Ophthalmic surgeons sutured the rectus muscles to the capsulated implant, and over time, growing tissue attached to it, giving the prosthesis more natural movement. In the 1980s the advent of hydroxyapatite, a porous material first used in orthopedic reconstruction, brought an even greater improvement in verisimilitude to artificial eyes. Implants made with hydroxyapatite or Medpor, a similar synthetic material, became integrated into ocular tissue and when combined with a pegged prosthesis, the result was remarkable.[39]

Following efforts to achieve natural motility, the next compelling issue in ocular prostheses is that of simulating sight. As the mechanical age ends, researchers are using computer technology with microsurgery to emulate the chemistry and biology of photoreceptors. The targeted locations for these new prostheses are the brain and nervous system, not Tenon's capsule and the eye socket. Neuronal prostheses, designed to re-create vision for blind people, stimulate neurons at either the retina or the visual cortex. Exceedingly small supercomputers, called neuromorphic vision chips, mimic the molecular structure of the retina. Consequently, the prostheses will not work without the eyeball or optic nerve in place. Another method for artificial vision employs a camera external to the eye that translates images into impulse patterns and transmits them to an implanted receiver.[40] These devices may eventually produce rudimentary sight. It remains to be seen if neuronal prostheses will become as controversial as cochlear implants, used to simulate rudimentary hearing. Certainly many of the cultural and psychological issues are similar for the two devices, such as how use might alter the client's identity.

The history of artificial eyes is both deceptively simple and infuriatingly complex. It is the story of how people have sought to produce a serviceable substitute for the living human eye. The mechanical and medical problems of creating an effective artificial eye are complicated enough without adding the cultural, economic, and aesthetic factors that shift over time and guide the research and science behind the prosthesis. Prosthetic eyes represent the confluence of several historical developments: refinement of medical techniques in ophthalmic and plastic surgery, early-twentieth-century plastics research, international exchange in design and expertise, and the vitality of craft work within industrial society, all leavened by the powerful yeast of individuals injured on the battlefield, at work, and at home.

NOTES

Thanks to the following for help with this article: Michael O. Hughes, the Schreiber and Spohn families, and the members of the Optical Heritage Society.

1. C. A. Lambert, "Injuries of the Eye," *Chicago Medical Journal and Examiner* 44 (1882): 139–41.

2. For a medical discussion of common injuries, see Henry Olin, "Foreign Bodies within the Eye," *Chicago Medical Times* 3 (1871): 193–96. For a twentieth-century discussion of industrial eye injuries, see George Cross, "Ophthalmology and Its Relation to Industry," *Delaware State Medical Journal* 13 (March 1940): 39–46; Hedwig Kuhn, *Industrial Ophthalmology* (St. Louis: C. V. Mosby, 1944).

3. For more on the history of ophthalmology, see Daniel Albert and Diane Edwards, eds., *The History of Ophthalmology* (Cambridge: Blackwell Science, 1996); Charles Snyder, *Our Ophthalmic Heritage* (Boston: Little, Brown, 1966); and the numerous monographs of Julius Hirschberg's *History of Ophthalmology* (Bonn, Germany: Wayenborgh, 1982 [1887]).

4. For background on these pharmaceuticals, see any of the versions of the United States Pharmacopoeia, including George Wood and Franklin Bache, *The Dispensatory of the United States of America* (Philadelphia: Lippincott, Grambo, 1854).

5. For more on the shift in the hierarchy of the senses and the importance of vision, see Jonathan Crary, *Techniques of the Observer: On Vision and Modernity in the Nineteenth Century* (Cambridge: MIT. Press, 1990); Martin Kemp, *The Science of Art: Optical Themes in Western Art from Brunelleschi to Seurat* (New Haven: Yale University Press, 1990); Chris Jenks, "The Centrality of the Eye in Western Culture," in Chris Jenks, ed., *Visual Culture* (New York: Routledge, 1995), 1–25; Barbara Maria Stafford, *Good Looking: Essays on the Virtue of Images* (Cambridge: MIT Press, 1996).

6. The contemporary term for many of these conditions would be uveitis. For typical medical descriptions of sympathetic ophthalmia, see G. E. de-Schweinitz, *Diseases of the Eye* (Philadelphia: W. B. Saunders, 1906), 418–30; or George Lawson, *Injuries of the Eye, Orbit, and Eyelids: Their Immediate and Remote Effects* (Philadelphia: Henry C. Lea, 1867), 289–321.

7. Dr. McGuire, "Extraction from the Eye of a Piece of Bone Which Had Remained Quiescent Fourteen Years," *Virginia Medical Monthly* 5 (1887): 216–17.

8. For a representative description of enucleation, see Casey Wood, "Enucleation of the Eye and Its Substitutes," in Casey Wood, ed., *The American Encyclopedia and Dictionary of Ophthalmology* (Chicago: Cleveland Press, 1915), 6: 4382–4475; Ernst Fuchs, *Text-Book of Ophthalmology,* trans. Alexander Duane (Philadelphia: J. B. Lippincott, 1908), 851–57. See also Charles Snyder, "An Operation Designated 'The Extirpation of the Eye,'" in *Our Ophthalmic Heritage,* 135–40.

Surgeons also performed evisceration, though less often than enucleation. In evisceration, only the contents of the globe are removed, not the globe itself. The sclera and recti remain intact.

9. A crucial piece of the puzzle was the structure of the capsule in which the eye resides. Jacques Tenon identified it in 1724, but no one paid much attention to it until Amedee Bonnet redescribed it in 1841. Tenon's or Bonnet's capsule was the primary location for surgery to remove the eye.

10. Joseph White, "Sympathetic Ophthalmia," *Virginia Medical Monthly* 6 (1879–80): 431–32.

11. Henry Williams, "Neurotomy of the Optic and Ciliary Nerves as a Substitute for Enucleation of the Eyeball," *Boston Medical and Surgical Journal* 102 (1880): 73.

For typical costs, see the 1908 catalog of the Philadelphia company McIntire, Magee, and Brown. Generic stock eyes cost $1.50 and custom eyes ranged from $5 to $25. Most made-to-order eyes cost about $10 and lasted about three years before the surface roughened. However, if the user dropped the glass eye, it easily broke.

12. "Artificial Eyes at the Paris Exhibition of 1855," *Lancet* 2 (September 13, 1856): 315.

13. Overviews of the history of artificial eyes have usually been written by makers themselves or physicians, rather than professionally trained historians. Consequently, dates, spellings of names, and other information can vary from author to author and should be used with caution. Such histories include J. H. Prince, *Ocular Prosthesis* (Baltimore: William Wood, 1946), 1–23; Carey McCord, "Artificial Eyes: The Early History of Ocular Prostheses," *Journal of Occupational Medicine* 7.2 (1965): 61–68; O. Martin and L. Clodius, "The History of the Artificial Eye," *Annals of Plastic Surgery* 3.2 (1979): 168–71; Lars Vistnes, *Surgical Reconstruction in the Anophthalmic Orbit* (Birmingham, AL: Aesculapius, 1987), 3–11; Den Tonkelaar et al., "Herman Snellen (1834–1908) and Muller's 'Reform-Auge,'" *Documenta Ophthalmologica* 77 (1991): 349–54.

14. M. Hazard-Mirault, *Traité pratique de l'oeil artificial* (Paris, 1818).

15. "Artificial Eyes at the Paris Exhibition of 1855." For numerous descriptions of prostheses made by and the skill of Boissonneau senior and junior, see Dr. Debout, "On the Mechanical Restoration of the Apparatus of Vision," *Dublin Quarterly Journal of Medical Science* 36 (1863): 67–105.

16. Debout, "On the Mechanical Restoration."

17. Tonkelaar et al., "Herman Snellen (1834–1908) and Muller's 'Reform-Auge,'" 351.

18. A. Boissonneau, "On the Mobility of Artificial Eyes," *Lancet* 1 (January 1852): 262; "Artificial Eyes at the Paris Exhibition of 1855."

19. See "Artificial Enamel Human Eyes," *New York American*, July 7, 1829.

20. P. H. Mules, "Evisceration of the Globe, with Artificial Vitreous," *Transactions of the Ophthalmological Society of the United Kingdom* 5 (1885): 200–206. Mules implants were made of glass, silver, aluminum, gold, rubber, and sometimes paraffin. For other descriptions, see Wood, *The American Encyclopedia and Dictionary of Ophthalmology*, 6: 4428–40; Thomas Bickerton, "The Operative Treatment—Past and Present—of Injured or Painful Blind Eyes, with Special Reference to Mules' Operation," *Medical Times and Hospital Gazette* 25 (1897): 272–73; 285–86, 301–2.

21. Interview by author with ocularist Margery Schreiber, November 22, 1999, Hazlet, New Jersey.

22. Details of the origins of plastic eyes are sketchy. They are mentioned in Paul Gougelmann, "The Artificial Eye Industry in America," *Eye, Ear, Nose, and Throat Monthly*, November 1941, 32.

23. Descriptions of the Valley Forge project can be found in Stanley Erpf, Victor Dietz, and Milton Wirtz, "Prosthesis of the Eye in Synthetic Resin: A

Preliminary Report," *Bulletin of the U.S. Army Medical Department,* July 1945, 76–86. See also *Valley Forge General Hospital, Plastic Artificial Eye Program* (1945), unpublished training manual, in the Milton Wirtz, D.D.S. Artificial Eye Collection, acc. no. 501, Archives Center, National Museum of American History, Smithsonian Institution; and Stanley Erpf, Victor Dietz, and Milton Wirtz, "Artificial Eye," U.S. Patent no. 2,497,872 (February 21, 1950).

24. Background on the thermoplastic of acrylic can be found in J. H. DuBois and F. W. John, *Plastics* (New York: Van Nostrand Reinhold, 1974), 59–62; Jeffrey Meikle, *American Plastic: A Cultural History* (New Brunswick: Rutgers University Press, 1995), 85–88.

25. The best source of information on the crafting of artificial eyes from acrylic is Vaune Bulgarelli and Carrie Messer, comp., *Apprentice/Associate Home Study Guide* (San Francisco: American Society of Ocularists, 1992). See also J. H. Prince, *Recent Advances in Ocular Prosthesis* (Baltimore: Williams and Wilkins, 1950), 100–125.

26. Interview by author with Barbara Spohn Lillo, an ocularist who uses the wax and ball bearing method, Littleton, Colorado, January 26–29, 1999.

27. The most accurate way to distinguish a glass eye from an acrylic one is to examine the edges of the sclera, where the outer laminate sheet is often visible.

28. For more on the presses used for multiple eye fabrication, see Prince, *Recent Advances in Ocular Prosthesis,* 105–17.

29. See George Tiemann and Company, *Surgical Instruments* (New York: C. H. Ludwig, 1889), 177, 754; Kny-Scheerer Company, *Illustrations of Surgical Instruments* (New York, 1909), 3045. Probably most nineteenth- and twentieth-century stock eyes were made by apprentices, as they learned their craft. Until the advent of acrylic eyes, Germany supplied the majority of stock glass eyes distributed in the United States.

Stock eyes today are commonly distributed in third world countries, where the craft of the ocularist is economically unfeasible and little known.

30. I interviewed both Walter Spohn and his daughter Barbara Spohn Lillo in Littleton, Colorado, January 26–29, 1999, while collecting materials from them for the medical collections at the National Museum of American History. Information about Spohn's life is based on those interviews and study of the materials collected.

31. It is important to note that other people, such as Lee Allen and Felix Weinberg, influenced the craft of eye making more than Spohn and Schreiber. Inclusion of their stories simply illustrates two aspects of the profession. Information about Earle Schreiber is based on an interview with his daughter Margery on November 22, 1999, in Hazlet, New Jersey, and study of materials collected from her for the National Museum of American History, Smithsonian Institution.

32. Peter Gougelmann's 1851 shop is usually credited as the first artificial eye business operating in the United States. Gougelmann may have operated the first business devoted solely to artificial eyes, but others dispensed eyes before him. For example, John Scudder, a New York "oculist" and eye specialist, sought clients for his highly polished, flint enamel eyes as early as 1829. See "Artificial Enamel Human Eyes." Thanks to Alan McBreyer for bringing this ad to my attention.

33. Literature on craft labor and artisans is vast and specialized. Basic works that aid in interpreting the history of ocularists are the classic E. P. Thompson, "Time, Work-Discipline, and Industrial Capitalism," *Past and Present* 38 (1967): 56–97; Jonathan Prude, *The Coming of Industrial Order: Town and Factory Life in Rural Massachusetts, 1810–1860* (Cambridge: Cambridge University Press, 1983); Herbert Gutman, *Work, Culture, and Society in Industrializing America* (New York: Knopf, 1976); David Montgomery, *Workers' Control in America: Studies in the History of Work, Technology, and Labor Struggles* (Cambridge: Cambridge University Press, 1979); W. J. Rorabaugh, *The Craft Apprentice: From Franklin to the Machine Age in America* (New York: Oxford University Press, 1986).

34. For background on the formation of the American Society of Ocularists, see Charles Workman, "American Society of Ocularists: Our Beginning, 1956–1962," *Today's Ocularist* 1.1 (1972): 7–9; Charles Workman, "American Society of Ocularists, 1963–1968," *Today's Ocularist* 1.2 (1972): 5–9; Charles Workman, "American Society of Ocularists, 1969–Present," *Today's Ocularist* 1.3 (1973): 4–6.

35. See letter about examinations of trainees, from John J. Kelley to Walter Spohn, January 18, 1973, Walter Spohn Collection, National Museum of American History, Division of Science, Medicine, and Society.

36. For more on postwar implants, see H. R. Alton, "Orbital Implants," *American Optical Vision* (1953): 16–17; Prince, *Ocular Prosthesis*, 16–63.

37. Anaplastology as a defined specialty dates from about 1980. According to the field's founders, it encompasses the making of eyes and also includes "treatment and care of patients through the design, fabrication, and repair of restorative appliances used primarily for cosmetic and semi-functional purposes." The anaplastologist works with artificial body parts of many sorts, such as eyes, ears, noses, hands, fingers, feet, and maxillo-facial appliances. See "The Anaplastologist: A New Member of the Medical/Surgical Team," unpublished manuscript, Walter Spohn Collection, National Museum of American History, Division of Science, Medicine, and Society.

38. Letter from Walter Spohn to Dennis Falk, 27 July 1981, Walter Spohn Collection, National Museum of American History, Division of Science, Medicine, and Society.

39. See, for example, Walter Johnson, "Analysis of the Experience of Oculists and Ophthalmic Surgeons Using the Bio-Eye Hydroxyapatite Ocular Implant: A Four-Year Retrospective Study," *Journal of the American Society of Oculists* 26 (1995–96): 17–19.

40. For more on optical prostheses, see "Optical Prosthesis: Visions of the Future," *Journal of the American Medical Association* 283.17 (May 3, 2000): 2297; "Special Report: Bioelectronic Vision," *IEEE Spectrum*, May 1996, 20–69.

6

Modern Miracles

The Development of Cosmetic Prosthetics

Elizabeth Haiken

IMAGINE AN ARCHEOLOGICAL dig some centuries in the future focused on medical practices of past times, a time when the term "primitive" is even more out of fashion than it is today. The dig site? One of the many cosmetic surgery centers that sprinkled the North American landscape in the late years of the twentieth century.

A core sample taken from the refuse pile reveals layer after layer of scientific and technological innovation. On top is Gore-Tex, that miracle fiber of "explornography," then, a layer of Teflon and several layers of silicone solids, underlain by a thick layer of still-viscous gel. Beneath these are several strata of what looks like compressed sponge of varying density and consistency. Below this is a frightening hodgepodge: "glass balls, terylene wool, ox cartilage."[1] At the very bottom is a thick layer of what looks like beeswax, embedded in which are chips of ivory, beef bone, and "quite a variety of foreign materials . . . bits of braided silk, bits of silk floss, particles of celluloid, gutta percha, [and] vegetable ivory."[2]

That a core sample—even an imaginary one—should suggest an increasingly synthetic environment is no surprise. Any landfill excavation, layer by layer, would similarly reveal the plastic (r)evolution that has fundamentally shaped the last one hundred years. What is striking about this sample are the shreds of human fat and flesh that have been preserved in paraffin and petrified sponge and liquid plastic—or (less so) what these materials have in common, which is that they have all been used to augment or reshape human flesh.

A prosthetic is generally defined as something created to replace a part of the body that has been removed, and by this definition the term "cosmetic prosthetic," in addition to being something of a tongue twister, is a misnomer. While an ivory or (later) latex or (still later) silicone strut needed to rebuild a nose destroyed by fire may, by this definition, be termed a prosthesis (as might a foam rubber– or silicone- or saline-filled breast implant needed to reconstruct a breast removed because of cancer), an implant designed and selected to create what did not exist in the first place (whether cheekbone, chin, pectoral, calf, buttock, or breast) cannot, strictly speaking, be called prosthetic.

Over the course of the twentieth century, however, "strictly speaking" has become increasingly difficult for practitioners as well as patients. The category of need, which once seemed self-evident (as well as strictly physical), became more difficult to define as psychological thinking was added to the mix. Furthermore, technological innovation has produced many more choices: an accident victim may "need" a prosthetic hand that enables him or her to grasp and manipulate objects, but does that hand "need" to be lifelike? Many of us can accept a breast cancer survivor's "need" for breast reconstruction, even with full knowledge of the fact that accepting this "need" pushes us closer to acknowledging all "needs" as valid. In the borderland between need and desire in which cosmetic surgery, as a practice and as a phenomenon, developed, the line between what is and what ought to be—that is, between the real and the imagined self—faded away, and the term "cosmetic prosthetic" began to make instinctive sense. And in the quest for the perfect prosthetic substance—one that could be easily inserted, injected, or implanted, that would not react or extrude itself or deteriorate or morph into something rich and strange, that would mimic (in texture, in movement, and in psychological effect) the "real thing" (whether bone or cartilage or soft flesh)—physicians and patients have collaborated in an endlessly inventive, and sometimes even dangerous, process of experimentation.

PREMODERN MIRACLE: PARAFFIN

Not until the late 1930s did plastic surgery become a recognized medical specialty, with its own organizations, publications, and standards of education, training, and certification. Until then, plastic surgery was an

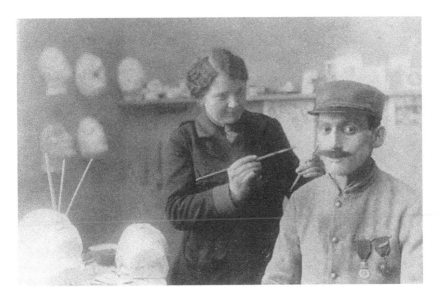

FIG. 6.1. Anna Coleman Ladd puts the finishing touches on a mask.

amalgam of dentistry, oral surgery, otolaryngology, and general surgery, as well as what was then called "beauty culture," though plastic surgeons are still loathe to admit this. Would-be plastic surgeons resembled, more than anything, pioneer scientists alone in their basement laboratories (think, for example, of Warner Brothers' *Young Tom Edison*), brewing and sculpting solutions to the perceived problem of human inadequacy.

One of the imagined, and ultimately (if imperfectly) realized possibilities with which early practitioners were concerned was building up the condition, much more common then than now, called "saddle-nose." A saddle-nose can be inherited or caused by trauma, an abscess, or infection, but more commonly scrofula, lupus, and especially syphilis were at fault. The Wassermann test, invented in 1906, provided a fairly reliable means of identifying syphilis, and arsenical compounds were used with some success to treat it after 1909, but not until penicillin was found to be effective against syphilis in 1943 was a simple and predictable cure found.[3]

Rebuilding a nasal bridge destroyed by syphilis would generally be classed as reconstructive, rather than cosmetic, surgery, but surgeons who attempted to correct depressed noses were aware that they were responding to a cultural as well as a medical problem. As the New York surgeon Joseph Safian observed in a 1926 radio address, "Many persons with a saddle nose . . . are suspected of having inherited disease and are greatly handicapped, both in their social and business relations." Dr. James T. Campbell of Chicago similarly noted, "The unfortunates with depressed noses are subject to remarks and stares of the thoughtless and the ignorant. . . . By shaping their features like those of normal men, we will earn their lasting gratitude."[4]

The "saddle-nose deformity" was a particular challenge because adding substance to the human body is harder than subtracting it. Some surgeons had recorded attempts to rebuild noses using bone and cartilage or internal prostheses of ivory or rubber, but these techniques were time-consuming and often unsuccessful. Grafts sometimes failed to take. The human body, they found, had an unfortunate tendency to reject foreign substances such as ivory, even years later. Paraffin, in contrast, seemed ideal. It was relatively easy to inject, it did not require troublesome incisions, and—at least initially—it appeared to remain inert once introduced into the body.

News of this apparently ideal substance began to spread through the medical community beginning in the late nineteenth century. In September 1903 F. Gregory Connell, a physician from Leadville, Colorado, noted cautiously that although the surgical use of paraffin was still "more or less" experimental, its potential was rapidly increasing: "prosthetic operations, undertaken solely for cosmetic effect," he forecast confidently, "should be absolutely harmless." Apparently successful in treating saddle-noses, paraffin quickly came to be seen, by some practitioners, as an instant panacea for soft-tissue defects: it was used to fill out facial wrinkles, in one case to create a testicle, and was rumored to have been injected into breasts.[5]

Physicians soon began to discover that paraffin was not the miracle solution originally described. Paraffin had a marked tendency to migrate, particularly if patients spent time in the sun, but even more alarming was the finding that many recipients began to develop paraffinomas, or "wax cancers." Removing paraffin proved to be much more difficult than injecting it; the process often left the patient severely scarred. Physicians were hesitant to abandon a practice that had seemed to hold such promise, and continued to experiment with different mixtures of substances and different methods and temperatures of

injection. Dr. J. Carlyle DeVries of Chicago described the use of unadul-
terated paraffin as "almost medieval in its brutality" and also advised
against mixing paraffin with either goose grease or white oak bark, recommending instead "a mixture of white vaseline, white wax, a shade of
glycerin and a shade of paraffin," all of which was to be boiled with car-
bolic acid "to render it antiseptic."[6]

By 1920, recipes like these also had proved problematic, and most
reputable physicians had abandoned the practice of injecting paraffin,
adulterated or not. Dr. Seymour Oppenheimer of New York, who that
year chronicled paraffin's rise and fall, tried to draw some lessons from
the episode. He attributed paraffin's meteoric rise in popularity to the
belief, common among even "skilled and well-recognized surgeons and
rhinologists," that "the operation was practically without pain, caused
no scars . . . and corrected nasal deformities that could not well be overcome otherwise." A more significant factor, however, was the combination of stereotype and stigma that drove public demand and made patients particularly vulnerable. As the surgeon Vilray Blair put it in 1936,
"the true syphilitic saddle nose is today a relatively rare deformity," but
because of its notoriety "it is nevertheless perfectly logical that the
bearer of a caved-in bridge . . . should be anxious to have the supposed
evidence of a syphilitic inheritance eliminated."[7]

The Chicago physician Charles C. Miller personified the experimental and entrepreneurial approach that continues to characterize this
specialty. Although he (presciently) eschewed paraffin, Miller was willing to utilize virtually any and all of the substances in his world to alter
the human face and form. Born in 1880 in New Albany, Indiana, Miller
graduated from the Hospital College of Medicine in Louisville, Ken-
tucky, in 1899. He set up practice in Chicago and taught clinical surgery
at a small medical college, and in 1906 began to publish articles on "featural surgery," a seemingly endless series of which appeared in county,
state, and some national medical journals. In 1907 alone he published
more than twenty articles, as well as a textbook entitled *Cosmetic
Surgery: The Correction of Featural Imperfections.*[8]

Between 1908 and 1923 Miller published little, but he reappeared in
1915 as editor of a lay publication entitled *Medicine and Health* and
opened a new office in Chicago's fashionable new North Side, to which
his tireless recruiting reportedly drew flocks of patients. His 1907 textbook was reissued in 1924, and in 1927 he began publishing his own

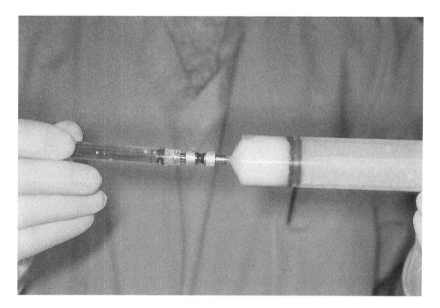

FIG. 6.2. Human fat, ready for injection. Courtesy of Dr. Michael Kaminer.

journal, *Dr. Charles Conrad Miller's Review of Plastic and Esthetic Surgery*. In addition to performing an astounding range of facial operations (including what he called the "subcutaneous dissection" of facial nerves and muscles to prevent formation of the "expression lines" to which he believed women were particularly prone), Miller spent a great deal of time and energy inventing prosthetic substances. He experimented with injections of autologous fat taken from the abdomen, and he concocted solutions of rubber suspended in ether (first ground in a food grinder) and gutta percha in glycerin. Miller's results were discouraging, and the 1924 edition of his text suggests that he abandoned his pathbreaking "featural" work in favor of a return to general surgery. In his "try, try again" approach, however, he personified the specialty.[9]

In many ways Miller was an aberration, and the practice of injecting paraffin is simply one of many footnotes to medical history, albeit one that foreshadowed the later experience with silicone. But these stories also suggest that well before the First World War, surgeons were beginning to identify and discuss issues we tend to assume are of more recent vintage: among them, the social value of beauty and the social cost of ugliness, the variety of ways the concept of "need" could be understood, and the clear financial potential of surgery with a cosmetic goal. In his many articles and books, Miller articulated the overwhelming contemporary concern with beauty and anticipated many of the themes that continue to shape the specialty, including the social and market value of beauty and the effect of aging on women's social, economic, and mental status.[10]

Some of those who served in the reconstructive ranks during the war continued to look askance at "beauty surgery." In 1926 the surgeon John Staige Davis declared that "true plastic surgery . . . is absolutely distinct and separate from what is known as cosmetic or decorative surgery." But the concept that would come to be called the inferiority complex, which crossed the Atlantic in the 1920s, transformed plastic surgery from vanity surgery to "psychiatry with a scalpel," and by the early 1930s even the most conservative of Davis's colleagues had to acknowledge, if grudgingly, that in the emerging consumer culture of urban North America, physical appearance was worthy of serious medical attention.[11]

MODERN MIRACLES: SILICONE

The physician Robert Gersuny of Vienna had augmented breasts with paraffin injections in the 1890s, with predictable results. In the 1920s and 1930s, some surgeons experimented with autologous fat transplantation—transferring fatty tissue from the abdomen or buttocks to the breast—but they found that the body tended to reabsorb fat quickly, sometimes in unshapely ways. In addition, surgeons found that the resulting lumps could impede early detection of cancer, and that the scarring of the donor sites was an unsatisfactory trade-off. As late as 1944, the *Archives of Surgery* recommended simply that surgeons learn how to construct "external prostheses of sponge rubber" for those women suffering from "congenital atrophy or absence of the breasts."[12]

Surgeons' attitudes, however, changed quickly after the war as women, inspired by movie stars like Jane Russell and Marilyn Monroe, clamored for new solutions. The Los Angeles surgeon H. O. Barnes, an early cosmetic surgery enthusiast, in 1950 explained to his colleagues that "Hypomastia [congenitally small breast size] causes psychological rather than physical distress. Its correction has been receiving increased attention only since our 'cult of the body beautiful' has revealed its existence in rather large numbers." He admonished them to search for new solutions. Bames himself did not find one—but the Los Angeles surgeons W. John Pangman and Robert Alan Franklyn did. In August 1953 the popular Sunday newspaper supplement *Pageant* boldly introduced "the operation that remolds flat-chested women," an original and unique (though unspecified) solution for the more than four million women in the United States who suffered from the serious disease of "micromastia."[13]

In his "as told to" autobiography, *Beauty Surgeon*, originally published in 1960, Franklyn explained that while his professional idols—Berlin's Jacques Joseph and New York's J. Eastman Sheehan—had lived in a time when small breasts were not regarded as problems, he lived in a time that "glorified the bountiful breast." Franklyn thus dedicated himself to solving the "new beauty problem" this glorification created. Like surgeons everywhere, he "rejoiced in the age of plastics," which by 1960 had largely replaced bone and cartilage as implant materials, but hard plastic was useless for soft-tissue augmentation. Franklyn's interest had been piqued by a German-made "imitation foam rubber" he had seen years before, and he eventually managed to import a sample and find a fabricator in the United States. "Endless hours, endless weeks" of tests later, "Surgifoam"—which, according to Franklyn, was lightweight, durable, resistant to bacteria and fungi, nonallergenic, easily sterilized, and easily shaped, and thus fulfilled all the crucial criteria for prosthetic material—was born.[14]

The manner in which Franklyn chose to publicize his discovery (trumpeted in the popular press rather than sedately reported in a peer-reviewed journal) probably accounts, at least in part, for his colleagues' reaction. A November 1953 column in the *Journal of the American Medical Association* dismissed the *Pageant* article as "basically self-promotion" and guessed that Franklyn's "Surgifoam" was probably the Ivalon (or polyvinyl) sponge with which other surgeons were already experimenting. In Los Angeles the surgeon W. John Pangman, who had been experimenting with sponge rubber (Ivalon) implants since 1951 and who by 1954 claimed to have implanted them in more than four hundred women, was particularly irked. "[I] began using plain Ivalon sponge . . . about one year before the blatant articles in the lay press by the Hollywood physician who claims to have devised the operation and developed the material," he wrote later. Unsatisfied with these results, Pangman went on to invent a compound prosthesis (an Ivalon shell around a polyethylene sac) that he had hand-sewn and implanted in 260 women and which, he claimed in 1955, had produced "excellent results without complication in over 90% of our cases."[15]

Less felicitous reports, however, were already beginning to emerge. In 1954, Dr. Walter C. Alvarez, an emeritus consultant to the Mayo Clinic, used the *Los Angeles Times* to warn women, "Operations on Bosoms Dangerous;" the Los Angeles plastic surgeon William Kiskadden carried the message to medical professionals in a January 1955 article by the same name. In 1958, two surgeons reported that whereas the fat grafts they had previously been using had liquefied, the Ivalon sponge had, at least for a time, seemed a satisfactory alternative: they were pleased to report "good results" in twelve women (a total of twenty-four breasts). They noted, however, that one patient complained of hardening, that all were disappointed at the 25 percent reduction in initial volume that occurred when the sponges shrank, and that the question of cancer risk remained open. Despite these and other cautions, however, sponges of varying synthetic sorts entered the arsenal of cosmetic surgery and were used throughout the 1950s and early 1960s.[16]

When he tried to explain why he had devoted so much time and energy to breast augmentation, Franklyn, like other surgeons, pointed directly to American consumer culture, which (in the years after World War Two) bestowed iconic status on the "sweater girl." The vogue of the "hourglass figure," Franklyn explained, meant that thousands of "girls and women whose neuroses had been traced definitely to the fact they were flat-chested" were desperate for new techniques that would release them from the bondage of inferiority. Popular magazine articles supported this interpretation. In 1956, under the heading "Monroes on the Increase," *Cosmopolitan* noted that the "[e]mphasis in our society on the beautiful bust has become so extreme that there was little surprise in psychological circles when a teen-aged girl just recently committed suicide because she was flat-chested. How much misery this condition causes is not known." A similar article in *Lady's Circle* entitled "Flat-Chested Females" marveled how "Women who feel socially inferior because of small breasts and flat chests have resorted to plastic operations in which resilient pads of inert plastic-foam sponge are placed beneath the wall of the chest and the glandular tissues. This builds up the breasts to satisfactory proportions." Both articles noted that breast augmentation techniques were still experimental: *Cosmopolitan* specifically advised women that while the new technique was generating "a great deal of excitement among lay people," it was unpredictable, while *Lady's Circle* recommended psychiatry as an alternative. At the same time, however, the articles expressed sympathy for women so afflicted, and hope that new solutions would be forthcoming.[17]

Some practitioners were satisfied with sponges, but others believed that the injection of liquid silicone held more promise. Breast augmentation with liquid silicone was largely an underground practice. Board-certified plastic surgeons seem not to have adopted the practice in large numbers, and they were among the most vocal and committed critics once problems began to surface. Patients and other doctors, however, perceived this practice as within the realm of cosmetic surgery, as part of the search for the perfect prosthetic.

Silicone was one of the wonder products of American industry that emerged from the Second World War. Chemists had been exploring the world of silicones for years, but in 1943, when the Corning Glass Works and Dow Chemical Company joined to form Dow Corning Corporation to make silicone materials needed for the war effort (such as an engine lubricant that would not break down at high temperatures), these products began to come of age. In 1946 it was reported that storage in siliconized bottles prolonged the clotting time of blood; in 1950 silicone rubber tubing was used to replace a damaged urethra; in 1955 Dow Corning used silicone rubber to manufacture the first successful shunt for draining excess cerebrospinal fluid in hydrocephalic children. Requests for samples and for specific products and information were so numerous that in January 1959 Dow Corning's board of directors established the Dow Corning Center for Aid to Medical Research to coordinate the diverse requests and the company's efforts.[18]

When, and by whom, liquid silicone was first used to enlarge small breasts is unclear. Most reports place it around World War Two, and many locate it in Japan, where Japanese surgeons allegedly used silicone to plump out legs withered by polio. The widespread publicity later accorded the Japanese Sakurai formula, invented in 1954, supports the attribution of this technique to Japanese physicians, although several other accounts place the invention earlier. According to the *New York Times*, Japanese cosmetologists pioneered the use of silicone to enlarge the breasts of Japanese prostitutes during the war, after such solutions as goats' milk and paraffin were found wanting.[19]

By the mid-1960s the practice of injecting liquid silicone was receiving widespread attention in the United States, much of it negative.

In 1964 a *Chicago Daily News* reporter found that doctors attending the annual meeting of the American Oto-Rhinologic Society for Plastic Surgery talked freely among themselves about liquid silicone, the "amazing liquid chemical that turns old faces into new." One conservative surgeon present at the meeting admitted, "It would appear to signal a definite revolution in the area of cosmetic surgery." But they also discussed the technique's drawbacks (primarily that long-range effects were unknown) and, fearful of publicity, clammed up when they found a reporter in their ranks. That same year, reports of negative sequelae had become numerous enough that Dow Corning voluntarily listed liquid silicone with the Food and Drug Administration as a drug rather than an implant material; the following year the FDA reclassified liquid silicone as a new drug in an attempt to restrict its use.[20]

The actions of Dow Corning and the FDA generated a wave of publicity about the silicone injection industry, particularly on the West Coast, where topless dancers and Las Vegas showgirls had enthusiastically adopted it. In November 1965, for example, the *San Francisco Chronicle* reported that a dancer named Carol Doda and another unnamed performer at Big Al's, a popular topless club, had each received weekly injections of a half ounce of liquid silicone over a period of about twenty weeks (in all, nearly a pint of liquid silicone in each breast). Both women were proud of their achievement. As Doda explained, "I believe in self improvement. If you don't make yourself better, you might just as well be dormant." And they were happy to share their experiences with others: "Why lots of times a man will come in here with his wife or date; she'll be kind of flat and I can see her looking at me all through my act," the other dancer explained. "Then she'll write me a letter—she's ashamed of her looks and wants to know who my doctor was. I always tell them."[21]

By the time this article appeared, however, Big Al's house doctor was the only San Francisco physician who would admit to having given the injections at all, and even he insisted that he had dropped the practice six months before. The surgeons Mark Gorney and Paul Schneider, with Dow Corning's Silas Braley, cautioned the paper's readers that with the exception of the seven physicians participating in a Dow Corning study group, anyone who was injecting liquid silicone was either using up medical-grade fluid that had been legally available until 1964, or using toxic or illegal substances (including, reports suggested, industrial-grade silicones, either alone or mixed with paraffin or vegetable or mineral oils). New side effects were still being discovered, but this at least was known: silicone, after injection, tended to migrate, turning up in lymph nodes and other areas of the body. Silicone could also form lumps (which surgeons, recalling paraffin's similar tendency, termed granulomas) that could mask and prevent early detection of breast cancer. At worst, silicone injections could result in amputation, and even at best all recipients were expected to have "pendulous breasts" by the time they were forty.[22]

But a lighthearted editorial entitled "Abreast of the Times" (published in *JAMA* in 1966) suggests that some medical practitioners had trouble taking the silicone injection industry seriously. "We live in a 'mammoriented' world," *JAMA* noted, "Breast size, within certain expanding limits, has become an aesthetic criterion." The editorial reminded doctors that due to "some evidence of problems," silicone was considered a drug and the practice of mammary injection was illegal, but concluded humorously, "the ladies must await either the clearance of the drug by the FDA . . . or a return to fashion of the less voluptuous figure characteristic of the 1920's and 1930's." Despite the growing stack of reports of rot, gangrene, amputation, and the like, women patients did not want to give up this modern miracle. As the *Chronicle* reported, women continued to demand and receive injections, often resorting to the flourishing black market that grew up in Los Angeles, Las Vegas, and, a few years later, Tijuana.[23]

Twenty-some years of less than satisfactory results might have persuaded everyone that women's breasts should be left alone, but patients continued to clamor for a solution and surgeons continued to search for one. In February 1961, disappointed with the results they had achieved and observed with sponge implants, the plastic surgeon Thomas D. Cronin, then chief of plastic surgery at St. Joseph Hospital in Houston, Texas, and his resident, Frank Gerow (recently both memorialized and satirized in the HBO film *Breast Men*), visited Dow Corning to discuss alternatives. The eventual result—the first Silastic® mammary prosthesis, a silicone rubber envelope filled with liquid silicone—was implanted in March 1962.[24]

New models (designed to address problems ranging from weight and hardening to palpability, which was a problem with early implants) were introduced almost yearly between 1964 and 1994, but the operation has remained substantially the same: incise (beneath the breast, around the areola, or in the armpit) and insert (either between

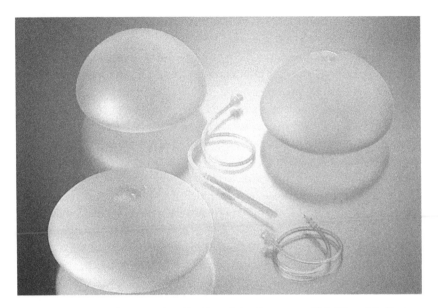

FIG. 6.3. Breast implants, styles 60, 64, and 68. Courtesy of McGhan Medical.

the pectoral muscle and breast tissue or beneath the pectoral muscle). And as early as 1965, in a widely publicized study, the surgeon Ralph Blocksma and Silas Braley of Dow Corning concluded that the silicone gel prosthesis fulfilled most if not all of the criteria defining the ideal soft-tissue substitute for which surgeons had long been searching: it was, they asserted, not physically modified by soft tissue, chemically inert and not carcinogenic; it produced no inflammation, no foreign body reaction, no signs of allergy or hypersensitivity. Unlike sponges, which surgeons had to carve and sterilize individually for each patient, silicone implants could be prefabricated and mass-produced; unlike the saline implants introduced later (and in use today), they didn't deflate. Reflecting America's postwar fascination with all things plastic, *Cosmopolitan* was even more enthusiastic: "The fact of the matter is that surgically augmented breasts have a *better* contour than the real thing. They stand up . . . will not sag or droop or get flaccid. They're firm and solid."[25]

Silicone solids are less amenable to mass production, but they have virtually replaced bone, cartilage, and ivory as firm-tissue substitutes and they are, according to the FDA, "in general . . . thought to be safe."

To date, while chin and cheekbone (malar) implants are mass-produced, pectoral and calf implants tend to be custom-made. Chin implants have become progressively more popular, and many patients report that surgeons suggest them as companion operations to nose jobs. Calf implants (solid silicone carved into a cigar shape) and pectoral implants (ditto, as a teardrop) are much less common: even Mel Bircoll, a Beverly Hills plastic surgeon who claims to have invented them, had done just two hundred pectoral sets in 1992. But while the implants themselves may be unusual, the constellation of needs and desires that produced them are almost banal in their familiarity. The process that begins with a yen for an ideal—a chest like Sylvester Stallone's, calves like Mel Gibson's, a chin like Arnold Schwarzenegger's—is made reality by one of the many products of the plastic century. And it is supported by a flexible, even expansive definition of need that, while mediated by the limits of technological achievement and the extent of medical bravura, is shaped primarily by the individual patient.[26]

POSTMODERN MIRACLES: HIGH-TECH AND NATURAL

In the United States, plasticization (or, as Stephen Fenichell puts it, the "national polymerization process") reached its apex in the years after World War Two. A flood of new, petroleum-based products—Naugahyde, nylon, polyester, Teflon, and silicone—bubbled up from basement laboratories and rolled off assembly lines, sealing American food, coating pots and pans, covering car seats and Barcoloungers, and clothing bodies. The continuing search for a permeable yet impermeable material—in other words, a substance that was waterproof but not airproof—however, was stalled: vinyl had replaced the rubber- and collodion-coated fabrics of the teens and twenties, but vinyl didn't breathe.[27]

In the early 1970s, Gore-Tex appeared to solve the problem. Invented by Bob Gore, son of Wilbert Gore (who for years had headed DuPont's Teflon division), Gore-Tex ("made from polytetrafluoroethylene, or PTFE, that is expanded to form a microporous structure") was hailed as the first polymer that breathed and immediately seemed to have medical applications: fibers were resilient, extremely strong, inert, and well-tolerated by the body, and Gore-Tex seemingly lasted forever;

it could be manufactured to fit a variety of needs, from very fine threads to sheets.[28]

Like virtually every other substance that has been used to augment the human body, Gore-Tex is not perfect—it works better in some areas of the body than it does in others, and physicians report varying results. Dr. Michael Kaminer, a Boston dermatologist, has found that unlike other implant materials (that "are temporary or create reactions to themselves by alerting the body's immune system to their presence, can be unpredictable, difficult to work with, stiff when implanted or that change their properties for the worse when in the body"), Gore-Tex produces predictably good results. Others have been less pleased; Dr. Sue Ellen Cox, for one, told *Dermatology Times* in 1996 that while Gore-Tex is "inert, bio-compatible, . . . causes minimal tissue reaction [and] is very easy to insert," it "is not the panacea we had hoped it would be"; potential problems include folding (causing lumps), migration, and suture extrusion.[29]

After nearly a century of searching—largely in vain—for the perfect biocompatible cosmetic prosthetic, it is not surprising that in recent years practitioners' sights have returned to settle on what would seem to be the most biocompatible of all: the human body itself.

Surgeons had attempted fat-transfer operations at various points during the century (and have recorded significant success in using flesh from the abdomen and back to rebuild breasts), but it was the advent of liposuction in the 1980s that reawakened their interest in using the body's own fat as a sculptural medium: Why couldn't fat that had been suctioned out of one part of the body, surgeons reasoned, be used to fill out another part? And didn't it make sense that transplants of fat taken from a patient's own body (autologous fat) would have a better chance of taking without rejection or infection? Thus was born the seemingly miraculous and simple technique of "microlipoinjection."[30]

Microlipoinjection, or autologous fat transfer, involves harvesting (suctioning fat from the body, usually out of the abdomen, buttocks, or thigh), washing (preparing the fat by removing blood and any remaining oils by techniques that physicians prefer not to divulge), and insertion. Whether or not the transfer "takes" depends both on the skill of the physician and on the target site for insertion: faces, in general, seem safer than bodies. When the FDA pulled silicone breast implants off the U.S. market in 1992, breast enlargement with autologous fat transfer spiked, as did warnings about scars, lumps, and the likelihood that future mammogram readings would be affected.[31]

The most dramatic episode, however, involved not breasts but penises. In the early 1990s, advertisements, toll-free numbers such as 1-800-U-DISTINCT and 1-800-680-MALE, and the World Wide Web broke down geographical barriers and connected anxious men all over the country with surgical centers largely located in Los Angeles, Miami, and New York and staffed by a variety of practitioners feeling the squeeze of managed care. In a 1994 interview in *Muscle and Fitness*, Melvyn Rosenstein, one of the most prominent advocates of the procedure, claimed to have enlarged 1,700 men (eight to ten a day) since 1991, increasing lengths by one and one-half to two inches, and width to "just beyond the maximum diameter of the head," with a complication rate of "about 5%." In advertisements, Rosenstein and others were even more enthusiastic. Promising significant increases in both length and girth, and using words such as "Medical Breakthrough," "Permanent Endowment," "Totally natural! No implants!" and "Most Patients appear as if they have doubled in size," the advertisements made the procedure sound too good to be true.[32]

And, of course, it was.

First, researchers found that while advertisements and before-and-after photo suites posted on the Web made glowing claims of significant size increase, results ranged, in most cases, from minimal to negligible. One year after injection, between 50 and 90 percent of fat had been reabsorbed into the body (a finding consistent with previous fat-transfer experiments).[33]

More significant was that just a few years after these procedures were developed, medical journals began publishing a number of articles that all began with the same words: "Complications of . . ." The complications were various and horrifying. Widening the penis with injections or grafts of fat resulted in "poor cosmetic appearance" at best; at worst, in painful nodules of fat that required surgical removal, chronic inflammation, spontaneous rupture, irregular reabsorption of fat (producing, in one case, "a bizarre mushroom-shaped penis"), necrosis (literally, "death") of grafted or injected fat (with consequent risk of infection, bacterial contamination, and gangrene), and decreased sexual function. Initial costs ranged from about $3,000 to $7,000; complications and subsequent operations could boost total cost well over

$20,000. All in all, not a terrifically impressive record, even for a technique explicitly described as "experimental."[34]

Given that previous experiments with injecting autologous fat had produced less than ideal results in breasts and faces, given that ten to fifteen thousand of these surgeries had been performed on American penises by the middle of 1996 and that reports of complications, some of them disastrous, were piling up, given that by this same date some eighteen attorneys had filed more than fifty lawsuits against Los Angeles doctor Melvyn Rosenstein alone for complications such as those described above, and given that men value their genitals, protecting them instinctively when threatened and giving them admiring nicknames when not, it seems bizarre that thousands of men were willing, even eager, to spend thousands of dollars and risk their physical and mental health for the chance of a slightly bigger penis. But they were: as a motivator, sexual performance was not nearly as important as appearance—looking good "at the gym, in swimsuits, in jeans," as the Washington, D.C., surgeon J. Howell Tiller put it. And as the Oklahoma City physician David Foerster noted, when he decided to take a chance on a new technique to enhance "overall penile thickness . . . a willing patient was not hard to find."[35]

The search for the perfect biocompatible prosthetic product continues, most notably with the engineered tissues that biotech companies are working on, but to date no one has been willing to go public with a market offering. [36]

THE QUEST FOR THE PERFECT PROSTHETIC

In 1915 the surgeon Ralph St. J. Perry decried the fact that the "advertising fraternity" was exploiting women concerned about their breasts, but proclaimed his faith in the future: "there is no doubt but that by proper methods the defective, deformed, deficient, or diseased breast can be made to take on most attractive features."[37]

For the rest of the century, physicians would attempt to fulfill such hopes. What drove them was, in part, deep sympathy for their patients combined with a conviction that their mission as medical professionals was to help those patients. In 1946 a New Jersey surgeon recommended chin implants because "chin malformations" (defined as those labeled "bird face" or "Andy Gump") "are a detriment . . . both socially and professionally." The plastic surgeon Milton T. Edgerton and the psychiatrist A. R. McClary, in 1958, supported breast implants for the same reasons: "Literally thousands of women are seriously disturbed by feelings of inadequacy. . . . Partly as a result of exposure to advertising propaganda and questionable publicity, many physically normal women develop an almost paralyzing self-consciousness focused on the feeling that they do not have the correct size bosom." In 1970 *Cosmopolitan* (in typical breathless style) reiterated this point: "Silicone breast augmentation is the operation that everybody whispers about. . . . yet it is actually among the leading 'cosmetic' operations today. . . . COSMO has received several hundred letters asking just these questions, usually from girls with fairly minuscule breasts. (Wouldn't *you* be concerned?)" In the 1980s, "increased awareness of this important aesthetic feature [cheekbones] . . . made correction . . . one of the goals of aesthetic surgery of the face," and malar implants more popular.[38]

Plastic surgeons were also driven by a vision of themselves—supported by their specialty's comparatively late start and by the suspicion with which early cosmetic practitioners had been regarded—as originals: as renegades, as artists, as inventors, as pioneers. Frankensteinish though it sounded, the goal on which they set their sights was the replication, through fabrication, of human flesh—the development of the perfect cosmetic prosthetic.

In this goal, they were both supported and driven by women and men who saw the world around them not just as a smorgasbord of raw materials meant to improve the human condition (as early conservationists had viewed the nation's timber and mineral stocks) but, increasingly, as an evolving supply of materials that could improve the human body itself. Thus in 1939, when the popular magazine the *Delineator* asserted that the day was not far off when stockyards would be able to supply the "right piece of bone, have it stuck in the man's face, and send him out handsomer than ever," the surgeon Albert D. Davis was troubled both because the story was ludicrous—and because so many readers believed it.[39]

The quest for the perfect cosmetic prosthetic was given impetus as well by a clear and instinctive, if not always rational, sense—articulated over and over by both patients and practitioners—of what was real and what was fake. W. John Pangman, in 1954, explained why he was drawn to Ivalon:

Ivalon is a white sponge material with the appearance of white bread and is [a] polymer of polyvinyl alcohol with formaldehyde. It is wetable, and when introduced into the body, the body fluids enter the sponge, fibroplasts and blood vessels grow into it, and unlike any other foreign substance it acts as a framework for living tissue while fibers remain strong but inert. Literally the mass becomes living and if cut into will bleed.[40]

It was precisely this quality of potential "humanness"—the capability of becoming human by being incorporated into a human—for which those intent on developing cosmetic prosthetics were searching. During the First World War medical practitioners noted that wounded soldiers would voluntarily undergo multiple experimental surgeries rather than settle for masks, because unlike masks surgery "does away with soldiers' intense dread of seeing themselves (or having others see them)" without masks. Edgerton and McClary found that while "falsies" had become common fashion accessories in the postwar years (Sears alone offered twenty-two varieties in its 1951 catalog), all of the thirty-two breast implant recipients who participated in their study shared a conviction that "wearing padded bras or falsies was 'phony', 'cheating', and made the feeling of inadequacy even worse." As one patient explained, "One might be in an accident and be found out and feel so ashamed that one couldn't face people again." In 1972 the plastic surgeon Kurt Wagner agreed that in cosmetic surgery, the result becomes reality. "Was Galatea any the less real," he asked rhetorically, "because Pygmalion had created her?" Trying to explain the growing popularity of hair transplants, the surgeon George Semel hit a similar note: "A man who wears a toupee is running, but the man with hair plugs is dealing with the problem. When you change your body, it becomes part of your body image and you accept it. A toupee is an appliance . . . it's never assimilated as part of a person." Dana Rogers, Miss Texas (1983) put it even more succinctly: "Some women wear their padding on the outside. Mine is on the inside."[41]

Patients and physicians, in other words, concurred that "looking" different was not the same as "being" (or becoming) different. Some voices cautioned against the use of experimental techniques. The surgeon John Goin, for example, in 1974 vehemently protested against silicone injections, insisting that "Facial 'furrows,' whatever they may be, are not cancer and do not need drastic remedies nor, for that matter, do

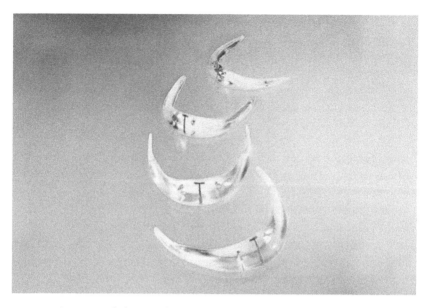

FIG. 6.4. Anatomical chin implant. Courtesy of McGhan Medical.

they *need* any remedy at all." But many others simply refused to take the question seriously. The humorous spin that Phyllis Diller, one of the few injectees willing to talk, put on her experience typified many commentators' attitude toward this practice. "It gave my psyche a big lift and helped my career," she told *Newsweek*. "I just hope to hell it isn't the type of silicone that travels. I don't want swollen ankles."[42]

Diller's jocular approach (unwittingly) reveals a great deal about what cosmetic prosthetics have meant in this country. Their hybrid status—as devices invented and selected for concerns with which many of us sympathize and yet at the same time view as suspiciously shallow, and at the same time as prosthetic devices that will live in the human body for years—leaves them (and those who implant and receive them) in a curious kind of limbo. This conflicted view is reflected in the amazingly cavalier attitude with which some practitioners have approached these substances and their incorporation into patients' bodies. In 1905 the Pittsburgh physician M. Delmar Ritchie proclaimed proudly that a series of experiments had "showed me conclusively that under no conditions will sterile paraffin act as an irritant when introduced into the healthy animal"; his conclusions (and his confidence) were based on a test period of thirty days. A thirty-day result would probably not now be published, but in the plastic surgical literature six-month to one-year results are common. Acknowledgments such as those with which Milton Edgerton and John McClary closed their 1958 article on Ivalon breast implants—the method was new, the possibility of a late unfavorable tissue reaction could not be excluded, and "any surgeon not willing to shoulder this responsibility should probably not use the material on patients with a long life expectancy"—are rare.[43]

On the other hand, if in their willingness to concoct, invent, develop, and insert, physicians are in some sense not only living out their Pygmalion fantasies but reflecting their own discomfort with the cosmetic project, they are in another sense merely responding to the world around them, and to patients who insist that the materials of that world be utilized to serve the ends that they themselves define. Consider the examples of the thirty-two-year-old nurse who in 1908 stole a syringe and injected her face with a substance of 60 percent paraffin and 40 percent olive oil to try to prevent the formation of wrinkles, and the forty-six-year-old man who almost a century later used a grease gun to inject commercial silicone into his own chest (through self-inflicted wounds in his pectoral muscles) in an attempt to enlarge it. These are extreme cases, clearly, but they can suggest the extent to which humans perceive the physical self as malleable and the desperate measures to which they will go to alter it.[44]

NOTES

1. Perras, 1965.
2. Miller, 1926; see also Miller, 1923.
3. Brandt, 1987: 10, 40, 161.
4. Safian, 1926; Campbell, 1904.
5. Goldwyn, 1980; Connell, 1903; San Francisco County Medical Society, 1903; see also Smith, 1903.
6. Goldwyn, 1980; DeVries, 1909; Beck, 1908; Rogers, 1971: 269.
7. Oppenheimer, 1920; Blair, 1936: 238. For examples of reports of negative results, see Davis (Benjamin Franklin), 1914 and 1920.
8. Mulliken, 1977; Rogers, 1971.
9. Mulliken, 1977; Rogers, 1971; also see Miller, 1923 and 1926.
10. Rogers, 1971: 267; Stephenson, 1970.
11. Goldwyn, 1980; Davis (John Staige), 1926.

12. Some surgeons, most neither members of the plastic surgical societies nor certified by the American Board of Plastic Surgery, did claim early successes in surgically treating small breasts. See Schireson, 1938: 218–26; and Broom, 1944; also see Schalk, 1988; Clark, 1948.

13. Bames, 1950 and 1953; Schalk, 1988. This operation has been "rediscovered" several times. In 1960 Dr. Morton I. Berson of New York recommended a "new derma-fat-fascia graft" at a congress in Mexico City. See *San Francisco Chronicle*, 1960; American Medical Association, 1953.

14. Franklyn, 1960: 15–22.

15. American Medical Association, 1953; Pangman and Wallace, 1954; Johnson, 1980; Pangman, 1955.

16. Alvarez, 1954; Kiskadden, 1955; Conway and Smith, 1958; Franklyn, 1960: 27–30; Schalk, 1988. In 1975 a Los Angeles plastic surgeon remembered Franklyn as having been one of "the ones everyone loved to hate." See Davis and Davis, 1975.

17. Franklyn, 1960: 27–30; Bailey, 1988: 73–74; Honor, 1956; Wade, 1965.

18. Braley, 1973.

19. Wagner, 1972: 126; Larned, 1977: 55; Bernstein, 1979; *New York Times*, 1992.

20. *Chicago Daily News*, 1964. Morini, 1972: 119–41; Stallings, 1977: 43.

21. *San Francisco Chronicle*, 1965a, 1965b.

22. *San Francisco Chronicle*, 1965a, 1965b; see also *Science News*, 1968.

23. American Medical Association, 1966; Ashley et al., 1967; Boo-Chai, 1969; Chaplin, 1969. No national statistics on complications are available, but one San Diego physician told a reporter that 20 percent of the approximately four hundred complications he saw between 1967 and 1974 required amputation. See Larned, 1977; *Science News*, 1968. Records showed that the recipient of one illegal silicone shipment was Harvey Kagan, a silicone pioneer (Larned, 1977: 55). M. E. Nelson responded to reports that criticized Dow Corning's distribution of silicone. According to Nelson, fourteen U.S. manufacturers produced industrial-grade silicone, and as for medical-grade silicone, Nelson stated that Dow Corning "always enforced rigorous controls to prevent unauthorized use of this material" (Nelson, 1978). Dow Corning later admitted that it should have made more of an effort to ensure that its product was not being used in humans; see *San Francisco Chronicle*, 1971; Braley, 1970; *San Francisco Chronicle*, 1974, 1975, 1976a; Reinert, 1975: 114; see also Moynihan, 1979: 102–3. According to *Ms. Magazine*, the problem in Las Vegas was so bad that in April 1975 Nevada enacted emergency legislation making it a felony; California made it a misdemeanor in 1976 (Larned, 1977: 55).

24. Schalk, 1988; Braley, 1973: 285–86; *New York Times*, 1988.

25. *Cosmopolitan*, 1970. Permeation by breast tissue was also a significant problem with the polyurethane-covered implants that were developed in an ef-

fort to solve the contracture problem. Schalk, 1988; Braley, 1973: 285–86; see also Blocksma and Braley, 1965.

26. Sherrill, 1992.

27. Fenichell, 1997: 209–10, 226–70.

28. Fenichell, 1997: 340; Siwolop, 1987; Stephens, 1991; Kaminer, 1999.

29. Moyer, 1996.

30. Alter, 1985: 889–90; Bannon, 1996.

31. Kaminer, 1999; Roan, 1992.

32. Bannon, 1996; Rosenthal, 1994; various advertisements clipped over the years in the author's possession (thanks to Doug Burnett for the first of these: U-Distinct, found in Los Angeles in 1994).

33. In 1987 the American Society of Plastic and Reconstructive Surgeons reported that in general only 30 percent of injected fat survived after one year (quoted in Alter, 1985: 890); in "Reconstruction of Deformities Resulting from Penile Enlargement Surgery" (1997: 2155), Alter cites a reabsorption rate of 50 to 75 percent. Other studies suggest that these are best-case scenarios. Wessells, Lue, and McAninch (1996) observe that "autologous fat transplants lose 55 to 90% of their volume by one year."

34. Trockman et al., 1994; Leithauser, Gilbert, and Barton, 1995; Holding, 1995; Perlman, 1995; Wessells, Lue, and McAninch, 1996; Alter, 1996 and 1997; Foerster, 1998. Thanks to Jesse Berrett for clipping the Perlman article.

35. Bannon, 1996; Stenson, 1993; Foerster, 1998.

36. *Medical Materials Update*, 1998.

37. Perry, 1915.

38. Eisenstadt, 1946; Edgerton and McClary, 1958; *Cosmopolitan*, 1970; Siemian and Samiian, 1988.

39. Perry, 1915; Davis (Albert D.), 1939.

40. Pangman and Wallace, 1954.

41. *San Francisco Chronicle*, 1916; Edgerton and McClary, 1958 (see also Edgerton, Meyer, and Jacobson, 1961); Wagner, 1972: 70; *San Francisco Chronicle*, 1976a, 1983. *Harper's Bazaar*, 1967; Morini, 1971; Kosover, 1972. A few articles were more cautious; see, for example, Hartley and Hartley, 1974.

42. Goin, 1974; *Newsweek*, 1972.

43. Ritchie, 1905; Edgerton and McClary, 1958: 300.

44. Beck, 1908, 104; Siemian, Bosse, and Bjerno, 1992.

REFERENCES

Alter, Gary. 1985. "Augmentation Phalloplasty." *Urologic Clinics of North America* 22.4 (November): 887–90.

———. 1996. "Re: Complications of Penile Lengthening and Augmentation Seen at 1 Referral Center." *Journal of Urology* 156 (November): 1784.

Alter, Gary. 1997. "Reconstruction of Deformities Resulting from Penile Enlargement Surgery." *Journal of Urology* 158 (December): 2153–57.

Alvarez, Walter. 1954. "Operations on Bosoms Dangerous." *Los Angeles Times*, January 11, 17.

American Medical Association. 1953. "The Business of Bolstering Bosoms." *Journal of the American Medical Association* 153.13 (November 28): 1200–1201.

———. 1966. "Abreast of the Times." *Journal of the American Medical Association* 195.10 (March 7): 863.

Ashley, Franklin L., Silas Braley, Thomas D. Rees, Dicran Goulian, and Donald L. Ballantyne Jr. 1967. "Present Status of Silicone Fluid in Soft Tissue Augmentation." *Plastic and Reconstructive Surgery* 39.4 (April): 411–17.

Bailey, Beth. 1988. *From Front Porch to Back Seat: Courtship in Twentieth Century America*. Baltimore: Johns Hopkins University Press.

Bames, H. O. 1950. "Breast Malformations and a New Approach to the Problem of the Small Breast." *Plastic and Reconstructive Surgery* 5.6 (June): 499.

———. 1953. "Augmentation Mammaplasty by Lipo-Transplant." *Plastic and Reconstructive Surgery* 11.5 (May): 404.

Bannon, Lisa. 1996. "How a Risky Surgery Became Profit Center in Los Angeles." *Wall Street Journal* (interactive edition) (June 6).

Beck, Joseph. 1908. "Chicago Laryngological and Otorhinological Society. Meeting of October 13, 1908." *Illinois Medical Journal* 15.1: 104.

Bernstein, Paul. 1979. "Newest Wrinkles in Cosmetic Surgery." *LA Magazine* 24.1 (January): 141.

Blair, Vilray P. 1936. "Plastic Surgery of the Head, Face and Neck: The Psychic Reactions." *Journal of the American Dental Association* 23 (February): 236–40.

Blocksma, Ralph, and Silas Braley. 1965. "Implantation Materials." In *Plastic Surgery*, ed. W. Grabb and J. Smith, 3–148. Boston: Little, Brown.

Boo-Chai, Khoo. 1969. "The Complications of Augmentation Mammaplasty by Silicone Injection." *British Journal of Plastic Surgery* 22.3 (July): 281.

Braley, Silas. 1970. "Letter to the Editor." *Plastic and Reconstructive Surgery* 45.3 (March): 288.

———. 1973. "The Use of Silicones in Plastic Surgery: A Retrospective View." *Plastic and Reconstructive Surgery* 51.3 (March): 280–88.

Brandt, Allan M. 1987. *No Magic Bullet: A Social History of Venereal Disease in the United States since 1880*. New York: Oxford University Press.

Broadbent, T. R., and Robert M. Wolf. 1964. "Augmentation Mammaplasty." *Plastic and Reconstructive Surgery* 40.6 (December): 517–23.

Broom, Adolph M. 1944. "Prosthetic Restorations for the Breast." *Archives of Surgery* 48.5 (May): 388.

Campbell, James T. 1904. "The Subcutaneous Injection of Paraffin More Particularly for the Correction of Nasal Deformities." *Illinois Medical Journal* 6.4 (September): 381.

Chaplin, C. Hal. 1969. "Loss of Both Breasts from Injections of Silicone (with Additive)." *Plastic and Reconstructive Surgery* 44.5 (November): 447.

Chicago Daily News. 1964. May 14, 3:25.

Clark, Marguerite. 1948. "Breast Surgery." *McCall's* 75 (April): 2.

Connell, F. Gregory. 1903. "The Subcutaneous Injection of Paraffin for the Correction of Deformities of the Nose." Parts 1 and 2. *Journal of the American Medical Association* 41.12 (September 19): 697–99; 41.13 (September 26): 781.

Conway, Herbert, and James Smith. 1958. "Breast Plastic Surgery." *Plastic and Reconstructive Surgery* 21.1 (January): 13–14.

Cosmopolitan. 1970. "Yes, You Can Have a Bigger Bosom!" *Cosmopolitan,* January, 66.

Davis, Albert D. 1939. "The Value and Limitations of Plastic Operative Procedures." *Medical Times* 67.4 (April): 158–63.

Davis, Benjamin Franklin. 1914. "Coal and Petroleum Products as Causes of Chronic Irritation and Cancer." *Journal of the American Medical Association* 62.22 (May 30): 1716–20.

———. 1920. "Paraffinoma and Wax Cancer." *Journal of the American Medical Association* 75.25 (December 18): 1709–11.

Davis, Ivor, and Sally Davis. 1975. "The Great Male Face Race." *LA Magazine* 20.2 (February): 63, 103–4.

Davis, John Staige. 1926. "Art and Science of Plastic Surgery." *Annals of Surgery* 84.2 (August): 203–10.

DeVries, J. Carlyle. 1909. "The Surgical Correction of Featural Deformities." *American Journal of Dermatology and Genito-Urinary Diseases* 13.9 (September): 427–28.

Edgerton, M. T., and A. R. McClary. 1958. "Augmentation Mammaplasty: Psychiatric Implications and Surgical Indications." *Plastic and Reconstructive Surgery* 21.4 (April): 279–300.

Edgerton, M. T., E. Meyer, and W. E. Jacobson. 1961. "Augmentation Mammaplasty II: Further Surgical and Psychiatric Evaluation." *Plastic and Reconstructive Surgery* 27.3 (March): 279–96.

Eisenstadt, Lester W. 1946. "Surgical Correction of Chin Malformations." *American Journal of Surgery* 71.4 (April): 491.

Fenichell, Stephen. 1997. *Plastic: The Making of a Synthetic Century.* New York: HarperBusiness.

Foerster, David. 1998. "Penile Enhancement: Another Wrong Way to Go." *Plastic and Reconstructive Surgery* 101 (January): 244–45.

Franklyn, Robert Alan. 1960. *Beauty Surgeon.* Long Beach, CA: Whitehorn.

Goin, John M. 1974. Letter. *Journal of the American Medical Association* 229.12 (September 16): 1581.

Goldwyn, Robert M. 1980. "The Paraffin Story." *Plastic and Reconstructive Surgery* 65.4 (April): 517–24.

Harper's Bazaar. 1967. "The Silicone Injection Story Updated." *Harper's Bazaar* 100 (May): 148.

Hartley, William, and Ellen Hartley. 1974. "How We're Saving Bodies and Psyches with Silicones." *Science Digest* 76 (August): 25.

Holding, Reynolds. 1995. "Physician Sued Over Penis Surgery." *San Francisco Chronicle,* April 24, A9–11.

Honor, Elizabeth. 1956. "Cosmetic Surgery." *Cosmopolitan* 141 (August): 28–31.

Johnson, Clare W. 1980. Letter to Garry S. Brody, December 16. Folder HMS c94 fd.1, National Archives of Plastic Surgery, Countway Library, Harvard University.

Kaminer, Michael. 1999. Personal communication. February 24.

Kiskadden, William S. 1955. "Operations on Bosoms Dangerous." *Plastic and Reconstructive Surgery* 15.1 (January): 79.

Kosover, Toni. 1972. "Fill Her Up." *W,* November 3, 20.

Larned, Deborah. 1977. "A Shot—or Two or Three—in the Breast." *Ms.* 6 (September): 55, 84–88.

Leithauser, Lance, Edward Gilbert, and Joel Barton. 1995. "Complications of Fat Grafting to the Penis." *Annals of Plastic Surgery* 34.2 (February): 173–75.

Medical Materials Update. 1998. "SwRI's Biocompatible Protein Filler." *Medical Materials Update* 5.11 (December).

Miller, Charles C. 1923. *Rubber and Gutta Percha Injections.* Chicago: Oak Publishers.

———. 1926. *Cannula Implants and Review of Implantation Technics in Esthetic Surgery.* Chicago: Oak Publishers.

Morini, Simona. 1971. "A New Aid to Plastic Surgery: Silicone." *Vogue* 157 (March 15): 84.

———. 1972. *Body Sculpture: Plastic Surgery from Head to Toe.* New York: Delacorte.

Moyer, Paula. 1996. "Goretex Tissue Implants Biocompatible but Not Perfect." *Dermatology Times,* September, 6.

Moynihan, Donald T. 1979. *Skin Deep: The Making of a Plastic Surgeon.* Boston: Little, Brown.

Mulliken, John B. 1977. "Biographical Sketch of Charles Conrad Miller, 'Featural Surgeon.'" *Plastic and Reconstructive Surgery* 59.2 (February): 175–84.

Nelson, M. E. 1978. Letter. *Ms.,* January, 4.

Newsweek. 1972. December 11.

New York Times. 1988. November 13, IV 9:1.

———. 1992. January 18, 1.

Oppenheimer, Seymour. 1920. "A Condemnatory Note on the Use of Paraffin in Cosmetic Rhinoplasty." *Laryngoscope* 30.9 (September): 595.

Pangman, W. John. 1955. Letter to Jerome Pierce Webster, November 10. Folder "P-Gen'l 1935–59," Jerome Webster Papers, Columbia University Special Collections.

Pangman, W. John, and Robert M. Wallace. 1954. "The Use of Plastic Prosthesis in Breast Plastic and Other Soft Tissue Surgery." Presented at Pan Pacific Surgical Association, Honolulu, HI. Folder HMSc94 fd.11, National Archives of Plastic Surgery, Countway Library, Harvard University.

Perlman, David. 1995. "Few Penis Enlargements Necessary, Doctors Say." *San Francisco Chronicle*, April 27, A7.

Perras, Colette. 1965. "Plastic Reconstruction of the Small Breast." *Journal of the American Women's Medical Association* 20.10 (October): 951–52.

Perry, Ralph St. J. 1915. "Cosmetic Surgery." *American Journal of Clinical Medicine* 22.1 (January): 51.

Reinert, Al. 1975. "Doctor Jack Makes His Rounds." *Esquire* 83 (May): 114–16, 160–63.

Ritchie, M. Delmar. 1905. "Paraffin as a Surgical Medium." *Pennsylvania Medical Journal* 8.5 (February): 277.

Roan, Shari. 1992. "Putting Extra Fat in Its Place." *Los Angeles Times*, November 10, E1.

Rogers, Blair O. 1971. "A Chronologic History of Cosmetic Surgery." *Bulletin of the New York Academy of Medicine* 47.3 (March): 265–302.

Rosenthal, Jim. 1994. "The Science of Size." *Muscle and Fitness* 55.11 (November): 220–21, 225.

Safian, Joseph. 1926. "Ethical Plastic Surgery vs. the Quack Beauty Doctor." Radio Lecture, Station WEAF, New York City, June 30. Given under the auspices of the Gorgas Memorial Institute. In Safian Correspondence, National Archives of Plastic Surgery, Countway Library, Harvard University.

San Francisco Chronicle. 1916. May 28, 34:2.

———. 1960. May 7, 18.

———. 1965a. November 15, 1:15.

———. 1965b. November 16, 1.

———. 1971. January 20, 4.

———. 1974. August 6, 16.

———. 1975. February 10, 34.

———. 1976a. January 30, 14.

———. 1976b. October 20, 4.

———. 1983. September 13, 5.

San Francisco County Medical Society. 1903. "Society Proceedings." *Occidental Medical Times* 17.10 (October): 393.

Schalk, Deborah N. 1988. "The History of Augmentation Mammaplasty." *Plastic Surgical Nursing* 8.3 (fall): 88–90.

Schireson, Henry Junius. 1938. *As Others See You: The Story of Plastic Surgery.* New York: Macaulay.

Science News. 1968. "Illegal, Immoral and Dangerous." *Science News* 93 (February 17): 173.

Sherrill, Martha. 1992. "Breast Him-Plants." *Washington Post,* March 8, F1.

Siemian, Peter A., P. N. Bosse, and T. Bjerno. 1992. Letter. *Plastic and Reconstructive Surgery* 89.6 (June): 1185.

Siemian, Walter, and M. Reza Samiian. 1988. "Malar Augmentation Using Autogenous Composite Conchal Cartilage and Temporalis Fascia." *Plastic and Reconstructive Surgery* 82.3 (September): 395–401.

Siwolop, Sana. 1987. "Spare Parts for the Battered Body." *Business Week,* May 18, 126.

Smith, Harmon. 1903. "Paraffin Injected Subcutaneously for the Correction of Nasal and Other Deformities." *Journal of the American Medical Association* 41.13 (September 26): 773–76.

Stallings, James O. 1977. *A New You: How Plastic Surgery Can Change Your Life.* New York: Mason/Charter.

Stenson, Jacqueline. 1993. "Cutting Edge." *Washingtonian,* May.

Stephens, Tim. 1991. "Prescription: Plastics." *Materials Engineering* 108.4 (April): 23.

Stephenson, Kathryn Lyle. 1970. "The 'Mini-Lift': An Old Wrinkle in Face Lifting." *Plastic and Reconstructive Surgery* 46.3 (September): 226.

Trockman, Brett A., Craig J. Berman, Karla Sendelbach, and John R. Canning. 1994. "Complication of Penile Injection of Autologous Fat." *Journal of Urology* 151 (February): 429–30.

Wade, Carlson. 1965. "Instant Beauty through Plastic Surgery." *Lady's Circle* 1.6 (April): 19. Folder HMS C87 no.403, National Archives of Plastic Surgery, Countway Library, Harvard University.

Wagner, Kurt. 1972. *How to Win in the Youth Game: The Magic of Plastic Surgery.* Englewood Cliffs, NJ: Prentice Hall.

Wessels, Hunter, Tom F. Lue, and Jack W. McAninch. 1996. "Complications of Penile Lengthening and Augmentation Seen at 1 Referral Center." *Journal of Urology* 155 (May): 1617–20.

7

Casing the Joint

The Material Development of Artificial Hips

Alex Faulkner

INTRODUCTION

Hundreds of thousands of people worldwide walk with the hidden aid of entirely artificial hips. Many have had artificial replacements installed for both of their hip joints. These devices, implanted by orthopedic surgeons in risky and expensive operations, restore locomotor function and reduce pain from arthritic or otherwise damaged joints. Indeed, artificial hips are perceived to be one of the success stories of modern technological surgery. Most people who function physically with these invisible aids, however, are unaware of their material composition, the process by which they have been manufactured, or even their brand name. For the user, their success is defined by their functionality: as long as it works and it reduces pain.

Today, total hip prostheses, as orthopedic surgeons and manufacturers call them, are one of the major products of multinational companies that specialize in medical technology. In contemporary medicine, designs and materials frequently change as innovating surgeons and manufacturers seek improved performance, a broader range of potential implantees, and improved profitability for their devices. Innovation in materials and designs should thus be understood in the context of a commercial environment as well as one in which medical practitioners and patients seek technologies to alleviate pain and improve physical functioning. This essay discusses the various materials used in modern devices that replace the hip joint completely. By tracing the range of materials used as the prosthetic technology has evolved, the essay will outline the materials used in the different types of designs produced today.

In medical terminology, the formation of an artificial joint between bones is known as arthroplasty. The hip joint is essentially a ball-and-socket joint, the "ball" being the rounded head of the thigh bone (femur), the socket being a cavity in the hip bone (acetabulum) itself. Human implant materials, to be successful, must exist in the tissue of the human body without causing adverse reaction, either to the tissue or to the materials. This means that the search for suitable materials is in part a search for "inert," biologically compatible materials as well as materials that will withstand the forces exerted on joints by physical activity. As this essay will show, surgeons and engineers have experimented with a wide variety of materials—including metals, plastics, and ceramics—during the evolution of this type of implant. Some of the major developments in industrial engineering and materials science in the twentieth century, as one might expect, have contributed to the history of artificial hips.

This essay divides its account of the development of artificial hips into four broad chronological stages: early history from the nineteenth century to the early 1940s; a "premodern" phase of accelerated activity from the mid-1940s to the mid-1950s; a "modern" phase from the mid-1950s through the 1970s; and recent developments over the last twenty years. Since clinical developments in artificial hip replacement were taking place around the world simultaneously, this historical account is organized around developments that involve similar materials and similar surgical techniques. It is worth saying that any study of the development of artificial hip implants must contend with the fact that whatever historical record already exists has been compiled primarily by members of the profession responsible for developing and implanting these devices. Thus, largely orthopedic surgeons and designers have determined the existing literature. By contrast, only now is a view of these devices emerging from the perspective of those who have received implants, especially as a result of multidisciplinary research into the efficacy of health care technologies in the West.

A leading commentator on the state of design and materials in hip implant technology at the end of the twentieth century has described the process of orthopedic innovation in hip prostheses as a "trial and error culture" (Huiskes, 1993). Thus, this chapter is concerned with the products of that culture, which is characterized by continual innovation and experimentation. It is easy to give the misleading impression that a technology has a clear, unilinear, predominantly technical and, with hindsight, predictable trajectory, in which one can discern the rational march of technological progress. And it is certainly the case, as noted above, that many perceive the artificial hip in its various forms to be a highly successful technology, the development of which is punctuated by heroic individuals and breakthrough moments. The literature on orthopedic research contains many examples of this type of history. From a sociological perspective, however, technological artifacts represent the product of networks of relations between groups of people who have been able to establish their stake in that technology. The "success" or "failure" of technological developments is of equal importance in seeking explanations for why some become dominant and accepted for routine use, and why others do not. The history of artificial hips has many examples of materials that did not "work" well, but also some where satisfactory explanations for changing material or design are less obvious.

The history presented here, then, is an account of the activities of a range of actors who have produced and used artificial hip replacement technology. Technology, in effect, is society made material, and the production of technologies is accompanied by the "production" of its markets and its users. The radical nature of total hip replacement and its general success in contemporary health care practice have created a high demand and indeed an increasingly large market for this type of prosthesis as both younger and older age groups with degenerative joint disease and other forms of joint damage are seen, or see themselves, as potential implantees.

In order to illustrate the perhaps unexpected variety in the material history produced by this trial and error culture, I chose the visual images presented in this essay in part simply because they show something of the range of the material technologies used over time. In addition to this, however, they draw attention to the different media in which these prostheses are represented within society. Normally, only the inhabitants of the confined worlds of biomechanical laboratories, manufacturing plants, or hospitals see artificial hips. But after looking at these images, one is reminded that these devices have been, or will be, inserted inside the human body in an attempt to mimic the function of human skeletal tissues. There is, surely, something rather unsettling about looking at body parts that are usually hidden from view. This raises questions about how we discuss the inner material and mechanics of the human body. Society's concern with technological medicine ensures that such images sometimes reach the public domain. But these images also challenge the conventional perception of the external fabric of human bodies, and thus challenge the material foundation of everyday life.

FIRST EXPERIMENTS WITH SURGICAL HIP IMPLANTS

The development of artificial hips is shared between Europe and the United States. In the late nineteenth and early twentieth centuries, a wide variety of materials was used in implant surgery generally, including metals such as zinc, copper, lead, and aluminum. However, none appeared especially suitable and it was customary to regard them as temporary measures, sometimes inserted into the body with the hope of stimulating self-repair by the body tissues. The first recorded successful arthroplasty of the human hip was carried out in 1822 in Westminster Hospital in London, but this did not involve any prosthetic components. The first known case of insertion of foreign material between bone ends occurred in 1840, when wood was used in an attempt to mobilize a stiff jawbone. In the late 1880s, experiments with hip joints were being conducted in France with techniques using muscle tissue as the implantation material, and in Germany with various natural and fabricated materials. Thomas Gluck in 1890 described ball-and-socket joints made from a luxurious, hard, natural material— ivory—and fixed internally with nickel-plated steel screws. He had also developed a glue made with colophony (a derivative of pine resin extract), pumice powder, and plaster to achieve fixation within the body tissue. Later, when this method led to extrusion of the joints, one surgeon employed gold foil.

In spite of Gluck's prophetic experiments, thirty years elapsed before the next significant development in prosthetic hip surgery. Sustained experimentation took place during the 1920s and 1930s, when surgeons used a variety of materials in an attempt to design a durable inverted cup—called a "floating cup" or mold—to fit over the shaped head of the thigh bone and between it and the acetabulum. This was the first type of hip implant to be used in any significant numbers. One surgeon, Otto Aufranc, was to report in 1956 that he had conducted over a thousand hip arthroplasties over a fifteen-year period. Aufranc asserted that the mold or cup method was the best solution to conditions of the hip resulting from rheumatoid arthritis and traumatic degenerative arthritis (Aufranc, 1957).

The floating cup was pioneered by Marius N. Smith-Petersen, an eminent surgeon from Boston, Massachusetts, whom Scales dubbed the "doyen of arthroplasty of the hip."[1] Smith-Petersen, an emigrant to the United States from Norway in his teens, made many innovations in orthopedic surgery and became a professor of orthopedic surgery at Harvard Medical School and chief of orthopedics at Massachusetts General Hospital. He was acclaimed in the United Kingdom, where he was elected an honorary member of the Royal Society of Medicine in 1952.[2] The principle of Smith-Petersen's mold was to restore function by introducing an artificial cup into the joint, rather than actually replacing a removed part of the joint. Experimenting with diverse materials, Smith-Petersen made successive use of glass, viscaloid, Pyrex, Bakelite, and Vitallium.[3]

Vitallium, a metal alloy of cobalt, chromium, and tungsten, appeared to be the most biocompatible material. By 1940 over 1,200 Vitallium floating mold operations by over sixty surgeons were presented to the Texas Surgical Society (Howmedica Inc., 1998). In fact, for the first—but not the last—time in the history of hip prostheses, this material was transferred to orthopedics from applications in the cognate fields of dentistry and dental implantation. As early as the 1870s, one of celluloid's applications also had been in the production of dental plates; indeed, Smith-Petersen borrowed Vitallium from his own dentist. While many of these materials appear with hindsight unlikely candidates for their intended function, they are extremely interesting for what they emphasize about the range of "man-made" materials, drawn from various embryonic or more established manufacturing industries, with which it was possible to experiment with the boundaries of the human body during the first decades of the twentieth century. Each of these materials, in fact, did have at least one attractive property to justify testing it in this environment. For example, after observing that glass stimulated tissue growth, scientists assumed that other related materials would be both inert and malleable under the appropriate manufacturing treatment.

The first recorded artificial *replacement* in a hip joint by a manufactured part occurred in 1922, when a forty-one-year-old man in

Britain suffered a fracture to the neck of the femur. A graft was taken from his other femur bone, and a head fashioned from ivory was attached to it before surgeons inserted it into the host hip socket.[4] More than a decade passed, however, before doctors implanted the first known, and soon the first successful, metallic replacement of the head and part of the neck of the femur.[5] Possibly the first artificial metal hip socket fixed into a human acetabulum was introduced by a German, E. Rehn, who inserted a steel cup with spikes on its outer surface to fasten the device into the refashioned host bone in cases of congenital dislocation. This was conceived as a temporary device that would enable new bone to form in the hip so that a secure joint would exist when the metal cup was removed. At about the same time perhaps the first metal acetabular cups, made of Vitallium, were introduced by Preston and Albee in the United States around 1940, which were known as the Albee and Albee-Preston cups (Howmedica Inc., 1998).

Meanwhile, in 1938 P. Wiles, a surgeon at Middlesex Hospital in England, had been experimenting for the first time with ground components of a stainless steel to replace both cup and ball elements of the joint, precisely engineered to fit each other, the first attempt at *total* hip joint replacement. Wiles inserted six such devices, bolt- and screw-fixed to the femoral and acetabular bone. At the same time, in the United States, E. J. Haboush in New York developed the concept of the mold arthroplasty further and introduced a hollow ball with a "skirt" that would fit around the shaped head and neck of the femur, made from Vitallium alloy. In the case of the Albee cup, fixation of the head to the prosthesis proved problematic; Haboush concluded that an artificial head and neck of the femur and an artificial socket were necessary. He organized tests in his New York laboratory using a Vitallium head and an acetabular socket made of acrylic. Unfortunately, excessive wear and abrading resulted from these tests.

The development of hip prostheses, therefore, through the early 1940s saw the birth of the trial and error culture in orthopedic implant surgery, in which a wide range of materials drawn from a variety of sources had been tested in different designs, producing a large number of "errors." Neither the mold nor partial joint bone replacement showed great success. The late 1940s and early 1950s, by contrast, were an especially fertile and productive period for the evolution of hip implant technologies—though not without error, of course—as new materials and modifications to known materials were brought into the test-bed of human hip implants.

EARLY MODERN DEVELOPMENTS

In the mid-1940s a new design signaled the first use of plastics in joint replacement technology, and brought with it the first biomechanically designed hip implant. In 1946 two Parisian brothers named Judet introduced this very influential innovation. The Judets believed that osteoarthritis was primarily a disease that attacked the femoral head; thus, because it was fitted to a diseased foundation, the "mold" arthroplasty was not a viable design. The brothers designed their prosthesis in methylmethacrylate polymer, a glassy thermoplastic that can be cast or molded, most commonly known as acrylic, but also produced under other proprietary names such as Perspex, Plexiglas, and Lucite. The material was first produced in Germany early in the century, but industrial production developed from 1932 onward when acrylic sheet and molding techniques became available. The acrylic industry progressed rapidly during World War II, when the material was used for glazing on aircraft bodies. Like Vitallium, acrylic was first used in medical treatment as a dental implant. Haboush had studied its wear-resistance properties in 1940 when considering his arthroplasty work, but had not used it in his surgical experiments. The Judet design in acrylic consisted of an enlarged hemispherical head and a short thick stem external to the neck of the femur, the design sometimes being referred to as a "mushroom." To insert it into the body, the surgeon needed to ream the socket into the recipient's hipbone.

The Judet acrylic hip joint was the first mass-produced surgical implant of any sort to use a thermoplastic. By 1952, surgeons had inserted more than four hundred Judet implants and the design became widely used throughout Europe. In spite of good biocompatibility of the material, however, the rate of subsequent fractures was high. To combat this, surgeons often embedded a rod of stainless steel or chromium-plated brass in the stem to reinforce the reconstructed hip. These modifications resulted in problems associated with the brittleness of acrylic resin; consequently, the device was produced in "block" or solid nylon. Although this reduced the occurrence of stem fractures, the particles of nylon material proved to be more destructive to the bony tissue of the hip than the acrylic had been. Some surgeons had similar designs made in cobalt-chrome alloys and stainless steels, but while again reducing fractures, and having improved wear characteristics at the articulating surfaces of ball and socket, it generally suffered from excessive loosening. Nevertheless, interest in this type of design still exists. In the early 1980s German surgeons implanted a version of the Judet-style endo-prosthesis (i.e., one that is used for repairing the head of the thighbone), the fair results of which were published in the orthopedic press in the 1990s (Bettin et al., 1993).

A well-known American surgeon, M. d'Aubigne, who produced his own design using acrylic resin material, also used the Judet prosthesis. This featured a very long stem for fitting inside the femur and—in a highly unusual departure—a flat plate as the weight-bearing part, which looks rather like a spatula. Solid resins were used in some later designs: in the early 1960s, for example, the socket component of a model produced in Italy used the polyacetal resin Delrin, which was in fact manufactured in the United States by DuPont. In general, however, despite the popularity of the acrylic resin Judet device, the general tide of opinion among surgeons turned against this material in the 1950s because of high levels of failure due to loosening caused by excessive wear. With hindsight, therefore, the Judet design is frequently regarded as a disaster in the orthopedic community, but it can be regarded as the first artificial hip to be implanted in numbers of patients sufficient to suggest that a totally artificial hip joint of some design could become a regular and accepted part of surgical treatment of joint disease and fracture in populations on a large scale.

The post–World War II years witnessed such an expansion in the development of polymer plastics for consumer goods that it is sometimes known as the "Age of Plastics." Orthopedic implants utilized solid nylon as a material in cup implants as well as in the Judet ball and stem device. The material was used for dry bearings in engineering applications, and its relative resilience was appealing as a possible means to spread the weight load through the femur. A small number of prostheses were implanted with this material; one design followed the Smith-Petersen model while another design was fixed to the head of the femur by three splines. Neither design was successful: like the Judet hip, both designs induced severe wear resulting in tissue reaction with abraded particles of nylon. In the late 1940s, polythene was used in a non–weight-bearing prosthesis and in a socket cup similar in design to the Smith-Petersen floating cup. The latter, which was weight-bearing, soon showed signs of deterioration and wear with the polythene, like nylon, reacting adversely and producing fine particles that were found embedded in body tissue.

At approximately the same time in 1950, there were major developments in the United States in the use of metals for the femoral component of the hip. Austin Moore, for example, a surgeon at the University of South Carolina, had been involved with the first known metallic replacement of the head and part of the neck of the femur in a human hip. Moore's name is closely linked with that of the surgeon F. R. Thompson in the United States. Both surgeons considered that a suitably shaped stem component could be inserted inside the upper section of the bone of the femur, in the relatively soft honeycomb-like bone of the "intramedullary canal" inside it. Moore's initial concept was of a "self-locking," straight device that achieved stability inside the slightly curved femur by the pressure of jamming it firmly in (later, such a method was to be termed "press-fit") (Moore, 1957). Moore, aided by a professor of engineering at the Austenal Laboratories in New York, produced the prototype of this design in cobalt-chrome alloy, probably Vitallium, and the design included a ball component that was offset from the top of the femoral stem. Figure 7.1 illustrates the design and its development. This type of collaboration between surgeons, engineers, and testing laboratories was to become increasingly crucial to future innovations in orthopedic implants.

The Moore device was technically successful in many ways, but implantees suffered from unstable movement at the hip and, although it did not completely loosen, in most cases "migration" of the device occurred. In closely related work, F. R. Thompson believed in the same concept of intra-femoral implantation. His 1951 design was quite similar in appearance to the Moore device, though Thompson feared breakage and difficulties of removing the stem if it was ingrown with bone tissue. Thompson also preferred cobalt-chrome to steel and used Vitallium for his devices. Haboush experimented further as well, and in 1951 he inserted a cast Vitallium ball and hip socket, fixed with dental acrylic cement, into a patient at the Hospital for Bone and Joint Diseases in New York.

While Vitallium had been the most promising metal alloy for hip implants during the 1940s, between the two world wars a large number

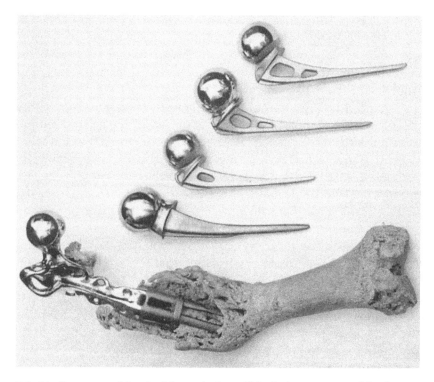

FIG. 7.1. Sequence of Austin Moore designs. This design was one of the first to use embedding of a tapered stem inside the bone of the femur. The first in the sequence shows the prosthesis emerging from the top of a retrieved, decayed thigh bone. The loops in the metal were intended for the attachment of muscle tissues. The material is cobalt-chrome alloy. The initial straight stem was soon modified. The windows in the stem—"fenestration"—were designed to enable the cancellous bone of the femur to grow through, thus fixing the device in position. From Moore, 1957. Reprinted by permission of the *Journal of Bone and Joint Surgery* (American).

of stainless steels and steel alloys were created and used in a wide range of engineering applications in the industrialized nations: "18-8" stainless steel (18 percent chromium, 8 percent nickel) had been first introduced into surgery in 1926 as an alternative to vanadium steel, while the addition of molybdenum produced an even more corrosion-resistant steel. Thus, the tensile strength and inertness of stainless steels helped them become, after World War II, the main alternative to cobalt-chrome alloys as the material for the load-bearing femoral component of artificial hips. In the United States in the early 1950s, stainless steel was used both in stem designs and in new designs of the mold or floating cup concept. For example, J. C. Adams produced first a hollow stainless steel cup, followed by a solid cup with a small aperture for tight containment of a reshaped femoral head and neck. The design proved to be unstable and bone was reabsorbed around the device. A Judet-style stem prosthesis also was conceived in stainless steel around this time, but failed to gain popularity, and Eicher produced a head-neck replacement, first in a stainless steel and then in cast cobalt-chrome alloy (Scales, 1967).

Stainless steels were also being used in England by G. K. McKee in Norwich in his first attempts to produce a design for a total ball and socket hip implant. McKee had designed and fabricated models of total hip prostheses as early as 1940. Like his counterparts in the United States, he found that his stainless steel devices quickly became loose in vivo, while a cobalt-chrome alloy version survived well for a period. Following a visit to the United States, McKee adopted the design form of the Thompson solid stem prosthesis. To this he added a three-clawed cup that was screwed into the acetabulum, all parts now made from a cobalt-chromium alloy called vinertia.[6] In spite of the developments in stainless steel alloys, McKee had come to the belief that this metal and its alloys were insufficiently inert for human implantation. He also believed that titanium had a tendency to "self-weld" (McKee, 1971: 50). Thus he used cobalt-chrome for cup and socket and femoral components that were produced as a pair for implantation in a single hip replacement, and he marked each component with a number for matching purposes.

Despite the fact that a long-lasting stable artificial hip remained on the horizon, knowledge of suitable materials—in terms of both biocompatibility and strength—had increased significantly by the 1950s. Vitallium and some forms of stainless steel were well established, and many of the trial and error designs described above were conceived in an attempt to preserve and utilize undamaged or reshaped hip sockets, where surgeons inserted them into either a replacement femoral neck and head or a head with a cup/mold positioned over it. On the other hand, the lack of successful hip replacement design was starting to lend support to the idea, already suggested by some surgeons, that for a hip implant to be functional without causing damage either to the human bone tissue or to the prosthetic materials themselves, surgeons would have to produce a design of highly wear-resistant components in which the articulating movement between ball and socket itself was achieved through the use of totally artificial materials. With benefit of hindsight, in the designs of Moore, Thompson, and McKee, the future of total hip replacement, the concept on which current artificial hip joints is based, can be discerned.

In reviewing these early hip implants we can see that they were pioneered typically by a single surgeon on a small number of patients using custom-made components. It is interesting to note the trend in naming devices after their surgeon-inventor, a trend that continued into the "modern" phase of development. The relative failure of some designs when implanted more widely, which may have seemed promising initially when implanted by the surgeon-inventor, might be explained to some extent by poorer manufacturing techniques used when the device was subjected to mass production techniques (Williams and Roaf, 1973). However, progress was being made in the understanding and production of orthopedic materials in spite of clinical failures.

"MODERN" HIP IMPLANTS

While stainless steels and Vitallium were established as leading contenders in artificial hip fabrication by the early 1950s, one metal—titanium—had yet to make an appearance. Although titanium is now a commonly used material in hip implants, its first recorded use in vivo was by Leventhal in 1957, six years after he had originally presented a case for its use in the *Journal of Bone and Joint Surgery*. Titanium has an oxide layer or film on its surface that reduces tissue reaction to a minimum, making it highly inert, like a ceramic. Titanium is also resistant to saline environments, which enhances its suitability for implantation inside the body. Cobalt-chrome and "316L" stainless steel are corrosion-resistant metal alloys with similar properties in this respect. Materials such as gold, silver, and platinum also have high corrosion-resistance but have poor mechanical properties, rendering them of little interest for heavy-duty implants. Titanium has less elasticity than cobalt-chrome alloys. In fact, titanium (and its alloys) is the only metallic material of significance to be introduced in implant surgery between 1950 and 1970. By contrast, many different plastics, rubbers, fibers, and fabrics were introduced during the same period. The U.S. Department of Defense supported the development of titanium technology, which required new melting and fabrication techniques, at its titanium metallurgy laboratory.[7]

Given its emergence at this time, it is striking that titanium alloys were not considered by the artificial hip's most successful surgeon-innovator, John Charnley, from Lancashire, England. Charnley is best known for integrating the scientific study of joint lubrication and biomechanics with the problems associated with prosthetic hip joint surgery. Indeed, in reviewing the "first 32 years" of total hip replacement in 1991, William Harris, a leading contemporary U.S. surgeon-designer, singled out Charnley in his appraisal of the progress of hip joint replacement technologies. Charnley had in fact developed a preliminary arthroplasty as early as 1946, but had abandoned the idea and throughout most of the 1950s had remained pessimistic about the prospects of a successful design. The main reason for his skepticism at this time lay in his view that the frictional properties of acrylic or metal in the prosthesis and bone and cartilage in the human body were incompatible. Cartilage lubricated with synovial fluid in human joints has an extremely low coefficient of friction, more slippery than a skate on ice (as his biographer notes), which artificial materials cannot match. With collaborators in engineering Charnley built rigs to gauge the friction in joints of bone and the artificial materials then mainly in use: stainless steel, cobalt-chrome, and acrylic (and perspex) (Waugh, 1990: 104). Friction was shown to be much greater with these artificial materials even when animal synovial fluid was used as a lubricant.

Charnley's aim thus became to find two different artificial materials for the ball and socket that would slide freely in contact with each other, but not require artificial lubrication. Charnley turned to manufacturers of synthetic plastics in a search for suitable socket material. He found a company in Bolton, Lancashire, that knew how to apply new polymers in engineering applications. Charnley believed that the best material for his purposes was polytetrafluorethylene (PTFE)—best known under the brand name Teflon, but sometimes marketed under the proprietary name Fluon—the same material now famous for its use in nonstick cooking utensils. Not only did it not stick, but Charnley believed it to be the most inert plastic then known; indeed, he tested this by inserting small pieces into his own leg. He experimented with a floating cup design combined with a socket cup, both in Teflon, but quickly moved on to a more radical approach: surgical removal of the femoral head, replacing it with a Moore-style femoral component, which was then fixed with the addition of "cement" inside the femur. Today this cementing principle is the mainstay of orthopedic hip replacement practice, especially for implants in elderly people. The Moore stem was the first to use the Teflon socket. McKee in Norwich and others, as we have seen, were using primarily metal, cobalt-chrome or stainless steel, for the femoral head, but this failed in patients with arthritic socket bones that could not withstand the abrasion of this material and design. In 1962, however, the PTFE sockets, made by Charnley himself and inserted into some three hundred patients, began to fail because bone tissue began to deteriorate in reaction to worn particles of the material. Charnley noted that the extreme gratitude expressed by his patients in the early stages following the operation delayed the recognition of the failure. Charnley sought more mechanically robust forms of polyethylene with high density, and the first high molecular weight polyethylene (HMWP) for the artificial hip socket was introduced at the end of 1962. Since that time, the development of the socket component forming the bearing surface with the ball has been dominated by the use of successive refinements of plastic materials.

Charnley's early total joint device appeared promising, and he accepted advice from mechanical engineers that a smaller femoral head would be an improvement, partly because it would enable a thicker, more robust socket cup to be used. This was the origin of his so-called low friction arthroplasty (Charnley, 1979). Charnley redesigned the Moore-style femoral component and had it manufactured in stainless steel by Thackrays, an engineering company from Leeds, Yorkshire, with experience in making surgical instruments. Although he believed that cobalt-chrome would prove to be the preferable metal, he never adopted it in his own surgical practice. Charnley's low friction design is illustrated in figure 7.2. It is worth noting that the two metals as produced at the time had different working characteristics: cobalt-chrome artifacts were cast, while stainless steel was wrought. This difference reflected different modes of production. Whereas cobalt-chrome required large numbers of relatively unskilled female labor, stainless steel was produced by "men who [were] true engineering craftsmen." The masculine image of stainless steel manufacture, a skilled engineering craft strongly associated with northern England, may have held some appeal for Charnley, and may partly explain why he continued to use artificial

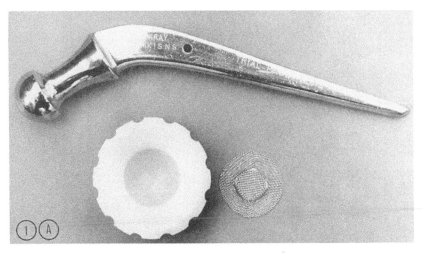

FIG. 7.2. Early Charnley prosthesis. The femoral component is in stainless steel, the cup in high-density polyethylene. The words "Trial prosthesis" are inscribed on the stem; the name of the manufacturers (Thackrays, the medical instrument engineering company in Leeds, England, bought in the early 1990s by DePuy International, one of the major manufacturers of orthopedic implants worldwide) is also legible. The "trial" prosthesis was in fact a manufacturer's model made to test the fabrication process, and would not have been implanted. As can be seen, the small femoral head was absolutely spherical and produced with a high degree of shine, which Charnley believed essential to low friction performance. From Owen, 1971, 69. Reprinted by permission of Professor Robert Owen.

hips produced in stainless steel, in addition to the fact that it was also cheaper. By the late 1960s, Thackrays was producing nine to ten thousand stainless steel artificial hips per year. In fact, the company did produce a cobalt-chrome version of the hip in the early to mid-1970s for the U.S. market, but the plan was not financially successful and was abandoned.

At the same time that Charnley was developing his designs, other surgeons in England were designing prostheses that were to be implanted very widely. For example, in the late 1950s and early 1960s the widely used "Stanmore" devices, named for a town in Essex where the country's National Orthopedic Hospital is located, used cobalt-chromium alloy as the material chosen for all related parts. Another

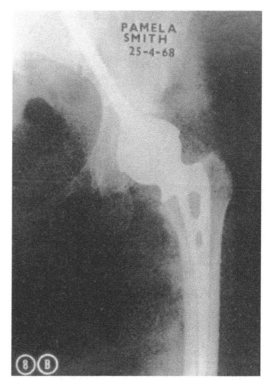

FIG. 7.3. The Ring hip prosthesis. Both components, including bearing surfaces, in cobalt-chrome. Note the very long socket screw fixed into the acetabulum. The name of the patient on the x-ray reminds us that these devices are implanted in the interior of a person's body, but the image is ambiguous in this respect, because, although the person is named, only part of the person is shown and the x-ray image is one generally available only to the specialist orthopedic surgeon and other hospital staff. While a large number of x-ray images of hip prostheses have been published in academic journals by orthopedic surgeons, it is relatively unusual to see the patient's name inscribed on them. From Ring, 1971. Reprinted by permission of Dr. P. A. Ring.

individual orthopedic surgeon, P. A. Ring, developed a cement-free prosthesis with a novel means of attaching the socket component. Again, in the Ring prosthesis, cobalt-chromium alloy was the material used. As can be seen from figure 7.3, the socket design featured a long screw for fixing the prosthesis up into the hip bone. As with the early

Charnley prostheses, clinical results of these implants are still being published today.

RECENT DEVELOPMENTS

Over the past ten to fifteen years, enormous institutional and financial resources have been marshaled for the purpose of exploring new materials and designs for artificial hips. In spite of the many apparent advances, the current state of implant technology has been described by one leading commentator as an "innovation impasse" and by another as having hit a "glass ceiling." The proliferation of new models, combinations of materials, and design variations, many of which are considerably more expensive than earlier models, has led some commentators to express concern about a trend toward "designer hips" (Bulstrode et al., 1993). In the 1960s most patients whom surgeons saw for replacements were relatively elderly people who suffered from severe joint pain due to arthritis. But this characterization of the end-user has been expanded as the technology, and demand for, hip prostheses has changed. The reports of good clinical results for prostheses fifteen years or longer after implantation has encouraged an expansion of the market to older and especially younger implantees, such as those who have suffered joint damage from sports-related injury or deterioration. Thus if artificial hips have reached a plateau in their current technological development, this may be because they fell victim to their own success during the 1970s and 1980s.

Perhaps the central issue in the contemporary development of hip implants is the division between those that are implanted with acrylic "cement" and those that are not. In spite of the success of cemented models, the development of cementless models has been spurred by two main factors. The first is the loosening of the components, which in the 1970s was attributed to "cement disease," a condition whose nature and existence are still disputed. It was believed that adverse reactions occurred between tissue and cement, causing particles of cement to aggravate the surrounding tissue, which in turn loosened the implant. Regardless of the veracity of this theory, it certainly is one of the forces behind the development of cementless models that, in turn, has encouraged a search for alternative materials with which to create adequate fixation to the host bone. The other main reason is the continued poorer performance of the socket components of cemented implants. More-over, there has been a trend toward dividing the prosthesis into sepa-rate functional parts. This is known as modularity, the prime example of which is the production of the head of the femoral component sepa-rately from its stem, which gives surgeons greater choice in seeking bet-ter anatomical fit of the device.

Surgeons and engineers have thus sought materials and designs that might improve the attachment of the implant to the host bone and tissue. A variety of techniques of encouraging the surrounding bone tis-sue to actually grow into the prosthesis, thus achieving what is known as "biological" fixation, have emerged. Surgeons did not introduce these uncemented "porous-coated" designs until the early 1980s, al-though the concept had been investigated as early as the 1960s. There are now more than twenty different models of this type of design on the market (Griffiths, Priest, and Kushner, 1995). The design usually con-sists of "micro-pores" of the basic implant metal added as a very thin layer to the basic device. The additional layer is formed of minute spherical beads in cobalt-chrome, or wire mesh or honeycomb-like lat-tice in titanium, requiring advanced production technologies to fix to the basic surface. The stem/head and the cup may be treated, usually all or part of the "shoulder" of the femoral component, and all of the outer surface of the socket. Such designs are increasingly widely mar-keted but remain somewhat controversial clinically, partly because of concerns about their longevity in the body and partly because pain in the thigh appears to be fairly common with this method of fixation of the femoral component (Faulkner et al., 1998).

The concept of biological fixation was tested in the laboratory as early as the late 1960s, as noted above. This has now been extended to the concept of a bond where, rather than simple ingrowth of bone into the inert prosthesis, a biological interaction between bone and prosthe-sis is sought. This represents the ultimate form of fixation within the body short of human cell-based tissue engineering. The bioactive mate-rial is applied as a further coating, usually in a ceramic material sprayed on to the surface of the porous coat. Hydroxyapatite (HA), a calcium phosphate ceramic, is of particular importance. This can be derived from natural bone, but can also be produced synthetically. Its chemical and crystalline structure is the same as the major mineral constituent of human bone. Dentistry again plays a part in the pedigree of the mate-rial, since it was originally used in oral and facial surgery, for example,

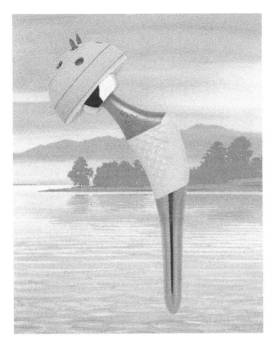

FIG. 7.4. ABG II hip with hydroxyapatite bioceramic coating. The stem is made from Vitallium cobalt-chrome-molybdenum alloy, and the socket and stem are coated with the ceramic hydroxyapatite (HA), characteristically white, for cementless fixation. Note the "macro-interlock" bobbling like fish gills on the upper part of the stem to enhance fixation. The image is from a 1998 advertisement. The backdrop of a calm scene of "Nature" emphasizes the appeal being made to smooth, organic, natural function. Reproduced by permission of Howmedica Osteonics.

as synthetic bone for artificial teeth, but it is unsuitable for weight-bearing because of its brittleness. Advanced forms of industrial technology are required for spraying HA, the coating being built up as a series of layers blasted on to the host metal by a computer-controlled robotic spray-nozzle. An example of an HA-coated device is in figure 7.4.

Long-term results of the performance of HA in the human hip are still awaited, but it is becoming increasingly widely used. Early studies suggest that it may be less associated with thigh pain than many of the earlier porous-coated devices (Faulkner et al., 1998). There is some technical controversy about the optimal metal to use with HA coating.

Titanium has higher elasticity than most other metals but is sensitive to the surface disturbance introduced with coating. Chromium-cobalt-molybdenum alloys remain stronger when coated (Learmonth and Spirakis, 1989), but on the other hand titanium may be preferable because it forms a chemical as well as a mechanical bond with HA coating (Geesink, 1990).

The materials used for the femoral stem and head in cementless implants in the recent period have been mainly stainless steel, cobalt-chrome-molybdenum alloy, and titanium aluminum vanadium alloy (Head, Bauk, and Emerson, 1995). However, stainless steels are much less used now for the stem. The orthopedic research literature disputes the relative advantages of the other two alloys. Again there is support for titanium alloy because of its biocompatibility, the degree of ingrowth of bone into the implant when porous-coated, and its elasticity, which is important for use in smaller stem sizes. Titanium was supported extensively in European centers of orthopedics during the 1980s (Stern et al., 1992). On the other hand, it is said to be an inferior material for the load-bearing surface of the head of the femur, is more prone to abrasive wear, and conveys greater stresses, making it less suitable for use with the particle-structure of acrylic cement (Head, Bauk, and Emerson, 1995). Ceramics and cobalt-chrome alloys are both superior in their wear properties. In fact, the most widely used cementless artificial hip in the United States—and probably worldwide—is the AML (anatomic medullary locking) device, produced by DePuy and manufactured in cobalt-chrome-molybdenum alloy. Where titanium stems are used they are generally combined now in modular devices with stainless steel or cobalt-chrome alloy heads, which are capable of taking a higher degree of polish and are less prone to scratching (Learmonth and Spirakis, 1989). The head component in modular designs may be coated in an attempt to achieve the smoothness of ceramic, for example by the use of titanium nitride.

Metal materials and surface finishes, therefore, especially for the femoral component of the artificial hip, are still being developed. "Superalloys" and composite materials are being tested in an attempt to achieve better biological and biomechanical matching to the flexibility of the femur. Polyacetal, polyethylene, carbon, and acrylic are among the materials that have been employed for this purpose in metal composites (Learmonth and Spirakis, 1994). In another technique to enhance fixation, the stems of devices for cemented implantation may be precoated with acrylic cement, added after either grit blasting to achieve a relatively rough surface or bead-blasting for a smooth surface.

A further major area of current debate and development in hip implant technology is the material used for the bearing surfaces between artificial ball and socket. Different combinations are in use and being tested, the major contenders being ceramics, metal, and polyethylene. Of the ceramics, alumina (the oxide of aluminum), titanium oxides, and zirconia (oxide of the rare crystalline element zirconium) are used and have good biocompatibility (Learmonth and Spirakis, 1994). Zirconia is a composite material, intermediate between metal and nonmetal, marketed as combining the advantages in wear and mechanics of both ceramics and the superalloys. The first all-ceramic (alumina-alumina) bearing in a total hip implant in a human had been implanted in 1970 in France (Nizard et al., 1992). Improved manufacturing after the mid-1970s enabled a smoother surface finish to be achieved, utilizing a dense alumina. In modular designs of implant, ceramic heads may be combined with high-density polyethylene, or alternatively modern cobalt-chrome for both surfaces may be used. McKee and others had used all-metal designs in the 1960s, but in general this was superseded by metal-polyethylene combinations. However, currently the metal-polyethylene bearing surface is seen as one of the weak points in the prosthesis design, and new metal-to-metal units have been developed again since the mid-1980s, for example by Müller in Switzerland, as illustrated in figure 7.5 (Head, Bauk, and Emerson, 1995). Müller's socket devices have a titanium outer shell inside that sits a polyethylene component that is lined with a cup in cobalt-chrome for the bearing surface of the joint. The femoral head is also of cobalt-chrome alloy. Maurice Müller is an extremely high-profile surgeon and orthopedic entrepreneur in Switzerland.

The advancing developments in materials and design appear to have brought their own problems in spite of the great clinical success of total hip implants. The earlier modern prostheses (1960s and 1970s) suffered from problems such as metal fractures and breakages, typically occurring five or more years after implantation. The arrival of superalloys and composite materials has almost eliminated mechanical breakage in normal usage of the artificial hip. The problems that these bring may appear only two or three years after implantation. Describing the effects of the new materials such as ultra-high molecular weight polyethylene, one surgical commentator has stated that "We have unleashed

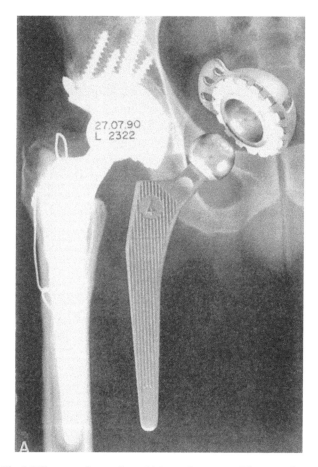

FIG. 7.5. The Müller metal-metal total hip replacement. The stem has vertical grooving for "macro-interlock" inside the thigh bone. The head of the Müller metal-metal model is much larger than the Charnley metal-polyethylene concept. The socket is comprised of three parts, the outer shell of titanium, the inner liner of polyethylene, and the cup, into which the head of the femoral component fits, of cobalt-chrome. In a previous design, now abandoned, the cup surface was treated with titanium nitrite for decreased friction, and the cobalt-chrome head of the femoral component was treated with a thin layer of titanium carbide (Head, Bauk, and Emerson, 1995). As can be seen, the socket is screwed into the hip bone, without cement. The design was developed in 1989 by Müller in collaboration with Sulzer Medical Technology. This distinctive image is unusual in depicting a photograph of the device superimposed upon an x-ray image of the same device in vivo. From Müller, 1995, 57. Reprinted by permission of *Clinical Orthopedics and Related Research*.

a torrent of particles into our joints, producing a devastation far exceeding simple prosthetic failure or fragmentation of parts" (Booth, 1994). While this may be a somewhat exaggerated account, it does appear to be the case that introduction of new materials within and adjacent to the tissue of the human hip and thighbone is a continuing cause for concern.

CONCLUSION

The early history of artificial hip technology was concerned with repair of conditions including fractured bones, congenital abnormalities, and ankylosis (joint stiffness)—conditions where disability was outwardly manifest. Even partial replacement technologies, especially those designed to position a bearing on the top of the femur, were designed primarily in these contexts. The concept of the total hip implant, however, allowed eventually for a relatively routine joint replacement operation, appropriate for people suffering from painful arthritic deterioration of the hip joint. This has turned out to be an enormous market, especially in an aging society, and the technology is now being extended to younger patients. Some of the newer designs, such as those featuring bioactive coatings, are being actively promoted particularly for this younger client group.

Technological medicine provides devices that can replace damaged or worn internal components of the human locomotor system. But in examining the design and material composition of artificial hips, we should not forget that we are peering into the normally hidden world of the human anatomy. Unlike external prostheses, these devices, once implanted, can be visualized only through x-ray and other imaging technologies. Since direct observation is not possible, the material properties of the devices are not part of the end-users' everyday social world. These technologies, then, are used and controlled by health professionals in the context of doctor-patient relationships. Implantees "consume" them only via their effect upon physical functions and experience of sensation such as pain or discomfort. Given their invisibility in the everyday life of implantees, the forms in which artificial hips are represented are of particular interest. The two most widely available sources of images of artificial hips are photographs and x-ray reproductions in clinical research articles in the academic orthopedic press, and in the advertising images of the orthopedic manufacturing companies. This chapter illustrates examples of these types of image. Orthopedic research articles focus primarily on performance of the prosthesis, defined in terms of technological and clinical criteria such as implantees' pain and physical function in the years following implantation, and the durability of implants. On the other hand, the manufacturers' portrayals focus upon two other key aspects of the prosthesis, its material properties and "operability" from the surgeon's point of view. As one might expect, some modern advertising representations of the devices attempt to incorporate images that express the strength, naturalness, and biocompatibility of modern materials.

Of course, as one would expect with devices that are usually hidden from view, hip prosthesis components in general feature little wording or iconography. Most, in fact, do have serial numbers and some, as seen in the Charnley example above, have the manufacturer's name(s) or lettering or other functional inscriptions. The representation of prosthetic devices within the orthopedic surgical and manufacturing communities has also been referred to in relation to the name, either conventional or legally trademarked, of artificial hips over the course of their evolution. In the 1940s and 1950s there was a strong tendency for hip implants to be known and named for the surgeon-designer responsible (e.g., the Judet, the Charnley) or, in some cases, the geographical origin (e.g., the Exeter, the Minneapolis). This tradition continues, to some extent, but has been joined now by designs that reflect a culture responding less to surgical ingenuity and more to global business and consumerism. This reflects the larger shift from surgeon-driven innovation to alliance with a competitive corporate environment of profit-related innovation where orthopedic implant manufacturers play a powerful role. Recent hip designs, for example, carry names that emphasize functionality and anatomical compatibility, such as the "Natural-Hip System," the "BioGroove Hip System," and the "Taper-Fit Total Hip System."

One can only speculate what these names convey in the marketplace of contemporary technological medicine. The term "system" perhaps suggests a product that has the capacity to fulfill a wide variety of consumers' needs and provides a variety of possible options from which the user can select. The images conjured by the words "Natural" and "Taper-Fit" clearly appeal to ideas about restoring natural and normal function. These appeals are as likely to be directed at surgeons and managed-care organizations as at the implantee-users for whom reduction in pain and restoration of function are generally the most important goals of prosthetic hip surgery. Thus by looking inside the body at these materials, we find ourselves looking also at the intersecting worlds of surgeons, engineers, and manufacturers. Decisions regarding choice of implant for different users rest essentially with surgeons, but these surgeons operate in an environment where they are exposed to manufacturing organizations that shape the prostheses that they will make available. Indeed, some of these practicing surgeons are surgeon-designers or surgeon-design consultants: the design of orthopedic implants now is the outcome of complex relationships between the clinical and bioengineering worlds.

When one contemplates a world in which such large numbers of people participate in "normal activities" with the invisible aid of such prostheses, one of the most striking features is the variety of materials and designs with which people have been provided. While this no doubt reflects the variety of shapes and sizes of the human body, it also reflects to some extent the inventiveness of designers and the competitiveness of manufacturing institutions. It is perhaps ironic to reflect that fashion is one of the driving forces behind an essentially invisible technology; the apparently late uptake of titanium alloys in Europe may be a case in point. The progression of materials and designs in artificial hip technology might be seen simply as the progressive, linear refinement of increasingly better-functioning devices—examples, in other words, of technical rationality in action. The shape and composition, however, of particular technologies might always have been different. Indeed, as this account demonstrates, the material development of artificial hips continues to be shaped by different forces of innovation in the context of contemporary orthopedics. Although some aspects of the design, such as the use of a stem sited within the femur, have achieved consensus among surgeons and engineers, there is no one single set of material technologies that can be said to dominate all areas of the design.

NOTES

1. In Scales, 1967, a survey of the early development of materials used in artificial hips.

2. An obituary of Smith-Petersen appeared in the *Harvard Medical Alumni Bulletin* 28 (October 1953): 36–37.

3. Viscaloid was a celluloid composed essentially of gun cotton and camphor; Pyrex is the borosilicate glass later used widely in heat-resistant cooking ware; Bakelite, a "thermo-setting" plastic, related to celluloid, was first patented in 1907 and used primarily in the development of electrical insulation and automobile parts as well as hundreds of household goods; Vitallium was a metal alloy of cobalt, chromium, and tungsten (tungsten was later replaced by the more easily obtainable molybdenum, which was available in Colorado from about 1918).

4. This was reported in the *British Journal of Surgery* by E. W. Hey-Groves in its 1926–27 volume, with an illustrative diagram (Hey-Groves, 1926–27, cited in Scales, 1967).

5. Implanted by the surgeon Dr. Bohlman of Maryland. Two such replacements failed, but the *American Journal of Surgery* later reported a successful, long-lasting result in one patient after ten years of implantation (Bohlman, 1952; cited in Scales, 1967).

6. See Waugh's account in his biography of John Charnley (1990).

7. See *Encyclopedia Britannica*, 1963.

REFERENCES

Aufranc, O. E. Constructive hip surgery with the Vitallium mould: A report on 1000 cases of arthroplasty of the hip over a fifteen-year period. *Journal of Bone and Joint Surgery* 39A, no. 2: 237.

Bettin, D., B. Greitemann, J. Polster, and S. Schulte Eistrup. 1993. Long term results of Judet's cementless total endoprosthesis of the hip joint. *Zeitschrift für Orthopädie und Ihre Grenzgebiete* 131, no. 6 496–502.

Bijker, W. E., T. P. Hughes, and T. J. Pinch, eds. 1987. The social construction of technological systems: New directions in the sociology and history of technology. Cambridge: MIT Press.

Bohlman, H. R. 1952. Replacement reconstruction of hip. *American Journal of Surgery* 84, no. 3: 1497.

Booth, R. E. 1994. Current concepts in joint replacement: The closing circle: Limitations of total joint arthroplasty. *Orthopedics* 17, no. 9: 757–59.

Bulstrode, C. J. K., D. W. Murray, A. J. Carr, et al. 1993. Designer hips. *British Medical Journal* 306: 732–33.

Charnley, J. 1979. Low friction arthroplasty of the hip: Theory and practice. Berlin: Springer Verlag.

Faulkner A., L. G. Kennedy, K. Baxter, J. Donovan, M. Wilkinson, and G. Bevan. 1998. Effectiveness of hip prostheses in primary total hip replacement: A critical review of evidence and an economic model. *Health Technology Assessment* 2, no. 6.

Geesink, R. G. T. 1990. Hydroxyapatite-coated total hip prostheses: Two-year clinical and roentgenographic results of 100 cases. *Clinical Orthopaedics* 261: 39–58.

Griffiths, H. J., D. R. Priest, and D. Kushner. 1995. Total hip replacement and other orthopedic procedures. *Radiologic Clinics of North America* 33, no. 2: 267–87.

Hahn, H., and W. Palich. 1970. W. Preliminary evaluation of porous metal surfaced titanium for orthopaedic implants. *Journal of Biomedical Materials Research* 4: 571.

Harris, W. H. 1992. The first 32 years of total hip arthroplasty: One surgeon's perspective. *Clinical Orthopaedics* 274: 6–11.

Head, W. C., D. J. Bauk, and R. H. Emerson. 1995. Titanium as the material of choice for cementless femoral components in total hip arthroplasty. *Clinical Orthopaedics* 311: 85–90.

Heck, C. V., and F. A. Chandler. 1954. Material failures in hip prostheses. *Journal of Bone and Joint Surgery* 36A: 1059.

Hey-Groves, E. W. 1926–27. Some contributions to the reconstructive surgery of the hip. *British Journal of Surgery* 14: 486.

Howmedica Inc. 1998. The Vitallium alloy story. <http://www. howmedica.com/book/vitall.htm>.

Huiskes, R. 1993. Failed innovation in total hip replacement: Diagnosis and proposals for a cure. *Acta. Orthop. Scand.* 64, no. 6: 699–716.

Learmonth, I. D., and A. Spirakis. 1989. Current status of total hip replacement: A review of biological and biomechanical factors. *South African Journal of Surgery* 27: 84–88.

———. 1994. Current thoughts on total hip replacement. *South African Medical Journal* 84: 88–90.

Leventhal, G. S. 1951. Titanium, a metal for surgery. *Journal of Bone and Joint Surgery* 33A: 473.

MacKenzie, D., and J. Wajcman, eds. 1985. The social shaping of technology: How the refrigerator got its hum. Milton Keynes: Open University Press.

McKee, G. K. 1971. McKee-Farrar total prosthetic replacement of the hip. In M. Jayson, ed., Total hip replacement. London: Sector Publishing, 47–67.

Moore, A. 1957. The Self-Locking Metal Hip Prosthesis. *Journal of Bone and Joint Surgery* 39(A): 811–27.

Müller, M. 1995. From *Clinical Orthopaedics and Related Research* 57.

Nizard, R. S., L. Sedel, P. Christel, et al. 1992. Ten year survivorship of cemented ceramic-ceramic total hip prosthesis. *Clinical Orthopaedics* 282: 53–63.

Owen, R. 1971. The Charnley total hip replacement. In M. Jayson, ed., Total hip replacement. London: Sector Publishing, 68–85.

Park, J. B. 1984. Biomaterials science and engineering. New York: Plenum.

Rang, M. 1966. Anthology of orthopaedics. Edinburgh: E. and S. Livingston.

Ring, P. A. 1971. Ring total hip replacement. In M. Jayson, ed., Total hip replacement. London: Sector Publishing, London 26–46.

Scales, J. T. 1967. Arthroplasty of the hip using foreign materials: A history. *Proceedings of the Institution of Mechanical Engineers* 181, no. 3: 63–84.

Smith-Petersen, M. N. 1939. Arthroplasty of the hip: A new method. *Journal of Bone and Joint Surgery* 21, no. 2: 269.

Stern, L. L. D., M. I. Cabadas, J. M. F. Fdez-Arroyo, J.M.F., R. Zarzoso, J. C. Sanchez-Barbero, and J. Granado. 1992. LD Hip arthroplasty: Design concepts and first clinical trials of a new modular system. *Clinical Orthopaedics* 283: 39–48.

Venable, C. S., and W. G. Stuck. 1947. The internal fixation of fractures. Springfield, IL: C. C. Thomas.

Waugh, W. 1990. John Charnley: The man and the hip. Berlin: Springer-Verlag.

Williams, D. F., and R. Roaf. 1973. Implants in surgery. London: Saunders.

8

"There's No Language for This"

Communication and Alignment in Contemporary Prosthetics

Steven Kurzman

THIS ESSAY IS about how contemporary lower-extremity amputees and prosthetists communicate with each other during the process of fitting and aligning a prosthesis in clinic. Amputees approach the use of prostheses from a subjective perspective, while prosthetists speak about fitting and aligning prostheses in the language of biomechanics. Since fit and alignment are essential to using a prosthesis, prosthetists and amputees must find ways to communicate with one another about prostheses and the subjective experience of using them. This essay describes how they collaboratively invent a language to do this.

I explore the clinical language, silence, and experience of prostheses in an effort to imbue this text with a flavor of these two perspectives and to show how they are in embodied dialogue with each other. I am both a cultural anthropologist and a below-knee amputee, and this dialogue also expresses my own peculiar position during my dissertation fieldwork in the prosthetics field in Chicago. Ultimately, I believe that juxtaposing the subjective experience of using a prosthesis and the clinical work of constructing bodies has potential to disrupt our habitus (in Marcel Mauss's terms), or learned techniques, of how we think about, talk about, and use our bodies, walking, and able-bodiedness (Mauss 1992).

THERE'S NO LANGUAGE FOR THIS

The process of fitting and dynamically aligning a prosthesis is integral to making and using one, and Kevin and I were ready to start. Kevin is a certified prosthetist who, during my fieldwork, worked at a prosthetics shop that served as one of my field sites. We were working on an informal experiment, a prototype for an inexpensive, easy-to-use below-knee prosthesis intended for geriatric amputees. It was a collaborative project in which Kevin designed the limb and did most of the fabrication, while I tested it and offered feedback. And now it was time to align the check socket.

As we entered the fitting room and closed the sliding door behind us, we shifted our roles from prosthetist and amputee/researcher to clinician and patient. Half kidding and half serious, Kevin began to speak in a more clinical tone, addressing me as "Mr. Kurzman" and giving me gentle but authoritative descriptions and instructions about how to use the new prosthesis. After removing my everyday leg, I pulled on silicone and cloth stump socks and donned the prosthesis. I stood up, shifted my weight around, and began to walk in the parallel bars. I didn't get very far, though, before the fiberglass tape binding the check socket to the pylon ripped with a loud cracking sound. After a quick repair, I walked in the bars for a few minutes and, quickly getting a feel for the limb, moved out of the fitting room and started trotting up and down the hallway. I tried to walk evenly and smoothly, looking straight ahead, and paying attention to where my body was and how it was moving. How were my feet rolling over during the gait cycle? Was my trunk leaning after heel-off? Meanwhile, Kevin gazed intently at my feet and body, asking himself similar questions, while Noah and Milton, the two shop technicians, cracked jokes about the prosthesis hurting.

After a few minutes of this, I informed Kevin that the prosthesis didn't feel right. He posed questions in an effort to pinpoint the problem: Where does it hurt? Does it feel like you're walking up a hill? Does it feel like you're walking into a hole? We moved to the workshop in the back of the facility, where I doffed the prosthesis and he made some adjustments. I was soon pacing the hallway again and we repeated the cycle of walking, feeling, observing, questioning, and readjusting. My attention focused on my legs and the effort of thinking about what it feels like to walk and how to articulate this feeling, while Kevin alternately observed my legs, face, and body language. We repeated the

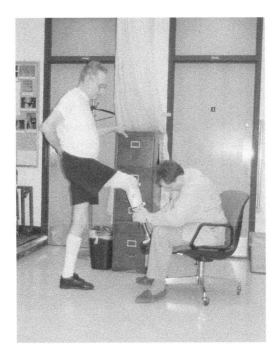

FIG. 8.1. Alignment. Mark, the senior instructor in prosthetics at Northwestern University Prosthetic-Orthotic Center, aligning Frank's leg during trials for Andy's experiment. Photograph courtesy of the author.

process over and over again, grinding out tight areas of the socket, plantarflexing or dorsiflexing the foot, adducting and a-b-ducting the socket, and toeing the foot in and out.[1] "Is that better or worse now? Or the same?" he asked after each adjustment.

Finally, we reached that moment when the prosthesis just felt right and I stopped thinking about walking because it no longer felt remarkable. I began walking at a faster pace and stopped looking at my feet. My face exuded the expression of one who has just figured something out. Kevin noticed this, as did Noah and Milton, especially when I cheered and raised my arms like a goal post. We got it right: the socket was comfortable and the prosthesis was aligned. Back in the fitting room, we were chatting about the process and its difficulties when Kevin remarked thoughtfully, "You know, there's no language for this . . ."

COLLABORATION

What Kevin meant is that there is no shared language available with which amputees and prosthetists can communicate about aligning or using a prosthesis. Kevin's comment points to the importance of communication in the prosthetics clinic, and implicitly, to the importance of amputees' subjective experience in the process of alignment. The process is so fascinatingly nuanced, so intimately customized, and the communication often so difficult, it was amazing that we could fit and align a prosthesis at all. A full day at a prosthetics shop participating in clinical situations usually left me completely stunned, and a lasting impression I carry from fieldwork is that it is a minor miracle that anything actually works in prosthetics.

Thus, the purpose of this essay is to explore how anything does work in a prosthetics clinic. I argue that lower-extremity amputees and prosthetists collaboratively communicate and, whether communicated verbally or through performance, amputees' subjective experience is crucial to this collaboration. Alignment itself is an important ritualistic performance of integrating or embodying a prosthesis, and the ability to communicate during and about the alignment process is a key to understanding how anything works in prosthetics, both inside the clinic and out.

Medical anthropologists often approach clinical communication in terms of the dichotomy between subjective experience and objective biomedical authority, and the difficulty of describing the experience of illness, pain, and suffering from within this dualism. In their essay "The Mindful Body: A Prolegomenon to Future Work in Medical Anthropology," Schepper-Hughes and Lock argue that the Cartesian dualism is so strongly embedded in biomedicine that it colors our attempts to describe the experience of illness (1987). They note that there is no language to describe this, and "[a]s both medical anthropologists and clinicians struggle to view humans and experience of illness and suffering from an integrated perspective, they often find themselves trapped by the Cartesian legacy. We lack a precise vocabulary with which to deal with mind-body-society interactions and so are left suspended in hyphens, testifying to the disconnectedness of our thoughts." (10).

It is indeed difficult to escape the material dualism of body and technology that permeates the prosthetics clinic, and, as Kevin pointed out, amputees and prosthetists do lack a shared vocabulary that fully describes body-prosthesis interactions. But amputees learn how to articulate their experience of prostheses, and good prosthetists tacitly recognize the importance of the subjective component of prostheses and often rely on their patients to help them understand problems in which the technical and the experiential blur together.

This may be due in part to a notable difference between the epistemologies of the biomedical clinic and the more biomechanical prosthetics clinic. Although the experience of aligning a prosthesis may involve pain and suffering for new amputees being fitted for their first prosthesis, the subjective experience of the prosthetics clinic is generally not about illness, but rather about integrating and embodying technology. As Martin describes it, biomedicine has long conceptualized the body as a fortress, or a closed system under attack from external contaminants (Martin 1994). But prosthetists tend to consider bodies as biomechanical systems in conjunction with prostheses, and are generally more interested in the interface between bodies and prostheses as a system, rather than in the body itself. They work within a tension between the claimed objectivity of biomechanics and the acknowledged relativity of prostheses to amputees' bodies. The technical and scientific influence of biomechanics is a key part of the increasingly medical and clinical quality of prosthetists' work, and is also important to speaking authoritatively to patients about treatment. But prosthetists believe that prostheses are relative to amputees' bodies and must be integrated into their subjective experiences of bodies and mobility. Since most prosthetists have not had this subjective experience, clear communication greatly facilitates this process.[2]

Prosthetists talk about bodies in terms of anatomy and physiology, and walking in terms of gait cycle and biomechanics. Many older prosthetists have learned gait analysis and alignment through apprenticeship and practice rather than formal education, but younger prosthetists learn these ideas as a didactic element of their increasingly medical prosthetics certification course as well as clinical practice. These terms are extremely precise and descriptive for discussing gait, but they obviously don't describe the subjective experience of walking. For instance, you can say that a foot is too plantarflexed, resulting in the patient vaulting over the foot and trunk leaning medially, and you can say that dorsiflexing the foot will probably help normalize gait. But this does not capture the feeling of walking over a plantarflexed foot, of trying to roll over toes that feel strangely resistant, or of vaulting over the foot and momentarily feeling your body catapulted just a bit higher—with just a slightly better view of things—and then falling back down onto your other foot. And while prosthetists would spot this particular example in their own terms, they rely on amputees at other times for subjective feedback in fitting and alignment.

Amputees, more frequently than not, have great difficulty articulating this verbally. The subjective experience of using a prosthesis disrupts language. This is especially true of new amputees, for whom an amputation is still a great shock to the body. Stumps are perplexing and delicate new body parts, and phantom limbs are somewhat disconcerting, distracting, and often painful at first. Compounding this problem, wearing a prosthesis is initially very uncomfortable. Part of your body, which was not evolutionarily designed to bear weight, is suddenly bearing your weight in motion, while your stump is encased in cloth socks and plastic. It is all so supremely alien that it is extremely difficult to describe the sensation at all, much less respond to the question as to whether it "feels right." Longer-term amputees learn from experience what feels right and what they like, and maybe even how to communicate that to their prosthetist. But for newer amputees, it's often frustratingly difficult to know, not to mention to articulate to the prosthetist, how it should feel.

And yet, despite the fact that "there's no language for this"—or, perhaps, that there are two languages for this—every time a prosthetist and amputee meet clinically, they must invent a way of communicating about the prosthesis and how it feels. Alignment and clinical interactions in general are interactive performances through which amputees and prosthetists communicate. The communication is important not only because fitting and alignment are crucial to a prosthesis being comfortable and easy to use, but also because such communication helps to negotiate clinical roles, bodily boundaries, and working rapport.

The vitality of clinical communication is most apparent when it goes wrong. In addition to Kevin's shop, I also fieldworked at another prosthetics shop, which was more working-class in flavor.[3] Don was working with a new patient named George and felt that his previous prosthesis, which had been made at another shop, was too short and caused gait problems. So he made his new prosthesis taller, at what he believed to be the correct height. George felt adamantly that his new leg was too tall but couldn't elaborate a more specific reason for not liking it. It didn't hurt; it was just too tall and didn't feel right. They were both getting a bit crabby when Don turned to face me and two physical therapy students visiting the shop for the day and hissed, "Half the difficulty of prosthetics is understanding *what the fuck* the patient is talking about."

This sentiment is sometimes mutual for amputees, and I will turn to a discussion of alignment in order to explain how they do manage to understand each other. Alignment refers to how a prosthesis is positioned and moves in relation to an amputee's body. It is the process of locating a prosthesis relative to an amputee's body and mechanically manipulating that relationship in order to facilitate the amputee's ability to comfortably integrate and embody the prosthesis. The mechanics and physical construction involved in integrating this technology into bodies are as important as the physical foundation of embodying prostheses. In other words, alignment involves physical as well as discursive construction of bodies.

ALIGNMENT

A certain degree of alignment of joints and limbs to each other is embodied common sense: it's difficult to walk with your foot pointing backward, and it's hard to feed yourself if your forearm is too long. Although dynamically aligning prostheses is basically a process of getting the foot pointed in the right direction, it is much more nuanced than this sounds. In theory, as prosthetists learn it in school, alignment is based in biomechanical principles and the concept of normal gait. But in clinic, normal gait is more of a guideline for how to observe patients and arrive at "good enough gait," an amalgam of normal gait, symmetry, and subjective comfort and satisfaction.

If we had gone through a formal patient exam, Kevin would have inquired as to my age, height, weight, cause and date of amputation, general health, illness complications, and physical activity level. Then he would have palpated my stump, checking for a number of physical landmarks and characteristics. On a below-knee amputee, for example, a prosthetist checks for stump shape, bony prominences, skin type, and other characteristics that figure into prostheses in terms of what areas of an amputee's stump will bear weight, what areas won't accept pressure without pain, and which kind of socket and suspension (method of keeping the prosthesis on the body) will best fit the person. For example, bony prominences such as the tibial tubercle and the fibular head are areas that suffer pain under pressure. Areas such as the patellar tendon, tibial flare, and interosseous region will comfortably support weight. Neuromas or "trigger spots" (balled up nerve endings near the end of the stump) are very intolerant of pressure.

The patient exam for prosthetists is a tactile process of mapping stumps and marking reference points for getting to know bodies. This tactile knowledge becomes a basis for deciding what is the most appropriate type of prosthesis for the patient, especially the socket and suspension. Bob, another prosthetist, one day pointed out to me how patients' bodies "indicated" or "contraindicated" certain styles of sockets and suspension. I didn't fully understand what he meant until later, when we were on a house call to one of his patients. Mr. Gambino was having difficulty donning his prosthesis. He was an above-knee amputee with a suction socket, which requires a good deal of pulling effort to don. You don a thin stump sock and then essentially pull your stump into the socket by pulling the sock through the socket and out a hole in the bottom. Bob pointed out that Mr. Gambino's effort to pull his stump into the socket was inappropriate because he had a heart condition and shouldn't be exerting himself that heavily. His health "contraindicated" this type of prosthesis, but the doctor, who lacked any expertise regarding prostheses, had written a very specific—and inappropriate—prescription.[4]

Since Kevin and I were already acquainted and even had a design in mind, we omitted the patient exam, normally the initial step, and proceeded directly to casting. Casting is a continuation of the exam, and is basically an opportunity for the prosthetist to make a visual and tactile inspection of his or her patient. Mapping landmarks prior to casting is essentially a way of knowing the body, reading its terrain in a very tactile sense, and then mapping it. Kevin had me don a thin cloth sock, called a casting sock, and made measurements of length and circumference at intervals along the length of the stump. Then, using a grease pencil dipped in water, he marked and defined landmarks on my stump. The pencil marks on the casting sock transfer to the inside of the cast and serve as guides for later modifications.

He grabbed a couple of rolls of plaster of paris bandage and, unwinding one and dipping it in warm water, began wrapping my stump and knee in warm plaster. When the cast had dried, we pulled it off and

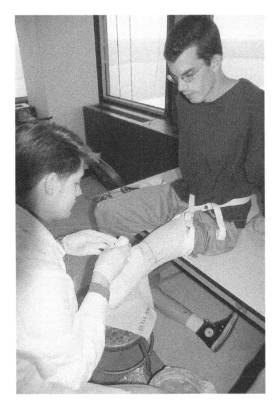

FIG. 8.2. Casting. The author being casted by a prosthetics student at the school. Photograph courtesy of the author.

checked to ensure that the grease pencil marks matched up with their corresponding landmarks inside the cast. Casting is important because it's surprisingly easy to mistakenly make bad markings or take wrong measurements, which can add to the difficulty of making an accurately fitting socket. It's an uncomfortable moment of crossing bodily boundaries: prosthetists and technicians have to learn to touch people in a way that would otherwise be inappropriate, and amputees have to get used to having their stump palpated, squeezed, and caressed. But it's also crucial to the process of knowing and mapping stumps and bodies and how they experience these tactile sensations.

Kevin filled the finished cast with plaster and, after it hardened, gave me the tedious chore of stripping the embedded plaster of Paris,

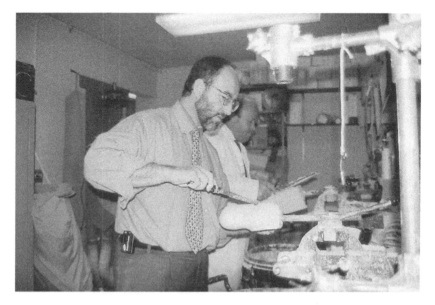

FIG. 8.3. Modifications. Kevin modifying a cast for a below-knee prosthesis. Photograph courtesy of the author.

leaving a solid, positive impression of my stump. He then modified the cast into a desirable negative image of the socket, using rasps and other tools to do the sculpting. The shop technicians made a check socket, or test socket, by wrapping the cast in an oven-heated piece of polyethylene plastic and applying a vacuum. They "broke out" the socket by using an airhammer to remove the plaster and Kevin attached a pylon (a hollow pole) and foot, and put the limb in bench alignment, a generic position for prostheses. We were ready for dynamic fitting and alignment.

I donned the prosthesis and stood up, shifting my weight back and forth to gauge the height and try to gain a sense of balance. I thought about how the socket felt and where it bore my weight as I shifted onto and off it. Kevin, sitting on one of the stools on caster-rollers that seem to occupy every prosthetics shop fitting room, checked my height, first visually and then by digging his fingers uncomfortably into the flesh above my hips. As I stood still, he scooted around me to check the pylon, making sure it was vertical in both sagittal and coronal planes. I began walking between the parallel bars. I focused on trying to walk consistently and paid attention to how the socket felt. Kevin hunkered down on his stool at the end of the bars and watched me walk toward him, looking at where the pylon was at mid-stance when the foot was flat on the floor bearing my weight. Then he scooted to the side and watched the pylon from the sagittal plane to assure that it was vertical at mid-stance from this view.

After a few minutes he had me sit down and doff the prosthesis. I peeled off the layers of socks and silicone, and Kevin inspected my stump for redness, a sign of excessive pressure and friction. He also used the back of his hand to check skin temperature on the weight-bearing areas. The fit was fine but the alignment was off, so Kevin made the adjustment using his allen wrench. In common endoskeletal prostheses, the socket and foot are connected using a hollow aluminum pylon and a pair of titanium pyramids, or mounts, one at either end.[5] By adjusting hex screws in the mounts, the prosthetist can move the foot and socket in relation to the body. The processes of casting, fitting, and alignment are physically customized techniques, intimately connecting bodies with prostheses.

COMMUNICATION

Whenever I have been fit for a prosthesis, whether in the United States, India, or Cambodia, the first question is always something to the effect of "Does it hurt?" Prostheses may be uncomfortable on occasion, especially at first, but they aren't supposed to hurt. Pain may be the fragmentation of language, but it is the opening of communication about how a prosthesis feels (Scarry 1985). If pain is "the unmaking of the world," alignment is one way of remaking the world for newly acquired amputees. New amputees know when their prostheses hurt and will call it to the attention of their prosthetist even when they are unable to articulate the cause. If they don't say anything, they still communicate through their performance of a painful socket. For example, an unwillingness of amputees to put their weight fully on the limb is often a sign of pain or of not yet trusting the prosthesis.

Although most lower-extremity amputees are interested in walking well and passing as non-amputees, they don't speak in terms of normal gait. From an amputee's perspective, dynamic alignment is about making sure the prosthesis feels right, learning how to walk again, and, on some level, beginning the process of embodying and habituating to a new limb. Amputees often speak metaphorically about their prostheses to describe what they feel like. The ultimate metaphor for many new amputees is their previous organic limb, particularly as it functioned and enabled them when they were younger. Lance, one of Kevin's patients, often compared his prosthesis to his organic leg, but differentiated between cosmesis and feeling. He and his wife were happy that his prosthesis resembled his leg, but he had difficulty adjusting to it, partly because it didn't feel like his old leg. In a variant on this, longer-term amputees often compare their new prosthesis to their last one. Amputees become strongly habituated to their prostheses, particularly to the fit of the socket and the style of suspension. This is an important issue for older men who lost limbs during World War Two and the Korean War, many of whom still prefer the style of limb they started wearing in the 1940s or 1950s. It is also a problem as older practitioners retire and are replaced by younger prosthetists who lack the woodworking and leatherworking skills to continue in this tradition. And both of these metaphors put prosthetists in somewhat of a bind, since no one can adequately replace an organic limb, nor can they exactly re-create the idiosyncratic fit of another prosthesis.

Longer-term amputees also share a few stock metaphors with prosthetists, who reproduce them in prosthetics school and clinic. For example, the feeling of "walking into a hole" corresponds to excessive dorsiflexion in the foot for prosthetists. Imagine that you are walking down a steep hill and think about the feeling of walking heavily on your heels and having your foot quickly slap down flat when your foot rolls down the hill—that is the feeling that walking into a hole describes for amputees. Likewise, the feeling of "walking up a hill" corresponds to excessive plantarflexion. Think about the feeling of walking up a steep slope and how you're pretty light on your heel, but spend a lot of time on your toes, maybe even actively pushing yourself off as you roll over your toes. This is the feeling described by walking up a hill for amputees, and means the prosthetist needs to dorsiflex the foot. These metaphors are interesting not only because of the easy correspondence between feeling and foot position, but because they make use of our common, nearly intuitive experience of walking on these terrains. Obviously, there's not actually a slope in the clinic, but the position of the foot comes to embody the landscape, and the prosthesis becomes a hill or a hole.

Other metaphors describe prostheses in terms of parts of the foot that may not even physically exist in the structure of the prosthesis, such as heel and toes. Both amputees and prosthetists often speak of prosthetic feet as having or not having toes, or as having soft or stiff heel or toes. During alignment, toes can also be turned too far in or out, giving one the odd sensation of rolling over a foot that isn't pointing in the right direction. At the prosthetics school where I conducted fieldwork, students gave professional patients a wide variety of feet in order to solicit diverse opinions from their patients during critique. One of the patients was trying a new brand of foot called Flex-Foot for the first time. Flex-Foot feet are renowned for their springy quality because they are basically a long keel of carbon fiber. The patient commented that he liked the foot because "it has toes." But this is always relative to the person using the component. Brian, an engineering graduate student at the lab and a bilateral above-knee amputee himself, didn't like the same brand of foot because he felt it had "too much toe" and made it difficult for him to roll over the foot.

Amputees are remarkably inventive in creating their own metaphors to describe prostheses, fit, and alignment. One of the professional patients at the prosthetics school, a young man who worked in construction, gave a funny running commentary one day on the practice prosthesis his student had just made him. As he paced back and forth between the parallel bars during critique, he described why he didn't like a certain new, lightweight prosthesis (which was interesting because lightness in a prosthesis is often equated with better quality). "It's like forks, you know? My normal leg, it's like a silver fork. It's solid. It's strong, sturdy, you can really feel it when you pick it up. But this thing," he waved the new leg dismissively, "just feels like a plastic fork. Like it might snap in half if I walked too hard on it." Upon completing his critique, the senior instructor took the opportunity to point out the importance of occupation (and implicitly, class as a factor influencing choice of occupation and physical activity level) as a consideration for prosthesis design.

This raises the issue of how to talk about feet. Longer-term amputees often compare different prosthetic feet using these metaphors, but this is largely a personal preference depending on many factors. While writing this essay, I realized that I've never actually had an extensive conversation with another long-term amputee about feet because we always speak in shorthand, metaphors, and nods. For example,

I've heard people refer to a type of foot called a SACH foot as "dead" or feeling "like a doorstop," and understood exactly what they meant: that the foot had no spring and rolled over with a particularly inactive feeling. I first became aware of the difficulty of describing what a foot should feel like while participating as a subject in an engineering experiment. Andy, one of the graduate students, was collecting data on the alignment of four different prosthetic feet for his M.S. thesis. Many trials were involved requiring me to walk on four very different feet, which Mark, the senior instructor at the prosthetics school, worked to align. Following the first trial, I wrote in my field notes that

> the Flex-Walk was intriguing, but not very appealing to me. It feels like a giant spring; I could feel it load and compress when I stepped onto the heel and then could feel it unload and propel me when I rolled over onto the toe. It didn't feel at all like a foot. This makes me think that the function and the sensation or experience of walking on a particular foot are two different things. The Flex-Foot is functionally attractive, but doesn't feel like a foot should feel, which I found disconcerting. Mark asked me if I felt like "the foot is walking me," and I said yes. It felt as though it were propelling me, and I felt compelled to walk faster. Part of this wasn't just the spring loading and unloading, but the very quick roll over.

I borrowed the Flex-Walk and learned how to use it for walking and bicycling. I grew to like it and, following the second trial, wrote in my notes that

> I also had a surprising reaction to the Flex-Walk this time: I liked it. I remember that I didn't like it last time because of the bounce, which was so severe that I felt a bit out of control of the foot. For whatever reason, the bounce wasn't that bad this time. In neutral, it did have a real strong kick to it, where my knee felt as though it were being pushed up and the foot kicked straight out when I was rolling off the toes. Apparently too much toe, but after Mark moved the knee and toed it out a bit, it felt pretty good. The bounce was nice and controllable, and worked together with a smooth roll-over to feel somewhat like a foot. Got some crazy compulsion to run on the thing and had a great time running in the halls and on E. Superior sidewalk. I can totally understand why athletes use Flex-Feet; it was amazingly easy to

run on. Sort of glided along on this very smooth foot with subtle heel and toe. After occasionally clomping along on my Carbon Copy 2, it was really fun. . . . My favorite overall would have to be the Flex-Foot, but how would I explain this turnaround in opinion? It definitely feels different from other prosthetic feet—I remember thinking this during the previous trials—and I think I was able to use that difference to my advantage this time rather than be annoyed by it. I didn't feel a distinct heel or keel or toe on it, whereas the other feet all have these identifiable foot characteristics. In some ways, it may be hard to judge as a prosthetic foot (e.g., there is no discernible keel).

At first, I had to resort to the concepts of spring from biomechanical engineers and roll over from gait analysis to describe how the foot felt. I was at a loss for embodied language except that it didn't feel like a foot and it felt external to me. After some practice and thought, I was able to describe how my body moved with the foot and why it didn't initially "feel like a foot should feel."

PERFORMING ALIGNMENT

Despite all these ways of talking about prostheses and how they feel, amputees are frequently rendered inarticulate about their prostheses. I have been in that position myself, and it is frustrating to walk back and forth, knowing that something just doesn't feel right, but not feeling able to describe what doesn't feel right. During one of my first days in the field, I observed a clinical interaction between Mr. Mitchell, a retired steel mill worker, and his prosthetist, Mark. Mr. Mitchell was actually Kevin's patient, but Mark was aligning him on his new prosthesis because Kevin was out of the shop. While Kevin is remarkably skilled in communicating with patients in lay terms, Mark deals with his patients much more clinically. The contrast was striking as he addressed Mr. Mitchell in clinical language while the latter responded in lay language about how his body felt. He felt the pressure in the back of the prosthesis was too tight, right where the shelf of the prosthesis presses against the gastrocnemius muscles, a key weight-bearing area. He couldn't pinpoint a problem but simply felt it was too tight, just a bit uncomfortable, and continued to pace back and forth between the parallel bars muttering to himself. Mark was uninterested in grinding out and irrevocably

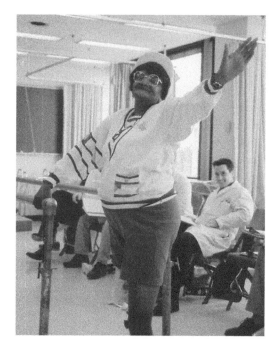

FIG. 8.4. Performing. Mrs. Hamill performing alignment for the prosthetics students during critique at the school. Photograph courtesy of the author.

loosening the socket so soon in the process, feeling that a new prosthesis was bound to feel a little snug. There was a stalemate in which Mr. Mitchell paced and muttered while Mark stood with his arms crossed. Though there was no mutually satisfactory resolution, Mr. Mitchell eventually agreed to give the prosthesis a spin in the outside world and return the following week.

Alignment and gait analysis are always performative, but even more so for inarticulate patients such as Mr. Mitchell. When the communicative performance of walking and analyzing gait break down, amputees and prosthetists utilize other means to perform alignment. One of these means is donning, using, and doffing the prosthesis. One day Bob and I went out on a house call to the home of Mr. Gambino, who was having difficulties donning his prosthesis (the same man mentioned earlier whose heart condition contraindicated his prosthesis). The first thing Bob did was have Mr. Gambino doff his prosthesis and then go through the process of donning it, standing and walking on it, and then doff it again. Bob noticed that because he failed to pull his stump deeply enough into the socket, the prosthesis wasn't totally secure. So he reviewed instructions on how to don it, and guided Mr. Gambino tactilely through the performance of donning his prosthesis correctly.

Another form of performance is much less conscious—on the amputee's part at least—and involves the prosthetist reading the amputee's body. Prosthetists read body language, facial expressions, and walking speed to gauge their patients' comfort with their alignment, and the color, texture, and temperature of skin on a stump to gauge socket fit. In an important sense, amputees' bodies perform and communicate through touch and without active intention.

TECHNOLOGIZATION

Prostheses are an important idiom for expressing emotions of loss, fright, and joy and negotiating issues such as body image, physical function, and the ability to live independently. Kleinman uses the concept of somatization to describe the use of bodies as an idiom for expressing personal, interpersonal, and social distress (Kleinman 1995). The analogous concept in the more biomechanical world of prosthetics is technologization, which describes how amputees and prosthetists use prosthetics technology as an idiom for expressing and dealing with personal and social distress. In fact, much of alignment and clinical interaction is about technologization, in which the prosthesis becomes a common ground for amputees and prosthetists to work through nontechnical issues.

An important factor in all of this is emotion. The majority of amputees I met in clinical situations were there for their first prosthesis, which meant they were also learning to walk again. This is an emotionally charged moment, especially for older amputees, many of whom, irrespective of amputation, have concerns about balance and stability and are afraid of falling. These concerns are exacerbated by the fact that they are essentially walking on stilts now. For example, Lance told me that walking was actually not the hard part for him, but getting his balance while standing—"getting his motor going," in his words. Once he started to walk, it became easier, but he still remained fearful.

Yet fright is often mixed with nervous excitement and joy. Mr. Konner, a patient of Don, was still fairly young but had a particularly brittle case of diabetes, which had led to bilateral below-knee amputations in his forties. He had spent an extensive postoperative recovery period in bed, and had recently started physical therapy. He was openly scared that he wouldn't be able to walk because it had been so long since he had been on his feet. Nervous, excited questions for me bubbled out of him as Don worked on his prostheses in the workshop. Do they leave the legs unfinished like they are now, or will they look more like real legs? When does it start to feel less weird and more comfortable? How long will it take to learn to drive a car again? Will I be able to walk up stairs again? Don sensed his nervousness and was firm with him, and commanded him to stand up and walk. As Mr. Konner stood and took his first steps, his face was beatific and beaming, and the electricity of his excitement at being able to walk was palpable in the room. Don was also pleased by the success, and I began to suspect that the thrill of enabling people to walk for the first time—again—is a powerful emotional draw for prosthetists.

Alignment and clinical interactions were highly emotional experiences for me, too. Prior to my fieldwork, I had forgotten how horribly uncomfortable prostheses are initially, how little sense it made to learn to adjust them, how alien they feel, and how disembodying it can be to try to pull a sock onto a foot that is no longer there during the first disoriented months following an amputation. Over the course of nearly a year and a half of fieldwork for my dissertation, I participated in dozens of these interactions and spent extensive periods of time with elders who had undergone recent amputations. I accompanied their prosthetist and dressed professionally, and fell into the role of "expert amputee." Nearly every day, I had to counter people's expectations for their prostheses by explaining to them that I walked relatively well because I was young enough to be their grandson and had had a decade of practice. I found this emotionally exhausting and frustrating. While many ethnographers face the classic challenge of how to get inside their field sites, I often faced the opposite challenge when working with other amputees: how to gain some distance from the outpouring of emotion.

Technologization is a syncretic mixture of somatization and medicalization. Somatization, borrowed from Kleinman, describes the use of bodies—and in this case, prostheses—as an important idiom for expressing individual and social distress. But prosthetics clinical interactions are also about the medicalization of amputation, and how distress becomes the object of treatment. It is not so much a dialogue, as it is a mode of communication about this experience that is expressed through verbal and physical performance. In a sense, technologization is about the embodied dialogue between the experience of prostheses and the observation of their biomechanical interaction with bodies, and how prosthetists and amputees communicate across this gap.

NOTES

Thank you to Katherine Ott, David Serlin, and Stephen Mihm for inviting me to participate in this volume, and to David for his editorial direction and patience. I am also grateful to Brendan Brisker, Nancy Chen, Tim Choy, and Cal Kurzman for reading earlier drafts of this essay, and to the U.C. Santa Cruz Anthropology Department for listening to and commenting on an earlier draft at a departmental colloquium. Support for my fieldwork was generously provided by the National Institute on Disability and Rehabilitation Research Mary E. Switzer Merit Fellowship H133F70011, Wenner-Gren Foundation for Anthropological Research Pre-Doctoral Grant 6235, and National Science Foundation Science and Technology Studies Doctoral Dissertation Research Improvement Grant 9710604.

1. Plantarflexing is bending your ankle to point your toes downwards, and dorsiflexing is pointing your toes upwards. Abduction and adduction are movements away from or toward a midline or reference point, respectively. Prosthetists frequently spell out the "ab" sound of abduction as "a-b-duction" to avoid confusion with the similar-sounding word "adduction."

2. There are actually a number of jokes in the field about whether amputee prosthetists are the best or worst prosthetists as a consequence of having had this experience. One opinion is that they are likely to be good out of empathy and the embodied knowledge that comes with wearing a prosthesis. The other side jokes that amputee prosthetists are horrible clinicians because they are jaded and don't communicate with or listen to their patients.

3. There is a subtle differentiation among prosthetists between practitioners and prosthetists. Practitioners are "old school," often having learned in apprenticeship or grown up working in their fathers' shops, while prosthetists are more academically trained. This also translates into a difference of emphasis on technical skill and craftsmanship versus theoretical knowledge and clinical skills, and a class division between working-class limb shops and more middle-class prosthetics clinics.

4. Prescriptions, which can be worded specifically or generally (e.g., left below-knee prosthesis), are de facto necessary for prostheses because third party payers require a prescription for reimbursement. Prescriptions also create a line of communication between prosthetists and doctors, and increasingly, a rehabilitation clinic team.

5. An endoskeletal prosthesis is an assemblage of the socket and connecting hardware, which may be covered with cosmetically shaped and colored foam and skin to resemble an organic limb. An exoskeletal prosthesis is a plastic shell incorporating the socket within the shell.

REFERENCES

Kleinman, A. 1995. *Writing at the Margin: Discourse between Anthropology and Medicine*. Berkeley: University of California Press.

Martin, E. 1994. *Flexible Bodies: Tracking Immunity in American Culture from the Days of Polio to the Age of AIDS*. Boston: Beacon Press.

Mauss, M. 1992. "Techniques of the Body." In J. Crary and S. Kwinter, eds., *Incorporations*. New York: Zone.

Scarry, E. 1985, *The Body in Pain: The Making and Unmaking of the World*. Oxford: Oxford University Press.

Schepper-Hughes, N., and M. M. Lock. 1987. "The Mindful Body: A Prolegomenon to Future Work in Medical Anthropology." *Medical Anthropology Quarterly* 1(1): 16–41.

PART III

USE AND REPRESENTATION

9

The Prosthetics of Management

Motion Study, Photography, and the Industrialized Body in World War I America

Elspeth Brown

I'D LIKE TO BEGIN with a familiar metaphor, first coined by Adam Smith and subsequently revised by many observers of business and economics. The metaphor is that of the "invisible hand," which Smith used to describe a capitalist market coherence driven by individual gain but resulting in common economic good.[1] Although this metaphor may have been persuasive to Smith's eighteenth-century mercantile audience, by the early twentieth century, social engineers and technocratic utopians began to reconsider the advisability of an "invisible" hand.[2] Rexford Tugwell, the Taylorite whom cultural historians remember for his role in fostering the Farm Security Administration's photography project, argued that Smith's invisible hand was a myth and that, instead, "a Taylor was needed for the economy as a whole." "The jig is up," he wrote. "The cat is out of the bag. There is no invisible hand. There never was. . . . instead, we must now supply a real and visible guiding hand to do the task."[3] To borrow the business historian Alfred Chandler's formulation, "the visible hand" of management would replace Smith's "invisible hand" of market forces.[4]

The visible hand of managerial reform, however, made the "hand," itself a synecdoche for the industrialized worker, increasingly invisible under scientific management, as the worker became abstracted as "the labor process" in the late nineteenth and early twentieth centuries.[5] As

managers sought to erase the worker and her "hands" from representation—visual, discursive, or political—they sought to insert themselves,
as engineers, efficiency experts, and industrial consultants, into the performance of work as the planners and publicizers of industry's managerial revolution.[6]

The question of the hand and its visibility under scientific management was an especially pressing one for the management consultant
Frank Gilbreth. Along with his wife, the industrial psychologist Dr. Lillian Gilbreth, Frank Gilbreth used photography and film to rationalize
industrial production both before and after World War I.[7] Motion study,
the umbrella name for their visually based technologies, enabled them
to analyze the precise trajectory of moving body parts, which in turn allowed them to redesign industrial work for increased efficiency. Although their consulting was primarily directed toward able-bodied
workers, during the war years the anxiety over "the problem of the crippled soldier" caused the Gilbreths to reassess not only motion study,
but also the assumptions underlying the relationship between the body
and the machine more generally. Their analysis of the human-machine
nexus led them to champion interchangeable prostheses, based on the
pioneering work of the French physiologist Dr. Jules Amar. Eventually,
however, the Gilbreths offered an alternative "American" approach to
human engineering, one that emphasized the redesign of work environments and machines over the design and use of artificial body parts.
In this formulation, motion study emerged as the key technology in analyzing the relationship between the individual and the workplace environment; managerial analysis, rather than artificial body parts, became the necessary "addition" for disabled veterans seeking reemployment after the war.

Like his onetime mentor Frederick Winslow Taylor, the "father of scientific management," Gilbreth shocked his middle-class family by donning overalls and pursuing an apprenticeship in the trades. He began as
a bricklayer, but by 1895 he had started his own contracting company,
eventually specializing in speedwork and running large-scale jobs
across the country.[8] Gilbreth's December 1907 introduction to Taylor
had a decisive impact on Gilbreth's career, as over the next several years
he introduced elements of Taylor's system to his construction jobs while
developing a very close relationship with Taylor and his management
ideas. At the same time, Gilbreth continued refining his own studies in

bricklaying efficiency, which—to carve out a market distinct from Taylor's "time study" and to sidestep labor opposition—Gilbreth had begun calling "motion study." By 1912, riding the wave of the era's popular efficiency craze, Gilbreth was ready to exploit the potentially universal applicability of motion study by starting his own consultancy business.[9]

Two threads mark Gilbreth's early work as a contractor: an increasing concern with system and efficiency in human motion, and a growing interest in the use of photographic technologies. Like many fellow Progressives, Gilbreth was infatuated with the promise that system and standardization offered for imposing order on what appeared to be an inefficient and disorderly world. The replacement of oral instructions with written rules, designed to be maintained uniformly despite local conditions, was part of a larger transformation toward "systematic management," which sought to replace the foremen's "rule of thumb" with uniform standards.[10] This shift toward system in managerial thought was in turn a response to what late-nineteenth-century industrialists saw as the high cost of American labor: if wages could not be effectively reduced, especially given the militancy of organized labor during these years, then perhaps costs could be reduced through what managers saw as more efficient production.[11] As the size of firms grew, managerial innovators in a number of industries turned their attentions toward appropriating craft knowledge, standardizing interchangeable parts, establishing an intensified division of labor, and coordinating the increasingly complex flow of goods and labor with newly developed instruction, routing, and accounting systems.[12] Systematic management emerged gradually over the years spanning the late nineteenth and early twentieth centuries, reconfiguring the way both goods and workers were organized in any number of industries and work sites.

Although Gilbreth, interested in system since his days as an apprentice, had institutionalized many aspects of systematic management in his contracting work, he did not turn his full attention to systematizing motion until he began construction on six brick buildings for the Atwood McManus Company, a massive wooden box factory, in 1909. As Gilbreth's business reputation was based on speedwork, the efficiency of the worker's motions in laying each brick became paramount. He analyzed the bricklayers' work, then codified these motions in a chart, delineating which motions were "right" and which were "wrong," noting on the chart which motions the bricklayer could omit; apprentices were to consult the chart and accompanying photographs to learn the correct method, and wages were tied to obedience.[13] Through this system, Gilbreth claimed to reduce the number of motions necessary to lay a brick from eighteen to four and a half while introducing an intensified division of labor; apprentices were expected to internalize these efficiencies by creating "charts representing their own motions."[14] The new use of scientific method, increasingly evident from 1909 forward, can be attributed to the increasing involvement of Lillian Gilbreth in both concept and analysis; she was responsible for much of the writing that appeared under Frank's name. Although her role in the photographic work was limited, it was her training in scientific method, as well as her superior writing ability, that provided scientific bedrock for some of her husband's more fanciful claims.[15]

Gilbreth's McManus job represented a shift not only in methods for laying bricks, but also in the possible role photography might play in generating efficiency in movement. In December 1908, Gilbreth began using the still camera to document each of a bricklayer's "right" motions, and organized these images into a sequence that told the story, Gilbreth hoped, of the body's efficiency.[16] Many of these images were later published in his 1909 book *Bricklaying System*, where they would serve the purpose of "teach[ing] apprentices that a brick can be laid with very few motions."[17] Gilbreth saw the bricklaying photographs as a beginning step in applying photography to work, writing in his 1908 diary, "Photographs of motions in all trades. Photographs of the right way and wrong way of doing it."[18] *Bricklaying System* represents Gilbreth's early foray into what would later expand into motion picture and chronophotographic technologies as methods of standardizing the motions of the working body.

The halftone illustrations in *Bricklaying System* represent what Gilbreth calls, for the first time, "actual motion studies," the visible hands (and usually only the hands) of bricklayers spreading mortar and laying bricks.[19] The first three images in figure 9.1, for example, show a bricklayer spreading mortar, cutting it off, and tapping down the brick. It is clear that Gilbreth is seeking to use the sequential arrangement of these still images to suggest a succession, in time, of the "right way" to lay bricks.

There are two ironies here, however, which suggest the tentative nature of Gilbreth's investigations at this point. First, these photographs, meant to teach apprentices the correct Gilbreth system, actually

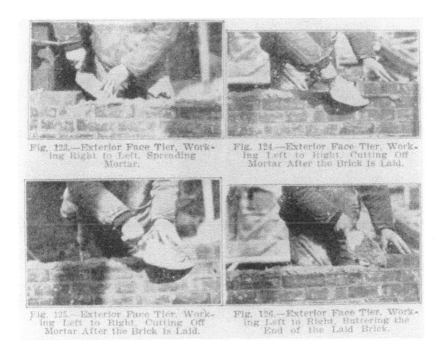

FIG. 9.1. From Frank Gilbreth, *Bricklaying System* (Easton: Hive, 1974 [1909]), 145.

show steps that Gilbreth sought to *omit*. In the chart that accompanies the images, Gilbreth lists these steps as operation no. 10 in "The Wrong Way," since "if the mortar is thrown from the trowel properly no spreading or cutting is necessary."[20] As it is difficult to photograph absence, lack, or omission, Gilbreth photographed excess—without, however, naming it as such in his caption. Second, the first three images here, representing the same worker at the same job with hands in similar but not identical poses, suggest a series, rather than a group—that is, the viewer is led to expect that the images depict one motion photographed over time and consecutively arranged.[21] Yet these halftone illustrations can only imperfectly convey the new series of motions required of apprentice bricklayers: not only are distinct steps in the process missing, but also who can say how much time has elapsed, or what has taken place, between the distinct frames? The cinematic imperative implied by a set of sequentially arranged images works against alternative interpretations for these images; we are not invited to speculate whether the worker had an extended lunch break or a work stoppage between exposures.[22] The still images and the static charts, while laying out a partial sequence of motions, are incapable of describing or prescribing the speed at which these discrete motions are performed. The photographs can only suggest a temporal continuity; they fail, ultimately, in documenting time or motion, the cornerstones of efficiency.

Nonetheless, these images represent a shift in Gilbreth's use of photography from a functional realism (where the image serves as an empirical substitute for the object, as a type of evidence) to an instrumental realism—in this case, using the realist promise of the photograph as truth to restructure the ways work is performed.[23] Here, Gilbreth shifts the role of his images from the generalized illustration of sites and buildings that pervades his earlier publications to a more specific focus on the human body in motion, with the goal of using these new images to intervene in the ways work is performed. Although his efforts here are tentative at best, his steps nonetheless suggest a new way for scientific managers to understand the relationship between visuality and the working body.

The corporeal logic underlying these bricklaying studies, however, suggests the extent to which Gilbreth's assumptions concerning efficiency and the body remained very much in step with Taylorist biases toward ideal bodies and "high-priced" man-machines. Gilbreth's work here is emphatically not with the physically disabled; masons without full use of their hands would not have been hired on any of these job sites. In restructuring the ways this highly skilled trade was performed, Gilbreth drained craft knowledge from workers while simultaneously positioning the manager as technological provider. Skill and brawn, mind and body had formerly worked together in the skilled work of bricklaying; Gilbreth divided these functions between worker and manager, with the manager providing the necessary knowledge to complete the job efficiently. The ideal of corporeal efficiency emerged as the new utopian standard; the camera and the manager became necessary additions, or prostheses, to the worker's radically delimited role.

Those familiar with the historiography of scientific management will recognize these years as marking a pitched battle between the Taylorites and organized labor. Recognizing that scientific management represented a radical appropriation of craft-based knowledge and control, workers and in some cases unions resisted its insidious encroachment throughout these years.[24] By 1911, when workers at the Watertown arsenal went out on strike over the issue of time study, the Taylor system—and, specifically, the practice of timing workers through the stopwatch—had become an issue of national visibility.[25] Organized labor succeeded in getting Congress to investigate the impact of the Taylor system on labor practices, and as a result, time study was banned in government installations.[26] By 1912, then, the stopwatch had become the contested symbol of an increasingly embattled scientific management movement. Gilbreth, recognizing the imbrication of the stopwatch with efficiency engineering, saw the camera as an opportunity to retain managerial prerogatives while convincing critics and workers that the Gilbreths were what he called "the good exception."[27]

For Gilbreth, motion study represented both a cost-controlling device and a means of distinguishing his management system in an ever more crowded field of competitors. In one of his early articles on the subject, Gilbreth joined a host of Progressive Era voices concerned about the prevalence of waste of American resources by arguing that workers' "needless, ill-directed and ineffective motions" represented one of the nation's great calamities.[28] Gilbreth compared the wasted labor represented by useless motions to the abuse of natural resources then consuming the attention of Progressive Era conservationists: as he argued, "while the waste from the soil washing to the sea is a slow but sure national calamity, it is of much less importance than the loss each year due to wasteful motions made by the workers of this country."[29] With this analogy, Gilbreth both allied himself with Progressive technocrats and rhetorically abstracted labor power from the human beings who produced it. Work was no longer subject to an individual worker's control and definition, but was instead an abstracted national resource threatened by waste and inefficiency. Workers became motors whose fuel was an abstracted form of labor power: "After all, a human being or a work animal is a power plant, and is subject to nearly all the laws that govern and limit the power plant."[30] Once Gilbreth had divorced labor from those who performed it, the motions made by workers could be objectified, analyzed, and standardized as simply another variable of the labor process.[31]

Although Gilbreth shared an enthusiasm widespread among engineers and managers for industrial standardization, his focus on the standardization of the "human element" through motion study (as opposed to the standardization of machine parts and products) was unique during these years. Through the analysis of individual motion, Gilbreth hoped to deduce a standard vocabulary of unchanging elements, which industrialists could craft into coherent and productive motive sentences. Since both good and bad habits were equally susceptible to what Gilbreth called "automaticity," correct training was necessary to ensure that the worker's "methods conform to standardized motions." Combinations of motions (or movement) could not be standardized, he argued, until the component parts, or motions, were each standardized individually; only then could they be strung together to create efficient, standardized combinations.[32] Gravity, the direction and path of motion, the relationship of the worker's body to necessary tools and materials, the role of inertia and momentum, and the relation between the ending of one motion and the beginning of the next (what Gilbreth, borrowing from billiards, called "play for position") were all factors influencing the efficiency of discrete motions.

Up through this period, however, Gilbreth's visual methodologies were rudimentary. As late as 1908 his initial explorations into what he was just beginning to call "motion study" made no reference to photographic technologies beyond the snapshot, relying instead on what the supervisor's eye could observe.[33] Gilbreth's opportunity to introduce more sophisticated visual technologies to an installation of scientific management came on May 13, 1912, when he signed a contract with the New England Butt Company, of Providence, Rhode Island. The company, which employed about three hundred workers, produced and assembled braiding machines for the manufacture of shoelaces, dress trimmings, and insulated wires. The contract represented Gilbreth's first as an independent management consultant, and marked his departure from the increasingly precarious construction business. Gilbreth's work with the company lasted about a year, and was marked by several overlapping stages: initial assessment and planning; the installation of industrial betterment elements as a means of securing employee cooperation; the preliminary introduction of an office efficiency system, again in the effort to defuse shop-floor suspicion of "Taylorist" managerial efforts; and the installation of a motion study laboratory, which the Gilbreths named the "Betterment Room."[34]

In the "Betterment Room," an experienced worker was chosen to perform a task, such as operate a drill press or assemble a machine, while speed and efficiency were recorded—usually simultaneously—by both stereographic and movie cameras.[35] With the motion picture camera the "micromotion expert" filmed the worker against a cross-sectioned background with two clocks in the viewfinder; the clocks, revolving at different speeds, allowed him to time motions to the thousandth of a second—what he later called "winks." The film enabled the motion study analyst to isolate and analyze the efficiency of individual motions through an analysis of the time (provided via the clocks as well as the speed of the camera) and through distance (provided through the cross-screened background). With the film, or "micromotion study," the efficiency engineer could examine the "minutiae of motions and the consequent resulting inventions from the synthesis of such selected subdivided motions."[36]

The purpose of these films was initially a replacement for stopwatch study: with the motion picture camera, Gilbreth argued, an observer could more "scientifically" analyze the work with the goal of setting times for discrete tasks, since the camera—running continuously throughout several cycles of repetitive motion—"objectively" recorded both the beginnings and endings of work cycles. The camera could "automatically" record wasteful movements, and "will detect instantly any attempt on the part of workmen to defeat time-study by soldiering, for while a workman may deceive a time-study man, he cannot deceive the camera."[37] Gilbreth relied on the realist promise of the photographic technology—the belief that the camera offered an unmediated access to an observable reality—to argue that the camera, not the motion study expert, timed and recorded the work process: the photographic record provided "indisputable evidence" of motion efficiency. In this analysis, Gilbreth presented his team as disinterested professionals utilizing a neutral technology to further the goals of both business and labor. They were not, as International Workers of the World organizers no doubt argued when they sought (unsuccessfully) to organize the New England Butt Company workers in August 1912, working against the interests of labor on behalf of management.[38]

Filming provided the efficiency expert and apprentice worker with most of the required visual data necessary to learn the Gilbreths' new sequence of industrialized motions, but film could not readily provide these data in three dimensions, nor could film represent, within one image, a continuous path of motion through space. In addition to slowing down the film, editing it into repeated motion cycle loops, examining it under a microscope, or projecting and therefore enlarging the image (all of which Gilbreth did with his motion films), Gilbreth sought an image that could capture the passage of time and the movement through space on a single, lengthy exposure.

The Gilbreths succeeded in their efforts in April 1913, when Gilbreth's micromotion specialist S. Edgar Whitaker successfully reported what was originally called the "orbit method" of motion study, later called the "cyclegraph."[39] Producing a cyclegraph involved attaching a mini electric light to the worker's moving body part (usually the hand and sometimes the head), and then photographing the worker while he or she performed the assigned task, using a long exposure (fig. 9.2). The result was an abstraction of movement through space where, as figure 9.2 demonstrates, the worker—as well as the hand—has become invisible, replaced by the hand's ghostly trace.[40] The following week, Whitaker reported that he had successfully interrupted the light's electric current, creating intermittent pulsations that could vary between 100 and 1,000 per minute.[41] The flashes were recorded as parsnip-shaped dashes which, when photographed against a cross-screened background, promised to map direction of movement as well as time.[42] The new dotted-line images Gilbreth called "chronocyclegraphs," as they represented time as well as motion. When motion cycles were photographed with a stereographic camera, as was usually the case so that worker and manager could see the depicted motion in three dimensions, the resulting document was called a "stereochronocyclegraph"; most of the time, however, the Gilbreths used the term "chronocyclegraph."[43]

Gilbreth began the cyclegraphic work with drill press operations, but almost immediately introduced the technology at a new contract with Hermann, Aukam, a New Jersey handkerchief manufacturer. And as he had argued with his work at the New England Butt Company, conducted at roughly the same time, the "chronocyclegraph" mapped inefficiency through a jerky, frenetic line, whereas the path of motion of an expert folder, using Gilbreth's standard motions, would be smooth. Gilbreth liked to use the example of handkerchief folding as a showcase for his motion study work since, he argued, "it is purely a case of reformed and selected motions. It has no belting to adjust; there is no case of standardizing machinery so that it will not break down." Instead, the workers themselves became standardized: as Gilbreth claimed, "another fine feature of this motion study is the benefits we obtain by having all operators habitually think in elementary motions."[44]

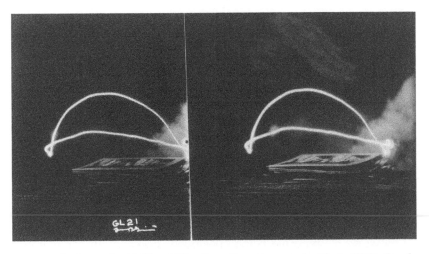

FIG. 9.2. Cyclegraph of Lillian Gilbreth sorting stereocards. Photo GL21, Frank and Lillian Gilbreth Collection, Purdue University Libraries Special Collections and Archives, N file 12/0031–19 (from the first cyclegraphs series).

An image, for example, depicting ten cycles of an expert folder is understandable only because Gilbreth, in his presentations and correspondence, deciphered the image for us. It seems unlikely that a careful observer would be able to detect ten distinct cycles of motion from the image alone, or that one would be able to detect time: counting individual dots and dashes with any accuracy is an impossibility, given the fact that the motions of an "expert" folder are meant to closely follow each other in space, thereby rendering each individual motion path less than distinct. The result of ten cycles of motion photographed on a single photographic plate was what Gilbreth, in his more conversational moments, jokingly referred to as a "plate of macaroni." Gilbreth's genius was his showmanlike ability to present these cyclegraphs as both photographic pasta and scientific documents, inviting the skepticism of a "humbug" only to win over his audiences through his mastery of the photographic sublime.[45] Gilbreth's introduction of moving pictures and photography to industrial efficiency was a public relations coup. His fledgling business, as yet dependent on Taylor without, however, Taylor's imprimatur as an approved installer of the "Taylor system," was a fragile enterprise; the use of the still and motion picture camera provided a way for Gilbreth to distinguish his work in the mushrooming field of efficiency engineers, a field increasingly marked by "charlatans, quacks and fakers."[46]

By January 1914, Gilbreth left day-to-day work at both New England Butt and Hermann, Aukam to pursue another, more lucrative, contract in Berlin.[47] Gilbreth's work in Berlin at the beginning of the war, well before the U.S. entry in April 1917, provided him with ample opportunity to observe the physical devastation wrought by the conflict. His surgery motion study work was taking him into German hospitals, where he saw "such terrible things you never heard of or could imagine," including amputations, infected wounds, and other evidence of the war's carnage.[48] His reaction is an odd mix of sincere horror and gleeful recognition of a unique business angle for his motion study work. He reported being "positively sickened" by the war and thought that a film showing a Bridgeport ammunition manufacturer, followed by images of operations and wound dressing, would make a "great hit."[49] Yet his outrage complemented his recognition that, in his opinion, the work on crippled soldiers represented the "greatest subject" he had ever had—"sob-stuff" that held his audience "spellbound."[50]

Gilbreth's drive to industrialize the movements of the working body converged with his public relations savvy in October 1915, when, while working in Germany, he developed a new motion study technology, which he promoted under the guise of rehabilitating the disabled soldier. The "simultaneous cycle motion chart," which Gilbreth presented to the public in October 1915, graphically displayed "the interrelation of the individual motions used in any method of performing any piece of work."[51] The chart required the isolation of individual motions that could be identified and charted, in their varying sequences, in relationship to time. With the "SIMO" chart, Gilbreth introduced these foundational motions, which he argued provided the basis of all work-related movement. The October 1915 list contained sixteen components: (1) search; (2) find; (3) select; (4) grasp; (5) position; (6) assemble; (7) use; (8) dissemble, or take apart; (9) inspect; (10) transport, loaded; (11) pre-position for next operation; (12) release load; (13) transport, empty; (14) wait (unavoidable delay); (15) wait (avoidable delay); (16) rest (for overcoming fatigue).[52] These foundational elements, later called "therbligs," a near anagram for Gilbreth, could be reconfigured into increasingly efficient combinations. They were assigned their own

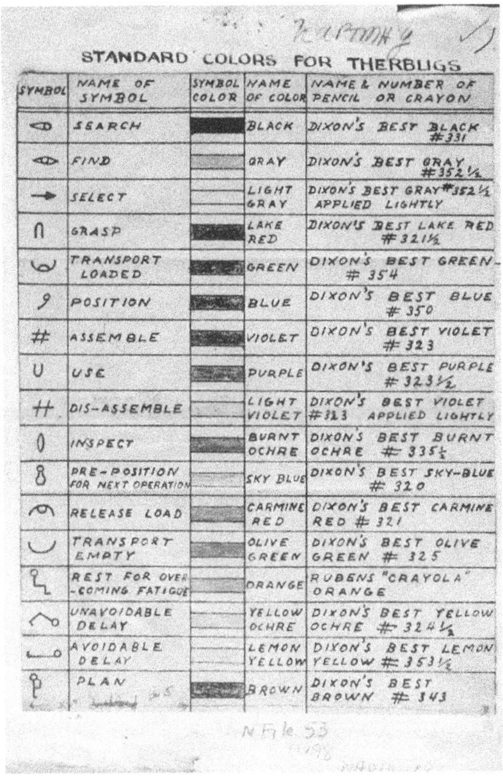

SYMBOL	NAME OF SYMBOL	SYMBOL COLOR	NAME OF COLOR	NAME & NUMBER OF PENCIL OR CRAYON
⊂D	SEARCH	⬛	BLACK	DIXON'S BEST BLACK #331
⊂D	FIND	▨	GRAY	DIXON'S BEST GRAY #352½
➔	SELECT		LIGHT GRAY	DIXON'S BEST GRAY #352½ APPLIED LIGHTLY
∩	GRASP	▨	LAKE RED	DIXON'S BEST LAKE RED #321½
∽	TRANSPORT LOADED	▨	GREEN	DIXON'S BEST GREEN #354
9	POSITION	▨	BLUE	DIXON'S BEST BLUE #350
#	ASSEMBLE	▨	VIOLET	DIXON'S BEST VIOLET #323
U	USE	▨	PURPLE	DIXON'S BEST PURPLE #323½
⫲	DIS-ASSEMBLE		LIGHT VIOLET	DIXON'S BEST VIOLET #323 APPLIED LIGHTLY
0	INSPECT		BURNT OCHRE	DIXON'S BEST BURNT OCHRE #335½
8	PRE-POSITION FOR NEXT OPERATION		SKY BLUE	DIXON'S BEST SKY-BLUE #320
⌒	RELEASE LOAD		CARMINE RED	DIXON'S BEST CARMINE RED #321
∪	TRANSPORT EMPTY	▨	OLIVE GREEN	DIXON'S BEST OLIVE GREEN #325
⌇	REST FOR OVER-COMING FATIGUE		ORANGE	RUBENS "CRAYOLA" ORANGE
⌒o	UNAVOIDABLE DELAY		YELLOW OCHRE	DIXON'S BEST YELLOW OCHRE #324½
⌐o	AVOIDABLE DELAY		LEMON YELLOW	DIXON'S BEST LEMON YELLOW #353½
φ	PLAN	▨	BROWN	DIXON'S BEST BROWN #343

FIG. 9.3. Therblig chart. Frank and Lillian Gilbreth Collection, Purdue University Libraries Special Collections and Archives, N file 53/0298.

standard color (matching those used in the SIMO chart) and symbol (which Gilbreth called a "hieroglyph") (fig. 9.3).[53]

Once Gilbreth had filmed a particular work cycle, he could then run the film slowly enough to isolate the individual "therbligs," which were then transferred to the SIMO chart (fig. 9.4). The chart was a means of visualizing the motions used for any type of work: the horizontal lines, reading from the top down, represent time, while the vertical spaces are divided into anatomical groups, such as right arm, with subgroups, such as wrists, thumb, and so forth. This anatomical map showed, Gilbreth argued, "which members of the human body are doing the work, [and which] are inefficiently occupied" during the performance of any task.[54]

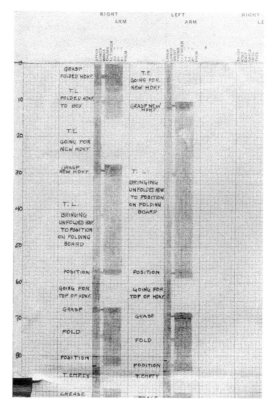

FIG. 9.4. SIMO chart of handkerchief folding. Frank and Lillian Gilbreth Collection, Purdue University Libraries Special Collections and Archives, N File 52/0297–5.

Just as Taylor introduced work functionalization to the industrial workplace by breaking down skilled work into component tasks, which he then reassigned to lower-paid workers, Gilbreth introduced work functionalization to the body itself. With the SIMO chart, Gilbreth could see at a diachronic glance evidence of soldiering limbs, and he reassigned tasks accordingly in order to make full use of the working body. With all limbs working to full capacity, he argued, the method of least waste would result, one best fitted to become the standard method. The standard method, in turn, would result in the least fatigue for the worker, as well as the greatest prosperity, he argued, for both worker and employer.[55]

Of course, for these returning veterans, soldiering limbs were often a result of absenteeism: over 247,000 Americans were eventually disabled during the war, and a large percentage of these disabilities were a result of loss of limb.[56] In a brilliant public relations move, Gilbreth introduced and popularized his SIMO charts, arguably the apotheosis of his efforts to industrialize the working body, initially only in the context of his work on behalf of disabled war veterans. By tying discussions of corporeal efficiency to an international concern for what was widely known as the "crippled soldier problem," Gilbreth invited—and received—unprecedented positive publicity for his motion study work. At a time when scientific management's reputation had been seriously undermined by years of sustained critique on the part of organized labor, Gilbreth effectively outflanked his critics by wrapping motion study in the patriotic flag of war hero rehabilitation.

Gilbreth's goal was to use motion study technologies, including film, photography, motion models, and SIMO charts, to reintroduce disabled veterans to productive employment after their release from convalescent hospitals. The SIMO chart, he argued, enabled the rehabilitation specialist to see, in graphic terms, which limbs were necessary for any given task; using such charts, the human engineer could reassign motions to accommodate the worker's disability. His plan was international in scope, both because he found a more sympathetic audience in Canada and Europe in the years before U.S. involvement, and because he sought to sell complete motion study outfits to hospitals, vocational therapists, and occupational therapists for $1,000 each.[57] His public discussions of the need to "solve the crippled soldier problem" quickly developed into a standard set of formulaic elements.

Gender, especially the perceived problematic masculinity of the disabled veteran, emerged as a key concern for most commentators on the topic, including Gilbreth. For many contemporary observers, the possibility of the veteran's economic dependence on the state or on his family threatened to undermine the veteran's masculinity, as manliness has been consolidated, in large part, around the role of the male breadwinner.[58] "The sudden drop from the strenuous life at the front to the inactivity of the hospital" appeared to threaten the soldier's masculinity both because the wounded veteran no longer retained the "fighting spirit of the trench" and because his disability prevented him from returning to "productive life."[59] Furthermore, the war years also saw the height of woman suffrage activism in the United States, especially after

Wilson's reelection in 1916: both the National American Woman Suffrage Association's (NAWSA) lobbying work and the direct action militarism of the National Woman's Party pointedly called into question contemporary definitions of American masculinity—in this case the assumed relationship between manhood and the vote. Battlefront disabilities combined with homefront suffrage activism engendered a "crisis of masculinity" in the wake of World War I, a crisis encapsulated by the "problem of the crippled soldier."

In his writings and lectures on behalf of the war-disabled, Gilbreth addressed these gendered anxieties to brilliant effect. Unlike many of the professionals whose rhetoric dripped with saccharine condescension for the "poor veteran," Gilbreth positioned himself as the veterans' manly champion, a fellow cripple disdainful of the rehabilitation experts' feminizing concern. "No man with red blood in his veins, no matter how disabled he may be, who has ever taken a man's part in the world's work is satisfied to become a national charge," is the declaration with which he opened one of his numerous lectures.[60] In other discussions, Gilbreth attacked the occupations that were being taught to disabled veterans during their rehabilitation. Many of those in charge of retraining veterans in the wake of the war were women who, Gilbreth claimed, taught only those occupations that they themselves knew best. "As the result," he argued, "many a strong hardy man became a weaver of baskets, a maker of toys, or a worker at some other feminine occupation."[61] Gilbreth advocated retraining for more manly pursuits—muscular work that could be commended as "a 'man's job,' the work of a producer, economically necessary, and therefore satisfying the social sense of the worker."[62] Paradoxically, the limited rehabilitation work Gilbreth documented features the disabled veterans in jobs that had, by this period, become predominantly female, including typing, retail sales, and a new job that Gilbreth tirelessly advocated in the cause of efficiency, that of the dental hygienist.[63]

Gilbreth needed to critique his contemporaries' pedagogical practices for two reasons. First, the way he wanted to make money was not by retraining the veterans himself, but by training the teachers of the disabled. In order to outfit convalescent hospitals with motion study equipment, he needed to argue that current vocational training was inadequate; exacerbating contemporary anxieties about the veterans' masculinity and then presenting himself as the instrument of remasculinization through providing more manly occupations was an effective rhetorical strategy. Second, Gilbreth sought to introduce motion study as a scientific technology, one that would make evident new occupations for the disabled. While claiming a role for motion study in determining appropriate occupations for the disabled, however, the Gilbreths argued that the technology had limitless applications. This flexibility was not so much due to the technology as it was to the continuity in the study subjects. "When we come to consider the subject closely we see that every one of us is in some way a cripple, either through being actually maimed or through having some power or faculty which has not been developed or used to its fullest extent." From an efficiency standpoint, any impediment to what the Gilbreths now called "the one best way to do work" represented a handicap of some sort, whether the disability was a corn on a policeman's foot or a typist's missing legs. "We can, then, think of every member of the community as having been a cripple, as being a cripple, or as a potential cripple."[64] With such a flexible definition of the disabled, the Gilbreths effectively collapsed the rhetorical distance that gives rise to the helping professions' pitying condescension toward the wounded veteran, while at the same time constructing a motion study audience limited only by the size of the industrialized world's adult population.[65]

Photography played an important publicity role in the Gilbreths' work with disabled soldiers. The first step in furnishing "real work to the cripple," the Gilbreths argued, was to illustrate, photographically, work currently being done by the disabled, or even work that looked *as if* it were being performed by crippled persons. Albert Jay Nock, the editor of *American Magazine*, who also circulated the Gilbreths' work in this area to *Scribner's* and *Scientific American*, was explicit on this point: "It is not important that the pictures be of actually crippled persons; the thing is to convey as strikingly as possible, a clear idea of what can be accomplished with cripples," wrote Nock.[66] He wrote the Gilbreths with an explicit shooting script: "What I want is this: Take a well man and make him simulate a cripple. Then take photographs of him showing just what you would do if he has lost a hand, and you are testing him out for certain work under this disability." "If you will just come through with illustrative photographs of the proper sort, for a popular magazine," he urged, "I will be able to get you very good publicity."

The Gilbreths responded with a series of photographs that imaged the "disabled" at work. Since the photographs were intended as a type of motivational image, designed to suggest the "possibilities and the

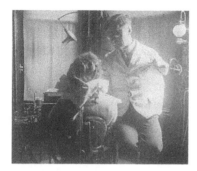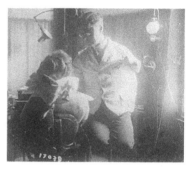

FIG. 9.5. Photo 17039, National Museum of American History, History of Technology, Gilbreth Collection, NMAH 318949.0654.

advantages of working," a photograph that featured an able-bodied person simulating a handicap had important pedagogical value. Figure 9.5, for example, shows what appears to be a disabled dentist working on a patient. A closer examination of the dentist's white coat, however, suggests the bulkiness of a stowaway limb. Indeed, Lillian Gilbreth's private correspondence concerning this image makes no attempt to pass it off as photographic evidence in the documentary sense: "one-eyed, one-armed, legless dentist engaged in cleaning the teeth. The subject of this slide is a well-known dentist who allowed himself to be crippled as seen in order to demonstrate that cleaning the teeth can be done with one hand and chiefly through the sense of touch."[67] As it doesn't appear that the Gilbreths actually worked with very many of the disabled themselves, simulating the disabled through photography became important if Nock's illustrations were to be provided.

Here, although photography's role is to provide visual inspiration rather than documentary evidence, the interpretive habit of seeing the photographic image as an index to a past "fact" adds evidentiary weight to what is, essentially, a publicity still, advertising new work possibilities for both the disabled and for Gilbreth, Inc. These early publicity photographs traffic in the interpretive habits of documentary realism, which explains their effectiveness, but their staged quality works against a documentary interpretation. Historically and aesthetically, they inhabit the liminal space between the social documentary rhetoric of early-twentieth-century reform photography and the capitalist realism of *Fortune* magazine photography in the late 1920s.[68] At the time, however, because of the effectiveness of photographic realism as an evidentiary tool in both magazine journalism and social reform movements, these Gilbreth images would most certainly have been understood as documentary evidence of the disabled at work. Regardless of the Gilbreths' intentions in producing the images, then, their publicity force stemmed in part from their *misreading* as documentary.

Once motion study had identified appropriate work for the disabled, the next step required "adjusting the cripple to the work." The fit between the disabled worker and the job could be approached from several directions. One approach was to understand the workplace as a standardized element not amenable to redesign or change, and to create prosthetic devices that would help the disabled veteran interact with this environment. One would expect American industrial engineers, reared on the gospel of workplace standardization, to pursue this approach. Surprisingly, however, despite their own emphasis on the standardization of the work environment, the Gilbreths eventually championed an alternative method, one that emphasized adaptation of the workplace, especially machinery, to the disabled worker's needs. The Gilbreths preferred to see the disabled worker (rather than the environment) as the "fixed element," around whom mechanical devices or machines would be adjusted in order to accommodate specific disabilities. They argued for the role of motion study in discovering exactly what motions are required to perform the activity, and then determining which of these motions managers could reassign or eliminate by altering the machine itself. The approach, innovative in its emphasis on environment over disability, was also designed to emphasize their motion study technologies, whose focus lay in the relationship between the individual body and its workplace environment.

The Gilbreths had been interested in the relationship between the worker and the surrounding environment since at least the early 1910s, stemming in part from Lillian Gilbreth's work on fatigue, and further energized by the Gilbreths' extensive familiarity with the European-based "science of work." As Anson Rabinbach has shown, an international scientific community of physiologists, physicians, and reformers had been engaged in understanding the physiology of labor power as a means of increasing industrial productivity while eliminating class conflict. Worker fatigue marked the limits of this utopian promise, and after 1890 a generation of European scientists sought to understand fatigue's physiological, ergonomical, and psychological causes. But whereas physiologists studied the human motor in the laboratory, the Gilbreths were the first Americans to consider the relationship of the body to the environment in the workplace—what became known after World War II as the field of "ergonomics."[69] Standardization of the work environment as well as of the body's working motions, the Gilbreths argued, reduced fatigue, positively affecting workers' moods, and therefore productivity. The Gilbreths redesigned stools, chairs, and footrests in order to reduce worker fatigue; they added springs, for example, to chair legs as a means of absorbing the vibrations caused by working machinery, and introduced adjustable-height stools to workers who had formerly been expected to stand at their workstations. One of the Gilbreths' many projects while working in Providence, Rhode Island, was to establish a "Museum of Devices for the Elimination of Unnecessary Fatigue," where they collected objects designed to reduce worker fatigue (mostly of their own design).[70] The museum never got off the ground in any serious way (in late 1914 the museum had six devices, mostly chairs, four of which the Gilbreths had designed), but the "museum" enabled the Gilbreths to publicize their interest in what progressive post-Taylor managers were increasingly calling the "human element" in production.[71]

When considering the plight of the war-disabled, the Gilbreths reintroduced their concern with the worker's environment to consider the ways it could be adjusted to meet the needs of the disabled. One of their most frequently used examples was provided by Mr. Casey, the "one-armed secretary" to the mayor of Boston. At the time the Gilbreths were introduced to Casey, he had already altered his typewriter by inventing devices to insert paper and to activate the shift key with a foot pedal. The Gilbreths elaborated on Casey's innovations by inventing an elaborate paper roller (thus eradicating the need to change paper), as well as advocating the use of a carbon ribbon and a double bank of keys (eliminating the necessity for the shift key) (fig. 9.6). Although it can be argued that Casey seemed perfectly able to accomplish his work through his own inventiveness prior to motion study, the Gilbreths nonetheless argued that motion study was still a necessity: "it is only through [motion and fatigue study] that one is able to classify completely the motions involved, and to discover which ones of these can be handed over to available, securable, or inventable devices."[72] Pho-

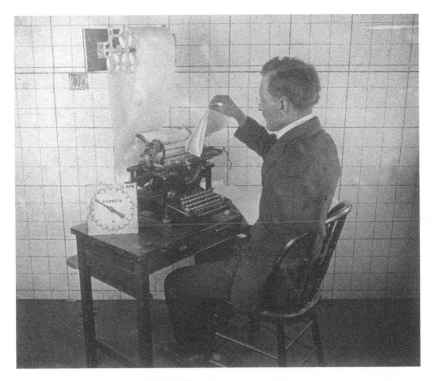

FIG. 9.6. Image 16269, National Museum of American History, History of Technology, Gilbreth Collection, NMAH 318949.0068.

tographs of Casey being motion-studied took their place alongside a series of related images of the disabled at work and were circulated throughout the periodical press, lectures, personal correspondence, and academic conferences. Through this photographic publicity, Gilbreth successfully fueled public concern for the disabled, as well as generated "personal publicity that will furnish jobs" for Gilbreth, Inc.[73]

The Gilbreths contrasted their approach of "adjusting the work to the cripple" to that of the French physiologist Dr. Jules Amar, who preferred the use of prostheses in reintroducing the disabled veteran or industrial worker to salaried employment. Whereas Gilbreth's approach entailed "adapting methods and devices to the cripple," Amar "adapted the cripple to existing methods and devices" (fig. 9.7).[74] Amar not only emphasized providing artificial limbs to the disabled,

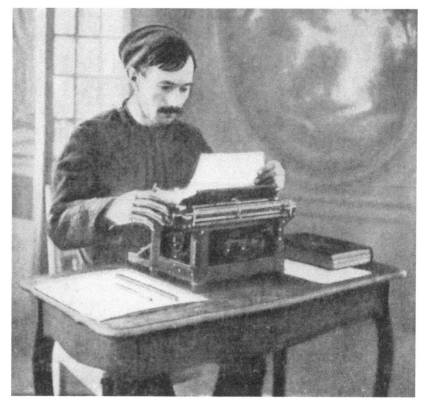

FIG. 9.7. From Jules Amar, *The Physiology of Industrial Organization and the Re-Employment of the Disabled*, trans. Bernard Miall (New York: Macmillan, 1919), 302.

but also invented an artificial "work arm" with a chuck, into which interchangeable hands or tools (for example, a file for work and an aesthetically pleasing hand for leisure) could be inserted.[75] For Amar, as for Gilbreth, the issue was not so much one of missing limbs as of missing functions, and his solution was to provide what the Gilbreths called "supplementary limbs," which could most effectively simulate missing functions such as grasp. The utility of such devices and the urgency of returning the disabled to productive employment outweighed any customary aesthetic considerations; the authors of one article, describing the special work appliances that could be fitted to an arm stump, declared that "drawing room considerations must be abandoned" in order to restore "the armless to a place in the industrial world."[76]

Frank Gilbreth was very much taken with Amar's approach, writing to Lillian Gilbreth, "I am glad that you appreciated the possibilities of the *re-design* as well as the re-education of the cripple. By making mechanical additions to his four *missing* or *present* or replaced limbs we can have a soldier with 10 limbs, adjustable, removable, replaceable, for special uses. A new line of possibilities without end for the crippled heroes."[77] This idea is clearly Amar's, and though the Gilbreths toyed with promoting replaceable limbs designed to accomplish specific work-related functions, in the end they advocated the "American" approach of redesigning machinery rather than artificial limbs. Their argument here was that since most artificial limbs and machinery were designed and built in the United States, Americans were better positioned to redesign machinery in order to accommodate the disabled veterans' special needs. The prosthetics, or additions, that the Gilbreths advocated were not limited to the material culture of artificial limbs. Instead, they argued for an environmental prosthetics, which required the adjustment of the environment to the needs of the worker. In this rarely heeded demand, the Gilbreths anticipated the call for "universal design" by some seventy years.[78]

There is no evidence that the Gilbreths did much work besides the rhetorical with the disabled during Frank's lifetime; the few examples that mark their work before Frank Gilbreth's death in 1924 represent disabled workers whom the Gilbreths came across in the course of their general motion study contracts, and most of these few disabled workers were not war-disabled.[79] The Gilbreths' efforts to industrialize the working body through motion study had both utopian and dystopic implications. If the visual analysis of the war-disabled promised a valorous return to productive life, it was as a human machine within industrial capitalism, a "hand" in an increasingly rationalized labor force. The visual technologies of motion study rendered the worker invisible while rendering Frank Gilbreth the increasingly "visible hand" of planning. As part of this visualizing process, what had been the visual hand of the laborer became the abstract trace of movement through space, a shift that metaphorically marks the transformation of labor during this period—at least from the perspective of scientific managers. If we were to return to the Greek etymology of "prosthesis" as "addition," we can

understand the Gilbreths' motion study as itself a prosthesis, a technological addition that replaced workers' control and craft knowledge
with the mind of management.

NOTES

I would like to thank Peter Liebhold, National Museum of American History,
Smithsonian Institution, for his considerable help with my investigation into
the Gilbreths' motion study work. Many thanks as well to Lillian Gilbreth's biographer, Jane Lancaster.

1. Smith, *Wealth of Nations* (New York: Modern Library, 1937), 423.

2. Frederick Taylor, for example, argued that "There was no 'invisible
hand' in the factory to bring order out of the complexity. This order was to be
discovered and realized by the systematizer." Taylor, *Principles of Scientific Management* (New York: Norton, 1967), 86, 140–41.

3. Tugwell, *The Battle for Democracy* (1935), 14, 245, quoted in John M. Jor-
dan, *Machine-Age Ideology: Social Engineering and American Democracy* (Chapel
Hill: University of North Carolina Press, 1994), 250. For a discussion of Tug-
well's relationship to the RSA/FSA photographic project, see Maren Stange,
Symbols of Ideal Life: Social Documentary Photography in America, 1890–1950 (New
York: Cambridge University Press, 1989), 89–133.

4. Chandler, *The Visible Hand: The Managerial Revolution in American Business* (Cambridge, MA: Belknap Press, 1977).

5. David Roediger, *The Wages of Whiteness: Race and the Making of the American Working Class* (New York: Verso, 1991), 43–64.

6. For the relationship between union representation and scientific management, see Robert Hoxie, *Scientific Management and Labor* (New York: D. Appleton [1915], 1921) as well as Milton Nadworny, *Scientific Management and the
Unions* (Cambridge: Harvard University Press, 1955); see also David Montgomery, *Workers' Control in America: Studies in the History of Work, Technology, and
Labor Struggles* (New York: Cambridge University Press, 1978).

7. Lillian Gilbreth's important career is beyond the scope of this discussion. She had a tremendous influence on her husband's work, especially concerning management questions, but was not as centrally involved with the photographing and filming of work. For more information about Lillian, see Sherry
E. Sullivan, "Management's Unsung Theorist: An Examination of the Works of
Lillian M. Gilbreth," *Biography: An Interdisciplinary Quarterly* 18, no. 1 (winter
1995): 31–41; Laurel Graham, *Managing on Her Own: Dr. Lillian Gilbreth and
Women's Work in the Interwar Era* (Norcross, GA: Engineering and Management
Press, 1998); and Jane Lancaster, "Wasn't She the Mother in *Cheaper by the Dozen*:

The Life of Dr. Lillian Moller Gilbreth, 1878–1972" (Ph.D. diss., Brown University, 1998).

8. Lillian Gilbreth, *The Quest of the One Best Way: A Sketch of the Life of Frank Bunker Gilbreth* (New York: Society of Industrial Engineers, 1925), 19–27; Edna Yost, *Frank and Lillian Gilbreth: Partners for Life* (New Brunswick: Rutgers University Press, 1949), 57–155.

9. Price, "One Best Way: Frank and Lillian Gilbreth's Transformation of Scientific Management, 1885–1940" (Ph.D. diss., Purdue University, 1987), 91. For a discussion of the pervasive appeal of efficiency in American culture more broadly during these years, see Cecilia Tichi, *Shifting Gears: Technology, Literature, Culture in Modernist America* (Chapel Hill: University of North Carolina Press, 1987); Martha Banta, *Taylorized Lives: Narrative Productions in the Age of Taylor, Veblen, and Ford* (Berkeley: University of California Press, 1993); Mark Seltzer, *Bodies and Machines* (New York: Routledge, 1992); and Samuel Haber, *Efficiency and Uplift: Scientific Management in the Progressive Era, 1890–1920* (Chicago: University of Chicago Press, 1964).

10. See Joseph A. Litterer, "Systematic Management: The Search for Order and Integration," *Business History Review* 35 (winter 1961): 461–77, as well as his "Systematic Management: Design for Organizational Recoupling in American Manufacturing Firms," *Business History Review* 37, no. 4 (winter 1963): 369–92.

11. "Efficiency," as a term, was hardly value-neutral; what is possible is not necessarily the same as what is desirable, and the conflict over the two was at the core of labor opposition to scientific management during these years. On this point, see Hugh Aitkin, *Taylorism at Watertown Arsenal* (Cambridge: Harvard University Press, 1960), 20–21.

12. Daniel Nelson, *Managers and Workers: Origins of the Twentieth-Century Factory System in the United States, 1880–1920*, 2d ed. (Madison: University of Wisconsin Press, 1995), 46–51, as well as his "Scientific Management, Systematic Management, and Labor, 1880–1915," *Business History Review* 48 (winter 1974): 480. See also David A. Hounshell, *From the American System to Mass Production, 1800–1932: The Development of Manufacturing Technology in the United States* (Baltimore: Johns Hopkins University Press, 1984). For a discussion of this transformation from the perspective of labor and management relations, see David Montgomery, *The Fall of the House of Labor: The Workplace, the State, and American Labor Activism, 1865–1925* (New York: Cambridge University Press, 1991), 9–58, 214–57.

13. Gilbreth had his own version of Taylor's differential piece rate, tied to the workers' adherence to Gilbreth's bricklaying methods. Those who followed the system received a "substantial increase over the minimum rate of pay"; those who could partly do it received "more money than the minimum rate"; those who made a good faith effort at the system but were nonetheless unable to learn it received minimum wage, while those who refused even a good faith

effort would not be hired on the job, unless no other bricklayers were available. Frank Gilbreth, *Bricklaying System* (Easton: Hive, 1974 [1909]), 142–43.

14. Ibid., 140–64. "At times individual records at the rate of 3,000 brick were made, and on the last two days of the contract the entire bricklaying gang averaged 2,600 bricks per day per man." L. W. Peck, "A High Record in Bricklaying Attained by Novel Methods," *Engineering News* 62 (August 5, 1909): 152.

15. Lancaster, "Wasn't She the Mother in *Cheaper by the Dozen.*"

16. See especially the series of images A49–111, 113, and 114, all made on December 22, 1908, in the Frank and Lillian Gilbreth Collection, Purdue University Libraries Special Collections and Archives, N file 10/0031–1 (hereafter cited "GPP"). Here, the hand of a well-dressed man demonstrates the proper way to reach for and pick up a brick. Most of the other images in this group of photographs record Gilbreth's site innovations designed to increase production speed, such as the conveyor belt, Gilbreth's patented scaffolding system, a pulley system for hauling bricks, and so forth. For a discussion of this aspect of Gilbreth's work, see Jane Morley, "Frank Bunker Gilbreth's Concrete System," *Concrete International* 12, no. 11 (November 1990): 3–62; and M. J. Steel and D. W. Cheetham, "Frank Bunker Gilbreth: Building Contractor, Inventor and Pioneer Industrial Engineer", *Construction History: Journal of the Construction History Society* 9 (1993): 51–70.

17. Gilbreth, *Bricklaying System*, 141.

18. Frank B. Gilbreth (FBG) diary, typescript November 23, 1908, vol. 2, p. 26, GPP, N file 109/808–3.

19. Gilbreth, *Bricklaying System*, 145.

20. Ibid., 148, 145.

21. For distinctions between a group, a series, and a sequence, see Keith A. Smith, *Structure of the Visual Book*, Book 95 (Rochester, NY: Visual Studies Workshop, 1984).

22. Indeed, the bricklayers had walked off Gilbreth's last job over a time study dispute; in a heated address to the strikers Gilbreth claimed legitimacy as a "union man." He more than likely undercut his efforts at solidarity, however, by exclaiming,"I will raise the pay of the bricklaying mechanics throughout the United States in spite of the interference of pig headed, ignorant men in Gardner." FBG diary, typescript, November 23, 1908, vol. 2, p. 26, GPP, N file 109/808–3. The unionized bricklayers struck Gilbreth's 1911 job at Glens Falls, New York, as well; they objected to having their output measured, and to Gilbreth's differential pay scale. Gilbreth capitulated on this job: he stopped measuring output, paid a uniform sixty-five cents per hour to all bricklayers, and stopped insisting on his bricklaying system. Price, "One Best Way," 84.

23. Allan Sekula, "Photography between Labour and Capital," in *Mining Photographs and Other Pictures, 1948–1968: A Selection from the Negative Archives of Shedden Studio, Glace Bay, Cape Breton*, photographs by Leslie Shedden, essays

by Don Macgillivray and Allan Sekula, introduction by Robert Wilkie, edited by Benjamin H. D. Buchloch and Robert Wilkie (Halifax, Nova Scotia: Press of the Nova Scotia College of Art and Design, 1983), 234.

24. Haber, *Efficiency and Uplift*; Montgomery, *Workers' Control*; and Harry Braverman, *Labor and Monopoly Capital* (New York: Monthly Review Press, 1974). For a different assessment, based on the experience of women workers, see Alice Kessler-Harris, *Out to Work: A History of Wage-Earning Women in the United States* (New York: Oxford University Press, 1982), 146–47.

25. Aitkin, *Taylorism at Watertown Arsenal.*

26. Hoxie, *Scientific Management and Labor*; Judith Merkle, *Management and Ideology* (Berkeley: University of California Press, 1980), 29.

27. Frank Bunker Gilbreth (FBG) to Lillian Moller Gilbreth (LMG), May 9, 1914, GPP N file 112/813–6.

28. "Waste" was the product of inefficiency, and Progressive Era reformers concerned with increasing any type of industrial or social efficiency identified and exhibited "waste" as a rhetorical strategy in numerous social and cultural debates. See, for example, Rudolf Cronau, *Our Wasteful Nation* (New York: Mitchell Kennerly, 1908); the Hoover-sponsored Committee on Elimination of Waste in Industry of the Federated American Engineering Societies, *Waste in Industry* (New York: McGraw-Hill, 1921); Stuart Chase, *The Tragedy of Waste* (New York: Macmillan, 1925).

29. Frank B. Gilbreth, "Economic Value of Motion Study in Standardizing the Trades," *Industrial Engineering*, April 1910, 265, GPP, N file 42/0265–2. For a discussion of the relationship between Progressive Era efficiency ideals and the early conservation movement, see Samuel Hays, *Conservation and the Gospel of Efficiency: The Progressive Conservation Movement, 1890–1920* (Cambridge: Harvard University Press, 1959).

30. Frank B. Gilbreth, *Motion Study: A Method for Increasing the Efficiency of the Workman* (New York: Van Nostrand, 1911; reprint, Easton: Hive, 1972), 76.

31. Anson Rabinbach discusses the ways nineteenth-century European scientists, borrowing from earlier discoveries in thermodynamics, reconceptualized work from an organic process connected to a discrete individual to a concept of "labor power," a distinct force that scientists could "objectively" identify, study, and control. The structuring metaphor for this conceptual shift became that of the human motor. Anson Rabinbach, *The Human Motor: Energy, Fatigue, and the Origins of Modernity* (New York: Basic Books, 1990).

32. Gilbreth, *Motion Study: A Method for Increasing the Efficiency of the Workman*, 65–70.

33. See, for example, "Decline of Brickwork," *Waterbury Republican*, August 2 1908, in Gilbreth microfilm roll 1, and Frank B. Gilbreth, "Systematizing a Contractor's Office," *Construction News*, November 7, 1908, microfilm roll 1, GPP.

34. Price, "One Best Way," 153–55. The term "Betterment Room" reflects the Gilbreths' increasing focus on post-Taylor modifications to scientific management, as they sought to introduce ideas of worker education and participation as a means of defusing worker antipathy. The classic discussion of what became known as "welfare capitalism" is Stuart Brandes, *American Welfare Capitalism* (Chicago: University of Chicago Press, 1976); but see also Andrea Tone, *The Business of Benevolence: Industrial Paternalism in Progressive America* (Ithaca: Cornell University Press, 1997).

35. Peter Liebhold, "Seeking 'The One Best Way'": Frank and Lillian Gilbreth's Time-Motion Photographs, 1910–1924," *Labor's Heritage* 7, no. 2 (fall 1995): 19–33, 56–61; Mike Mandel, *Making Good Time* (Santa Cruz, CA: University of California, 1989).

36. "Description of Photographs Sent to Mr. Robert Moulton," caption for no. 1109, GPP, N file 1/0019, vol. 3. Gilbreth began telling colleagues of this technique, which he called micromotion study, in early March 1912; by April he had filed patent claims. Gilbreth to Butterworth, March 4, 1912, GPP, N file 118/0816–54. For patent claims, see N file 117/0816–44.

37. Robert Thurston Kent, "Micro-Motion Study in Industry," *Iron Age* 91 (January 2, 1913): 34–37; see also Robert Thurston Kent, "Micro-Motion Study: A New Development in the Art of Time Study," *Industrial Engineering* 13, no. 1 (January 1913): 1–4.

38. Whitaker to Gilbreth, August 2, 1912, GPP, N file 159/0952–2. For more on the relationship between the I.W.W. and time study, see Mike Davis, "The Stopwatch and the Wooden Shoe: Scientific Management and the Industrial Workers of the World," *Radical America* 8, no. 6 (January–February 1975).

39. On April 2, 1913, Whitaker wrote FBG that on "Tuesday afternoon, at 71 Brown Street, the first trial of the Orbit method of motion study was made; the second study was made at the New England Butt Co. on the third floor later in the afternoon." Brown Street was the Gilbreth residence, where some of the photographic work was being experimented with; the third floor of the New England Butt Company was the "Betterment Room." See Whitaker to FBG, April 2, 1913, GPP, N file 159/ 0952–2.

40. For an early description of the cyclegraph process, see "Cymography: The New Efficiency Science," *Coal Age* clipping in GPP, N file 5/0030–28A. This article reprinted two cyclegraph images from the *American Machinist*, which had also covered the story. Almost all of the Gilbreths' published writings and business correspondence highlight the development of cyclegraphy after April 1913. For a representative discussion of the technology and its applications, see Frank B. Gilbreth and L. M. Gilbreth, "Motion Study and Time-Study Instruments of Precision" (paper to be presented at a meeting of the International Engineering Congress, San Francisco, September 20–25, 1915), GPP, N file 42/0265–4.

41. Later, the pace of pulsations was increased to as much as 3,000 per minute. See, for example, the caption to image 1028, a chronocyclegraph of a turret lathe operator. GPP, N file 01/0019, vol. 1.

42. The direction of movement could be detected from the shape of the dashes, as the narrow end represented the slowly lingering light pulsation, and therefore the direction from which the body part had traveled. In Gilbreth's formulation, the cyclegraph "shows intermittent electric lights with the filament and the current so proportioned that the light brightens quickly and dies out slowly. This gives us a photograph of time in that the number of flashes per second is known. Moreover, the point on the spot shows the direction of the motion." GPP, misc. captions (this is for 618–G68–2, N file 1/0019, vol. 3). See also Frank Gilbreth and Lillian Gilbreth, "Chronocyclegraph Motion Devices for Measuring Achievement" (paper presented at the Second Pan-American Congress, Washington, D.C., January 3, 1916); reprinted in *Efficiency Society Journal* 5, no. 3 (March 1916): 137–49. They created the effect of a cross-screened background by photographing chalk lines on a blackboard and then using the same plate to photograph a worker's motions. The resulting image was a double exposure. Muybridge used a cross-screened background (constructed through white threads) at the University of Pennsylvania as early as 1885; this innovation was borrowed, in turn, from J. H. Lamprey's ethnographic photography work. See J. H. Lamprey, "On a Method of Measuring the Human Form," *Journal of the Ethnological Society* 1 (1869): 84–85.

43. Gilbreth's main source of inspiration in this appropriation of visual technologies was the work of Etienne-Jules Marey, the French research scientist who spent his life recording motion: first through various graphic inscription machines of his own invention (such as his 1860 sphygmograph), then through photography (especially after seeing Muybridge's photographs of the horse in motion in 1878), and finally through film (after 1890). As Marta Braun has convincingly argued, Gilbreth's chronophotographic method of "attaching light bulbs to the subject and using a still camera to track their movement was an exact emulation of the system [Etienne-Jules] Marey had devised" over twenty years earlier. Marta Braun, *Picturing Time: The Work of Etienne-Jules Marey, 1830–1904* (Chicago: University of Chicago Press, 1992), 344. The Gilbreths, however, took great pains to distance themselves from Marey's accomplishments, not only through arguing the precedence of their own investigations but also through the management of their own carefully constructed archive.

44. Microfilm rolls of Gilbreth papers, Cyclegraph Book, November 1, 1913, roll 2, GPP.

45. For P. T. Barnum's sophisticated manipulation of audience gullibility and skepticism, see Neil Harris, *Humbug: The Art of P. T. Barnum* (Boston: Little Brown, 1973).

46. Kent, "Micro-Motion Study in Industry," 34.

47. The shift of his energies and personnel away from Hermann, Aukam caused considerable acrimony among the company directors, who eventually sought Taylor's help in rescuing the fraying installation. Taylor's involvement in the contract infuriated Gilbreth, who irrevocably severed his relations with Taylor and his associates. There are many conflicting stories about this break, but see Milton J. Nadworny, "Frederick Taylor and Frank Gilbreth: Competition in Scientific Management," *Business History Review* 31 (spring 1957): 26; FBG to LMG, May 9, 1914, GPP, N file 112/0813–6; Charles D. Wrege and Ronald G. Greenwood, *Frederick W. Taylor: The Father of Scientific Management: Myth and Reality* (Homewood, IL: Business One Irwin, 1991); Yost, *Frank and Lillian Gilbreth: Partners for Life*, 257; Price, "One Best Way," 256–63.

48. FBG to LMG, May 1, 1915, and April 5, 1915, GPP, N file 112/813–4.

49. FBG to Prof. William Stewart Ayars, October 28, 1915, GPP, N file 0019–5; FBG to LMG, May 1, 1915, GPP, N file 112/813–4.

50. See FBG to LMG, October 6, 1915, where he describes a talk he gave on the crippled soldier before the Buffalo Society of Engineers, GPP, N file 112/813–4.

51. F. B. Gilbreth, "Motion Study for the Crippled Soldier," *Journal of the American Society of Mechanical Engineers*, December 1915, 671.

52. By the end of the year, Gilbreth had added a seventeenth motion: "transport, loaded" was added a second time, to position 7. See Frank B. Gilbreth and L. M. Gilbreth, "Motion Study for Crippled Soldiers" (paper presented at a meeting of the American Association for the Advancement of Science, Columbus, Ohio, December 27, 1915–January 1, 1916), 4, Morley Papers, Division of the History of Technology, National Museum of American History, Smithsonian Institution. My thanks to Jane Morley, who donated her extensive Gilbreth research and materials to NMAH. (Hereafter cited as Morley/NMAH.)

53. Frank B. Gilbreth and L. M. Gilbreth, "Applications of Motion Study: Its Use in Developing the Best Methods of Work," *Management and Administration* 8, no. 3 (1925), GPP, N file 53/0298. By 1915 Gilbreth was an avid moviegoer, watching one or two films daily while working in Berlin; he was no doubt familiar with Vachel Lindsay's *Art of the Moving Picture* (1915), where Lindsay compared moving images to Egyptian hieroglyphs. See also Michael O'Malley, *Keeping Watch: A History of American Time* (New York: Viking, 1990), 237–38.

54. Gilbreth, "Motion Study for the Crippled Soldier," 672.

55. Gilbreth and Gilbreth, "Motion Study for Crippled Soldiers," 5; Frank B. Gilbreth and L. M. Gilbreth, "The Engineer, the Cripple, and the New Education" (presented at the annual meeting of the ASME, December 4–7, 1917), 5, Morley/NMAH.

56. "Crippled Soldiers Disheartened by Delays," *New York Times*, August 24, 1919, 7; "Provision for Disabled Soldiers," *Monthly Review of the Bureau of Labor Statistics*, October 1917, 683–94.

57. FBG to LMG, October 12, 1915, GPP, N file 112/813–4. For Gilbreth's interest in Canadian rehabilitation efforts, see his correspondence with William Stewart Ayars, as well as his extensive newspaper clipping files concerning Canadian, French, English, and German rehabilitation work. GPP, crippled soldier files.

58. Nancy Bristow, *Making Men Moral: Social Engineering during the Great War* (New York: New York University Press, 1996); Roxanne Panchasi, "Reconstruction: Prosthetics and the Rehabilitation of the Male Body in World War I France," *differences* 7, no. 3 (1995): 109–40.

59. This language is from Henry A. Whitmarsh, "Rehabilitation of the Crippled Soldier," *Journal of the American Institute of Homeopathy*, October 1918, 397, but see also Douglas C. McMurtrie, "The War Cripple," *Columbia War Papers* series I, no. 17 (1917): 5.

60. Frank B. Gilbreth and L. M. Gilbreth, "Motion Study and the Mutilated Soldiers" (unpublished typescript), 2, GPP, f.78–3. See also Frank B. Gilbreth and Lillian M. Gilbreth, "Measurement of the Human Factor in Industry" (to be presented at the National Conference of the Western Efficiency Society, May 22–25, 1917), 7, Seeley G. Mudd Library, Yale University.

61. Frank B. Gilbreth and L. M. Gilbreth, "First Steps toward Solving the Crippled Soldier Problem" (unpublished typescript), 7, GPP, f.78–1. Ironically, during these same years the Gilbreth children were themselves taking basket-weaving classes. My thanks to Jane Lancaster for this observation.

62. FBG to Lt. Colonel James Bordley, Director, Red Cross Institute for the Blind, Baltimore, December 24, 1918, GPP, f.696–4.

63. For the gendered transformations of office work during these years, see Angel Kwolek-Folland, *Engendering Business: Men and Women in the Corporate Office, 1870–1930* (Baltimore: Johns Hopkins University Press, 1994); for retail sales, see Susan Porter Benson, *Counter Cultures: Saleswomen, Managers, and Customers in American Department Stores, 1890–1940* (Urbana: University of Illinois Press, 1986). For the dental hygiene work, see Frank B. Gilbreth and Lillian M. Gilbreth, "The Conservation of the World's Teeth: A New Occupation for Crippled Soldiers," *Trained Nurse and Hospital Review*, July 1917, NMAH/Morley "pamphlets."

64. Gilbreth and Gilbreth, "The Engineer, the Cripple, and the New Education," 6.

65. The experience of reintroducing disabled veterans to productive employment after the war served to join those working on behalf of the veterans with the Safety First, or industrial safety, movement. For a discussion of the

movement to reduce industrial accidents and safeguard workers' health, see Mark Aldrich, *Safety First: Technology, Labor, and Business in the Building of American Work Safety, 1870–1939* (Baltimore: Johns Hopkins University Press, 1997).

66. Albert Jay Nock to LMG, January 29, 1916, and February 7, 1916, GPP, 816–22.

67. LMG to Bradley Stoughton, February 15, 1918, GPP, crippled soldier files.

68. For social documentary reform photography, see Stange, *Symbols of Ideal Life;* for a discussion of "capitalist realism" as an American advertising aesthetic that simplifies and typifies, see Michael Schudson, *Advertising: The Uneasy Persuasion: Its Dubious Impact on American Society* (New York: Basic Books, 1984), 209–33; for *Fortune* magazine (founded in 1929), see Terry Smith, *Making the Modern: Industry, Art, and Design in America* (Chicago: University of Chicago Press, 1993), 159–98.

69. "The word 'ergonomics' comes from the Greek: *ergos*, work; *nomos*, natural law. The word was coined by the late Professor Hywell Murrell, as a result of a meeting of a working party, which was held in room 1101 of the Admiralty building at Queene Anne's Mansions on 8 July 1949—at which it was resolved to form a society for the 'study of human beings in their working environment'." See Stephen Pheasant, *Bodyspace: Anthropometry, Ergonomics, and the Design of Work,* 2d ed. (London: Taylor and Francis, 1996 [1986]), 4; Amit Bhattacharya and James D. McGlothlin, eds., *Occupational Ergonomics: Theory and Applications* (New York: Marcel Dekker, 1996).

70. The museum was partially a result of discussions stemming from the Gilbreths' Summer School in Scientific Management, which they began in 1913 and which continued for several summers thereafter.

71. In addition to the letters, the Gilbreths used the photographs of the chairs as evidence of their interest in the workers' welfare, distributing them to newspapers as well as to professional colleagues and potential clients. The Gilbreths continued their interest in creating museums for their work well after their work at New England Butt Company. In the winter of 1915 they tried to get the National Museum in Washington (now the National Museum of American History, Smithsonian Institution) to start a national fatigue department, but were unsuccessful. The National Museum did collect, however, several wire motion models, which have since been lost. In 1917 they called for a government-sponsored museum that would include models of artificial limbs and appliances for the disabled. See Gilbreth and Gilbreth, "The Engineer, the Cripple, and the New Education"; Frank B. Gilbreth and L. M. Gilbreth, *Fatigue Study: The Elimination of Humanity's Greatest Unnecessary Waste* (New York: Sturgis and Walton, 1916); Frank B. Gilbreth and L. M. Gilbreth, *Motion Study for the Handicapped* (London: Routledge, 1920), 100.

72. Frank B. Gilbreth and Lillian M. Gilbreth, "How to Put the Crippled Soldier on the Payroll," reprinted from *Trained Nurse and Hospital Review*, May 1917, and delivered before the Economic Psychology Association, New York, January 26–27, 1917, 5, Morley/NMAH.

73. Frank B. Gilbreth, "Third Summer School of Scientific Management," typescript of discussions taking place on the afternoon of August 13, 1915, in GPP, f.104–2. For further discussion of the positive publicity generated by the crippled soldier work, see correspondence between the Gilbreths and Dr. Ing. Georg Schlesinger, Germany's foremost advocate of scientific management, from June 6, 1915, through July 13, 1916 (especially FBG to Schlesinger, December 6, 1915), GPP, f.816–139.

74. Gilbreth and Gilbreth, "The Engineer, the Cripple, and the New Education," 6; "How to Attack the Problem of the Crippled Soldier," GPP, 104–1. This typescript appears to be a draft of "The Engineer, the Cripple, and the New Education."

75. Jules Amar, *La Prothèse et la Travail des Mutilés* (Paris: H. Dunod et E. Pinat, 1916), 8–10; Jules Amar, *The Physiology of Industrial Organization and the Re-Employment of the Disabled*, trans. Bernard Miall (London: Library Press, 1918), 66–73, where Amar briefly references both Marey and the Gilbreths (73). The Gilbreths owned two editions of Amar's *Le Moteur Humain*, one from 1914 and a personally inscribed 1923 edition: "á mes chers amis Fr. B et L. Gilbreth cordial hommage par Jules Amar Paris 7 Juin 1923 62 Blvd. St. Germain." Gilbreth Library, Engineering, Purdue.

76. Waldemar Kaempffert and A. M. Jungmann, "Crippled but Undaunted," *Popular Science Monthly*, November 1918.

77. FBG to LMG, July 12, 1917, GPP, N file 112/813–4.

78. The term "universal design" originated in the United States, where the architect Ronald Mace and others grounded their design work in commitment to the civil rights of people with disabilities. Since the 1980s, the concept has grown to include designing with the needs of a varied population in view, not just the standardized "Joe and Josephine" of mid-twentieth-century industrial design. See James Mueller, "Towards Universal Design," *American Rehabilitation* 16, no. 2 (summer 1990): 15–19; Abir Mullick and Edward Steinfeld, "Universal Design," *Innovation*, spring 1997, 14–18.

79. For another assessment, see Frank T. Lohrke, "Motion Study for the Blind: A Review of the Gilbreths' Work with the Visually Handicapped," *International Journal of Public Administration* 16, no. 5 (1993): 667–782. After Frank Gilbreth's death in 1924, Lillian Gilbreth continued work with the disabled; see Edna Yost and Lillian Moller Gilbreth, *Normal Lives for the Disabled* (New York: Macmillan, 1944).

10

"A Limb Which Shall Be Presentable in Polite Society"

Prosthetic Technologies in the Nineteenth Century

Stephen Mihm

THE DISPLAY OF the A. A. Marks Company must have been one of the more memorable at the Columbian Exposition of 1893 (fig. 10.1). In an impressive bid to capture visitors' attention, the firm had constructed four large display cases roofed by a gilded dome and a "colossal golden leg" that towered over the surrounding exhibits. Each glass case, the company's pamphlet patiently explained, "contained artificial legs and arms for amputations in the hips, thighs, knees, legs, ankles, feet, shoulders, arms, elbows, forearms, wrists, hands, and fingers"—over fifty limbs in all. Though the Marks Company took home the highest award on this occasion, it was not for a lack of competition. In a testament to the demand for prostheses, no fewer than nine manufacturers of artificial limbs had assembled on this occasion to display their wares.[1]

Aside from selling artificial limbs, the company's monument silently commemorated the grim toll of the industrial age. The flywheels and pulleys of the new mills and factories severed arms and legs with alarming frequency throughout the nineteenth century, as did the wheels of railroad locomotives, particularly at perilous grade crossings in urban areas. Most destructive, however, was the Civil War, which marked the first sustained use of accurate, breech-loading firearms. Unlike earlier guns, these weapons fired so-called minie balls, expansive bullets that lost their shape upon contact with a target. They usually shattered two to three inches of bone, and carried bits of skin and cloth-

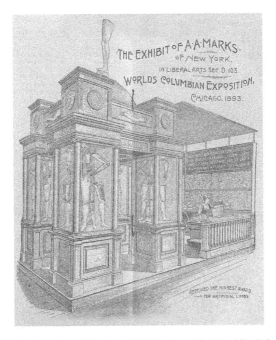

FIG. 10.1. *From Highest Award for Artificial Limbs at the World's Columbian Exposition, Chicago, 1893,* pamphlet in "Artificial Limbs," box 1, folder 10, Warshaw Collection of Business Americana, National Museum of American History, Washington, D.C.

ing deep into the wound, increasing the possibility of infection if the victim was fortunate enough to survive the initial impact.[2] Doctors in field hospitals, overwhelmed with the wounded, usually opted to amputate the limb rather than reconstruct it.

All the carnage did not go unnoticed. One writer captured the state of affairs when he noted that "there are few of us who have not a cripple among our friends, if not in our own families. A mechanical art which provided for an occasional and exceptional want has become a great and active industry."[3] Indeed, the scale of this mutilation seems to have prompted an outpouring of invention: between 1846 and 1873, Americans submitted some 167 patents for prosthetic devices.[4] Manufacturers turned out ever more sophisticated models throughout the nineteenth century, making the United States the preeminent supplier of artificial limbs in the world.

The limbs exhibited by the Marks Company represented a tremendous advance in design over earlier prostheses; most artificial legs from ancient times onward consisted of crude pegs. Though some craftsmen did experiment with more intricate devices beginning in the sixteenth century, few of these models found much of a following. The most famous of these was the "Anglesey leg," developed in Britain in the late eighteenth century. It depended on cogs and gears to approximate the movement of an actual arm or leg. Unfortunately, this model, like those that preceded it, broke down, made considerable noise, and required frequent oiling; indeed, amputees often carried an oil can with them to prevent the gears from binding.[5]

More troubling, however, was the fact that, for all their mechanical sophistication, these more advanced models did not move in tandem with the body; they did not complement the rhythm and gait of the wearer. If anything, these early limbs had a mind of their own. One commentator observed that these "jerking, clapping, snapping and rattling" contraptions inevitably exhibited "many unreliable and *uncontrolable* [sic] gyrations"—they simply failed to respond reliably and predictably to the movement and weight of the body.[6]

Things began to change around the mid-nineteenth century. The typical limb was made of a light and flexible wood, such as willow or bass, and colored, as one manufacturer claimed, "so natural that the most delicately wrought hose and slipper are sufficient to conceal the work of art."[7] Yet unlike earlier models, this emphasis on mimicking the natural limb extended to the internal design of the prosthesis. It was not enough to craft artificial limbs that *looked* like real arms and legs; manufacturers spared no expense in producing artificial limbs that actually *moved* like real arms and legs. They increasingly sought to replicate the workings of the human body, where, as one pamphlet put it, "levers and pulleys are found more perfect than in machine shops and valves more perfect than in steam engines."[8]

Illustrations of the so-called Bly prosthesis, popular in the 1860s, reveal the extent to which these devices mimicked the anatomical structure of the leg (fig. 10.2). Bly was an anatomist and supplier to the U.S. army who spent his spare time building artificial limbs. Having observed that "nature used not bolts or pins to bolt or fasten the foot to the leg, but that she nicely rounded the bones at the joint, and held them in place by means of ligaments, tendons, and muscles," Bly set out to "Reproduce Nature in Art." The ankle joint of his prosthesis was thus

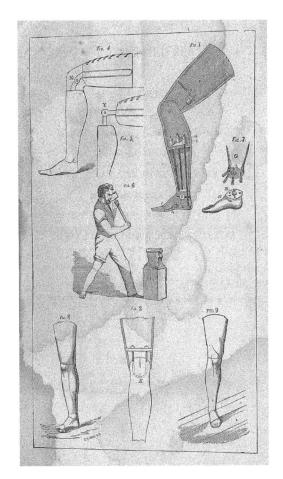

FIG. 10.2. From John McGuire, Supplier of Bly's Artificial Limbs, *Descriptive Catalogue of Artificial Limbs* (St. Paul, n.d.), 18, pamphlet in "Artificial Limbs," box 1, folder 4, Warshaw Collection of Business Americana, National Museum of American History, Washington, D.C.

formed by a ball of polished ivory that fit into a socket of vulcanized rubber. This joint, Bly claimed, "admits of motion in all directions like the natural ankle joint," while the cords within the lower leg "assume the position and function of the natural tendons." The knee cords, the pamphlet noted, "take the place of the crucial ligaments of the natural knee," and rubber springs, "made of rail-road car spring rubber and used by compression," functioned as "artificial muscles" that contracted and expanded as the wearer walked on the leg. "Instead of the mechanical motions given a limb by metallic springs," Bly asserted, "rubber springs impart easy, uniform motions to the limb, like those of the natural muscles, which give it, when in use, a remarkable life-like appearance." These springs could also be adjusted to suit the gait of the wearer.[9]

Claims that such limbs supplied "a successful imitation of the natural limb in symmetry and motion" might easily be dismissed as inflated advertising rhetoric were it not for corroboration from other sources. A prize committee at the 1858 New York State Fair contrasted the Bly limb with earlier prostheses, asserting that it "is a nearer approach, in its anatomical structure and motions, when in use, to its 'model,' the natural Leg." An 1876 exposition circular offered a similar assessment on the efficiency of the Clement artificial leg: "the anatomical structure of the natural limb is closely studied and perfectly reproduced; springs, bands, and other mechanical contrivances . . . serving in place, and readily fulfilling without an effort of the wearer every purpose of muscles, sinews, tendons, and joints in the natural limbs of flesh and bone."[10] Surgeons and doctors also submitted testimonials that stressed the "life-like motions of the joints" and the "naturalness of form and movement" that this new generation of prostheses afforded.[11]

This sort of rhetoric, much less the alterations in the actual design of the limbs, is curious. Certainly, the phenomenal increase in the number of amputees, the development of new materials, and perhaps most important of all, the allocation of government funds to subsidize military amputees' purchase of limbs helped to usher in this new generation of articulated prostheses. But none of these factors satisfactorily explains the revolution in prosthesis design. Generations of amputees had managed well enough with pegs and other crude contrivances. Why the sudden interest in developing lifelike limbs?

Such a question might seem insignificant and uninteresting at first glance. But there is more here than meets the eye. Though one would not suspect it, these mute pieces of machinery, rusted and relegated to collections in the basements of hospitals and medical schools, are in fact the emblems of a new social order that emerged in the burgeoning cities of the industrial era.[12]

It is difficult for us to appreciate the dramatic changes that urban life brought to a population accustomed to living in the relatively closed communities of the late eighteenth and early nineteenth centuries. As a character in George Lippard's popular novel *The Quaker City* (1845) observed of urban life, "Every thing is fleeting and nothing stable, every thing shifting and changing, and nothing substantial!"[13] His lament betokened the interpretations of modern historians and sociologists, who have argued that the rapid transition to a modern, urban, and industrial society eroded the traditional means by which individuals defined themselves and recognized one another. The emergence of a society of strangers, in other words, transformed the rules of social interaction.

In the process, the importance of personal appearance underwent a profound transformation. Earlier, preindustrial societies had placed a premium on appearance, especially members of the upper classes, whose continued control of the local social hierarchy depended on the ritual expression of power in the form of dress, speech, and bodily comportment. The carefully orchestrated presentations mounted by aspiring aristocrats in the eighteenth and early nineteenth centuries did not aim to impress strangers, but rather, the community over which they ruled.[14]

In the increasingly anonymous urban milieu of the nineteenth century, appearance no longer functioned as a confirmation and expression of acknowledged social hierarchies and privileges. Instead, the wealth, mobility, and anonymity of the modern city enabled individuals to assume new guises through the adoption of manners, diction, and dress. Indeed, this was the very foundation of an emergent middle-class identity. Membership in the middle classes, historians like Karen Haltunnen have observed, did not rest on birthright, but on acts of self-fashioning. Men who could cultivate an appearance of probity and industry, and thus command the respect and trust of strangers and acquaintances, might succeed in the world of business and beyond.[15]

Yet the ethos of the self-made man had a more sinister side, enabling social climbers and confidence men to assume the appearance of respectability. Members of the middle classes thus became obsessed with making sure that those with whom they conducted business, socialized, and married had the proper qualifications. To buttress their precarious social status and police the boundaries of their class, they developed an elaborate array of social rituals to sort out the truly respectable from those who were merely putting on airs and manipulating appearances. Unfortunately, as so many etiquette writers bemoaned, such social niceties could be faked. The social conditions of modern urban life inevitably enabled individuals to make what some perceived as spurious claims regarding their social stature. Authority was no longer a function of fixed social status, but of fluid self-promotion.[16]

In such a treacherous environment, members of the middle classes turned to a curious array of strategies to divine the true, inner nature of the people with whom they dealt. Foremost among these was the "reading" of a person's physical appearance to determine their inner character. Middle-class writers, such as phrenologists and the authors of popular etiquette books, placed great emphasis on the ability to read temperament and character from the appearance of the body.[17] Diction and dress could be faked and affected. But the bumps on one's head, the shape of one's body offered, it seemed, some insights into a person's real character, a reliable marker in a time when all else disappeared into the play of appearances.

This tendency to equate external, bodily appearance with internal character presented extraordinary problems for the amputee. In a remarkable article on prosthetic limbs published in the *Atlantic Monthly*, Oliver Wendell Holmes made clear the nature of the dilemma that faced the maimed. He cited one such "cripple" who, while otherwise attractive, faced great difficulties in the culture of his day: "just at the period when personal graces are most valued, when a good presence is a blank check on the Bank of Fortune, with Nature's signature on the bottom, he found himself made hideous." Holmes put the matter even more directly to his readers elsewhere in the article. Surveying the increasingly urban, anonymous society of the 1860s, he asserted that in "an age when *appearances are realities* . . . it becomes important to provide the cripple with a limb which shall be presentable in polite society." "Misfortunes of a certain obtrusiveness may be pitied," observed Holmes, "but are never tolerated under the chandeliers." The truth was inescapable, for as Holmes put it, "there is an absolute demand for a certain comeliness of person throughout all the decent classes of our society."[18]

In an age of appearances, members of the middle classes necessarily hid their deformities and weaknesses, for fear that first impressions might deny them opportunities in marriage, employment, and social advancement. Concealment, as much as detection, became a requisite in the urban milieu, particularly for those who had something to hide. Many activities assumed a new importance in this context, among them the simple act of walking. "A man's walk," declared one etiquette manual, is "an index of his character and of the grade of his culture," while another guide asserted that one could "know the character of a man by his walk."[19] The sight of a man, however respectably dressed, hobbling down the street on an "odious peg" would inevitably lead strangers to judge him in a negative light, as a "cripple." He might even call to mind the figure of the limping criminal who became a stock character in the fiction of the era. Manufacturers, not surprisingly, played on these fears. One advertising pamphlet beseeched parents of children with missing arms and legs to purchase an artificial limb, or face "its growing up in your sight a constant spectacle of regret, and sorrow to yourself." Though the limb enabled a child to walk, its true value lay in its ability "to remove an almost certain barrier to its proper place in society, and its lasting welfare in mature years."[20]

The emergence of this new generation of prosthetic devices—with their ability to not only restore mobility but actually mimic the movements of the missing limb—must be understood as part and parcel of these anxieties. Indeed, judges and journalists writing on artificial limbs focused not so much on the improved mobility these "lifelike" models offered, but rather, on their capacity to conceal the condition of the amputee. The Franklin Institute, in a report on the Palmer leg, asserted that it enabled the wearer "to walk without a cane in such a manner as to deceive one not acquainted with the facts of the case." Similarly, a British newspaper noted of the celebrated Clement leg that "the materials employed are selected and finished . . . with such care as not only to give entire freedom of action, but in appearance, to deceive the sense of sight in other persons." Of the same limb, the *Philadelphia Inquirer* observed that it "may be walked, ridden, and sat upon, without revealing to curious eyes its artificial structure," or as another journalist put it, "without for an instant disclosing to the shrewdest of observers the remotest hint of [its] artificial structure." Doctors relayed similar sentiments; one surgeon wrote of a Civil War amputee who worked as a clerk in the War Department that "in every appearance—standing, locomotion, dancing—he passes for a whole man."[21]

Letters written by amputees corroborate this emphasis on its ability to conceal the "hideous" stump. As one satisfied customer wrote, "I frequently attend balls, parties, &c., and dance as long as most of them, and no one but those who know I use the leg even suspect such a thing." Another related that "many who are acquainted with me, are at a loss to distinguish the real from the artificial limb." On the same note, one man wrote that "I frequently meet my old acquaintances whom I have not seen for several years, and they do not believe that I have lost my legs. . . . I can now fully appreciate that it is 'the perfection of art to conceal art,' and that you have fully accomplished this is practically demonstrated in my own case."[22]

Whether these claims are "true" in the sense that the writers' friends really could not detect the artificial limb matters very little; indeed, it is possible that they sometimes indulged the amputee. What matters is that these devices allayed the anxieties of the maimed and enabled them to navigate the increasingly judgmental world of the urban middle class. One satisfied patient put it well when he gave thanks that the amputee might "again pass in mixed assemblages of his fellow citizens without being gazed upon or pointed at, or, what is still worse, to hear that harsh, but oft-repeated exclamation, 'There is a cripple!'"[23]

This emphasis on concealment rather than mobility confirms that there is more to these devices than meets the eye. The more flexible design of the limbs and the elimination of noisy machinery, while enabling amputees to walk with greater ease than if they wore a simple peg leg, was the source of less tangible, but no less important, dividends in a culture that increasingly passed judgment on the so-called cripple.

Additional, visual evidence confirms this point. Many of the manufacturers of prosthetic limbs extensively illustrated their advertising literature with engravings and photographs of their customers. In their depiction of middle-class amputees, companies made a point of showing off how well the limb concealed their condition (fig. 10.3). Typically, they presented a "before and after" series of images that showed the amputee seated on a chair, and then standing without evidence of the leg. The trade cards of the A. A. Marks company took this method to new levels (fig. 10.4). On one side, the cards depicted the emblem of the company, while on the obverse, they reproduced photographic images of amputees both with and without their artificial limbs. Superimposed onto one frame, these photos offered dramatic evidence of the ability of these prostheses to make a man "whole" again. The man depicted in figure 10.4 stands erect, with hat on, next to his "crippled" counterpart, whose mangled legs provide a stark contrast.[24]

The middle-class obsession with concealment becomes all the more obvious in an examination of the next largest group of artificial limb recipients: urban laborers.[25] Unlike illustrations of the more wealthy patrons, who merely stood as testament to their improved condition, depictions of these other amputees deliberately called attention to their

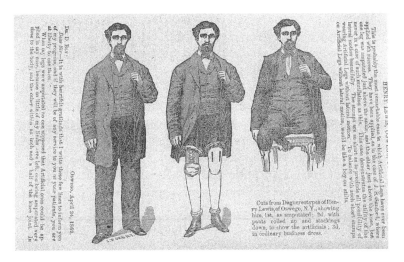

FIG. 10.3. From Douglas Bly, M.D., *A New and Important Invention* (Rochester: Curtis, Butts, and Company, 1862), 24, pamphlet in "Artificial Limbs," box 1, folder 4, Warshaw Collection of Business Americana, National Museum of American History, Washington, D.C.

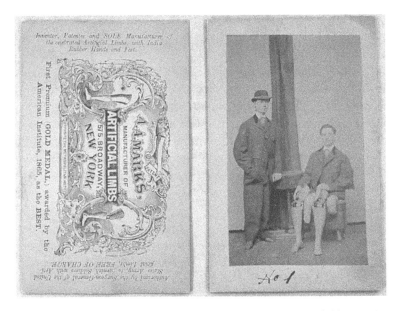

FIG. 10.4. Trade card of the A. A. Marks Company, n.d., box 1, folder 11, Warshaw Collection of Business Americana, National Museum of American History, Washington, D.C.

prostheses, and implicitly, to the different social functions that they performed. In countless engravings, manufacturers did not depict a "before and after" sequence, but instead showed the laborer at work in some job, with the artificial limb prominently displayed (figs. 10.5, 10.6). As these illustrations suggest, the limb, at least as understood by manufacturers of prostheses, functioned not as a means to conceal, but rather, as a means to ensure continued employment.[26]

Given this emphasis, it is not entirely surprising that the limbs designed for "persons of limited means" lacked certain amenities so central to the middle-class culture of concealment. Oliver Wendell Holmes observed that "a plain working-man, who has outlived his courting-days and need not sacrifice much to personal appearance, may find an honest, old-fashioned wooden leg, cheap, lasting, requiring no repairs, *the best thing for his purpose.*" While more expensive prostheses might be "*soft* to the touch, as in nature," and "covered with a delicate skin, which is enameled with the most delicate flesh-colored enamel, shaded to suit each particular case," working-class limbs lacked such details. For example, the limbs for "persons of limited means" designed by Douglas Bly had a "plain and substantial" exterior, for "nothing is spent in showy finish—the main object being to produce great durability with but little cost." These legs, he claimed, "make it to the poor, what my 'Ball and Socket' joined Leg is to the rich."[27]

It is difficult to determine whether the working-class wearers of these limbs shared their sentiments, though the few testimonials written by laborers generally suggest as much, or at least indicate that the utility of the limb had more to do with the fact that it enabled them to keep their jobs and avoid the fate of the unemployed. Stevedores, machinists, ship's carpenters, and other members of the working class relayed their thanks; one man employed at the loading docks of the Central Railroad of New Jersey wrote that "In going to and from work I have to go on ferry-boats and cars, which I do with perfect ease. Had it not been for you, I should have been a helpless cripple all of my days." Another laborer, one Tom O'Donnell, wrote that "Its [the limb] out of sight. It would cork a mule to see me get there on the dump boards. I am driving a team on city work, and can hold my job."[28]

Among urban laborers, this new generation of prostheses fulfilled a more obvious function—namely, enabling them to walk and work again. Yet if the writings of manufacturers, inventors, and other commentators are any indication, the revolution in prosthesis design did

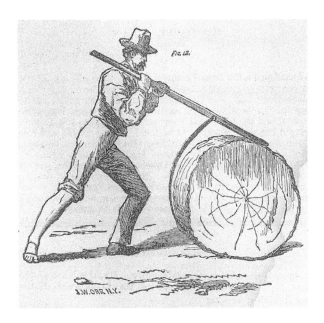

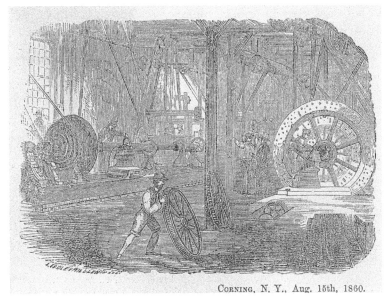

FIGS. 10.5 AND 10.6. From Douglas Bly, M.D., *A New and Important Invention* (Rochester: Curtis, Butts, and Company, 1862), 10, 19, pamphlet in "Artificial Limbs," box 1, folder 4, Warshaw Collection of Business Americana, National Museum of American History, Washington, D.C.

not derive from an interest in assisting this particular group of amputees. If anything, working-class amputees were instead the beneficiaries of developments spurred on by a middle-class obsession with appearances and concealment.

The only amputees who did not benefit from these innovations—and this is suggestive in and of itself—were amputees in the rural South. In the wake of the Civil War, the thousands of amputees who returned home made do with more traditional limbs, or quite often nothing at all. In the North, a sleeve without an arm might inspire revulsion and cries of "cripple," but in the South it could be a badge of honor. While "American taste," by which Oliver Wendell Holmes meant the taste of "respectable" northerners, "was offended, outraged, by the odious 'peg' which the Old-World soldier or beggar was proud to show," southerners living in agrarian communities felt otherwise.[29]

In "First Impressions," a forgotten piece of poetry from the antebellum era, a writer observed that the inner character of strangers may best be "read" in a person's looks, "just as one reads in plainly written books."[30] The subject of her verse—the peculiar social relations of that era—left their mark in unlikely places. Prostheses from that time, far from being mere markers of technological progress, remain emblems, largely forgotten, of the demands posed by an "age of appearances" in whose shadow we continue to live today.

NOTES

1. *Highest Award for Artificial Limbs at the World's Columbian Exposition, Chicago, 1893*, pamphlet in "Artificial Limbs," box 1, folder 10, Warshaw Collection of Business Americana, National Museum of American History.

2. Laurann Figg and Jane Farrell-Beck, "Amputation in the Civil War: Physical and Social Dimensions," *Journal of the History of Medicine and Allied Sciences* 48 (1993): 455. On the distinctly "modern" carnage of the Civil War, see Charles Royster, *The Destructive War: William Tecumsah Sherman, Stonewall Jackson, and the Americans* (New York: Vintage, 1991).

3. Oliver Wendell Holmes, "The Human Wheel, Its Spokes and Felloes," *Atlantic Monthly*, May 1863, 574.

4. On patents for artificial limbs, see *Subject-Matter Index of Patents for Inventions Issued by the United States Patent Office from 1790 to 1873, Inclusive* (New York: Arno, 1976; original edition, 1874).

5. Historical treatments of prosthetic limbs are almost nonexistent. Developments in the Italian Renaissance are documented in Vittorio Putti, *Historic Artificial Limbs* (New York: P. B. Hoeber, 1930). A more anecdotal treatment may be found, appropriately enough, in a book published by A. A. Marks, a manufacturer of artificial limbs. See A. A. Marks, *A Treatise on Artificial Limbs with Rubber Hands and Feet* (New York: A. A. Marks, 1901), esp. 11–17.

6. *Scientific American*, April 15, 1865, 4, quoted in A. A. Marks, *Marks' Patent Artificial Limbs, with India Rubber Hands and Feet* (New York: William B. Smyth, 1867), 13, emphasis in original, pamphlet in "Artificial Limbs," box 1, folder 11, Warshaw Collection of Business Americana, National Museum of American History. Several of the American models developed in the 1840s and 1850s, especially the "Palmer leg," exhibited at the Crystal Palace in 1851, represent an intermediate stage in the development of prosthetic technology. Such limbs relied on systems of gears, but made these more responsive to the movement of the body.

7. *Palmer and Company, Manufacturers of "Palmer's Patent Leg,"* pamphlet in "Artificial Limbs," box 1, folder 13, Warshaw Collection of Business Americana, National Museum of American History. A step-by-step account of the manufacture of artificial limbs may be found in the chapter of Marks's 1901 *Treatise on Artificial Limbs* entitled "From the Stump to the Limb," 348–68.

8. Douglas Bly, M.D., *A Description of a New, Curious, and Important Invention* (Rochester: Union and Advertiser Printers, 1860), in the Toner Collection, Division of Rare Books and Special Collections, Library of Congress, Washington, D.C. For a fascinating account of the larger shift from mechanical to organic technologies, see David F. Channell, *The Vital Machine: A Study of Technology and Organic Life* (New York: Oxford University Press, 1991).

9. Douglas Bly, M.D., *A New and Important Invention* (Rochester: Curtis, Butts, and Company, 1862), 2–5, pamphlet in "Artificial Limbs," box 1, folder 4, Warshaw Collection of Business Americana, National Museum of American History; Bly, quoted in John McGuire, *Descriptive Catalogue of Artifical Limbs* (St. Paul, n.d.), 14–17, pamphlet in "Artificial Limbs," box 1, folder 4, Warshaw Collection of Business Americana, National Museum of American History.

10. Bly, *A New and Important Innovation*, 6; *Centennial Testimonials to the Clement Artificial Leg*, 3–6, pamphlet in "Artificial Limbs," box 1, folder 17, Warshaw Collection of Business Americana, National Museum of American History.

11. DeForrest Douglass, *Reporter of the New Patent Artificial Leg* (Springfield, MA: J. F. Tannatt, 1861), 11. Similarly, the Union nurse Adelaide Smith commented on the quality of the artificial limbs in her memoirs: "It was surprising how many were well fitted with the limbs, and they could walk so well that only a slight limp betrayed them." One of her patients wore a limb that

"fitted so well that he could jump off a moving car." Adelaide W. Smith, *Reminiscences of an Army Nurse during the Civil War* (New York: Greaves, 1911), 129, 189, quoted in Figg and Farrell-Beck, "Amputation in the Civil War," 462.

12. This essay derives much of its theoretical force from much of the recent studies in the social construction of technology. See, for example, Wiebe E. Bijker, *Of Bicycles, Bakelites, and Bulbs: Toward a Theory of Sociotechnical Change* (Cambridge: MA: MIT Press, 1995), esp. 1–17; W. E. Bijker, T. P. Hughes, and T. J. Pinch, eds., *The Social Construction of Technological Systems: New Directions in the Sociology and History of Technology* (Cambridge: MA: MIT Press, 1987).

13. George Lippard, *The Quaker City, or The Monks of Monk Hall* (Philadelphia, 1845; reprint, New York: Odyssey Press, 1970), 23.

14. On the nature and function of personal appearance prior to urbanization, see Richard L. Bushman, *The Refinement of America: Persons, Houses, Cities* (New York: Vintage, 1992), 1–203. See also Norbert Elias, *The Civilizing Process: The History of Manners and State Formation and Civilization*, trans. Edmund Jephcott (Cambridge, MA: Blackwell, 1994).

15. Karen Halttunen, *Confidence Men and Painted Women: A Study of Middle-Class Culture in America, 1830–1870* (New Haven: Yale University Press, 1982).

16. John F. Kasson, *Rudeness and Civility: Manners in Nineteenth-Century Urban America* (New York: Hill and Wang, 1990); Halttunen, *Confidence Men and Painted Women*, esp. 1–55. See also David Scobey, "Anatomy of the Promenade: The Politics of Bourgeois Sociability in Nineteenth-Century New York," *Social History* 17 (1992): 203–26.

17. Kasson, *Rudeness and Civility*, 96.

18. Holmes, "The Human Wheel," 574, 578.

19. Thomas Embley Osmun, *The Mentor: A Little Book for the Guidance of Such Men and Boys as Would Appear to Advantage in the Society of Persons of the Better Sort* (New York: Funk and Wagnalls, 1885), quoted in Kasson, *Rudeness and Civility*, 123; Samuel R. Wells, *New Physiognomy* (New York: American Book Company, 1871), 321. Etiquette manuals abound with these sorts of references.

20. Holmes, "The Human Wheel," 578; Marks, *Marks' Patent Artificial Limbs*, 16.

21. *Palmer's Patent Artificial Leg Reporter and Surgical Adjuvant* 2 (1850): 8; *Centennial Testimonials to the Clement Artificial Leg*, 6; Erasmus Darwin Hudson, *Mechanical Surgery as a Specialty* (New York, n.d.), 41, pamphlet in the Toner Collection, Division of Rare Books and Special Collections, Library of Congress, Washington, D.C.

22. Marks, *Marks' Patent Artificial Limbs*, 25, 29.

23. Marks, *Marks' Patent Artificial Limbs*, 29

24. Trade card of the A. A. Marks Company, n.d., box 1, folder 11, Warshaw Collection of Business Americana, National Museum of American History. Interestingly, the man's posture belies his condition. Unable to hold still for the

camera, he leans on the table in the center of the photograph. This is not especially surprising; double amputees generally used a cane in addition to the limbs.

25. Judging from the advertising literature and testimonials, these individuals seem to be a minority of the total number of customers, despite the probability that the majority of amputees were members of these "lower" classes. Farmers and other rural inhabitants appear much less frequently in the literature, a fact that has much to do with the limited accessibility these social groups had to artificial limb manufacturers; also, as this essay suggests, these amputees could make do with more primitive limbs without the stigma that their use entailed in urban milieus. Finally, it should be noted that women of any social class rarely appear, primarily because they had little exposure to gunfire, heavy machinery, and other such perils.

26. For a discussion of limbs and employment of the laboring classes, see James A. Foster, *James A. Foster's Illustrated Circular* (n.d.), 2, pamphlet in "Artificial Limbs," box 1, folder 6, Warshaw Collection of Business Americana, National Museum of History.

27. Holmes, "The Human Wheel," 574; Salem Leg Company, *Circular Number Four* (n.d.), 2, pamphlet in "Artificial Limbs," box 1, folder 15, Warshaw Collection of Business Americana, National Museum of History; Bly, *A New and Important Invention*, 5, 26.

28. McGuire, *Descriptive Catalogue of Artificial Limbs*, 79; Erasmus Darwin Hudson, Surgical Speciality. (New York, n.d.), 31, pamphlet in the Toner Collection, Division of Rare Books and Special Collections, Library of Congress, Washington, D.C.

29. Holmes, "The Human Wheel," 574.

30. Blanche Bennairde, "First Impressions," *Godey's Magazine and Lady's Book* 47 (September 1853): 228.

BIBLIOGRAPHY

Primary Sources

Special Collections

Warshaw Collection of Business Americana, National Museum of American History
Bly, Douglas, M.D. *A New and Important Invention*. Rochester: Curtis, Butts, and Company, 1862. Pamphlet in "Artificial Limbs," box 1, folder 4.
Centennial Testimonials to the Clement Artificial Leg. Pamphlet in "Artificial Limbs," box 1, folder 17.
Foster, James A. *James A. Foster's Illustrated Circular*. N.d. Pamphlet in "Artificial Limbs," box 1, folder 6.

Highest Award for Artificial Limbs at the World's Columbian Exposition, Chicago, 1893. Pamphlet in "Artificial Limbs," box 1, folder 10.

Marks, A. A. *Marks' Patent Artificial Limbs, with India Rubber Hands and Feet.* New York: William B. Smyth, 1867. Pamphlet in "Artificial Limbs," box 1, folder 11.

McGuire, John. *Descriptive Catalogue of Artificial Limbs.* St. Paul, n.d. Pamphlet in "Artificial Limbs," box 1, folder 4.

Palmer and Company, Manufacturers of "Palmer's Patent Leg." Pamphlet in "Artificial Limbs," box 1, folder 13.

Salem Leg Company. *Circular Number Four.* N.d. Pamphlet in "Artificial Limbs," box 1, folder 15.

Trade card of the A. A. Marks Company. N.d. box 1, folder 11.

Toner Collection, Division of Rare Books and Special Collections, Library of Congress

Bly, Douglas, M.D. *A Description of a New, Curious, and Important Invention.* Rochester: Union and Advertiser Printers, 1860.

Hudson, Erasmus Darwin. *Mechanical Surgery as a Specialty.* New York, n.d. Pamphlet.

———— *Surgical Speciality.* New York, n.d. Pamphlet.

Additional Books and Articles

Bennairde, Blanche. "First Impressions." *Godey's Magazine and Lady's Book* 47 (September 1853): 228.

Douglass, DeForrest. *Reporter of the New Patent Artificial Leg,* Springfield, MA: J. F. Tannatt, 1861.

Holmes, Oliver Wendell. "The Human Wheel, Its Spokes and Felloes." *Atlantic Monthly,* May 1863.

Lippard, George. *The Quaker City, or The Monks of Monk Hall.* Philadelphia, 1845; reprint, New York: Odyssey Press, 1970.

Marks, A. A. *A Treatise on Artificial Limbs with Rubber Hands and Feet.* New York: A. A. Marks, 1901.

Osmun, Thomas Embley. *The Mentor: A Little Book for the Guidance of Such Men and Boys as Would Appear to Advantage in the Society of Persons of the Better Sort.* New York: Funk and Wagnalls, 1885.

Palmer's Patent Artificial Leg Reporter and Surgical Adjuvant 2 (1850): 8.

Wells, Samuel R. *New Physiognomy.* New York: American Book Company. 1871.

Secondary Sources

Bijker, Wiebe E. *Of Bicycles, Bakelites, and Bulbs: Toward a Theory of Sociotechnical Change.* Cambridge: MIT Press, 1995.

Bijker, Wiebe E., T. P. Hughes, and T. J. Pinch, eds. *The Social Construction of Technological Systems: New Directions in the Sociology and History of Technology.* Cambridge: MIT Press, 1987.

Bushman, Richard L. *The Refinement of America: Persons, Houses, Cities.* New York: Vintage, 1992.

Channell, David F. *The Vital Machine: A Study of Technology and Organic Life.* New York: Oxford University Press, 1991.

Elias, Norbert. *The Civilizing Process: The History of Manners and State Formation and Civilization,* trans. Edmund Jephcott. Cambridge, MA: Blackwell, 1994.

Figg, Laurann, and Jane Farrell-Beck. "Amputation in the Civil War: Physical and Social Dimensions." *Journal of the History of Medicine and Allied Sciences* 48 (1993).

Halttunen, Karen. *Confidence Men and Painted Women: A Study of Middle-Class Culture in America, 1830–1870.* New Haven: Yale University Press, 1982.

Kasson, John F. *Rudeness and Civility: Manners in Nineteenth-Century Urban America.* New York: Hill and Wang, 1990.

Putti, Vittorio. *Historic Artificial Limbs.* New York: P. B. Hoeber, 1930.

Royster, Charles. *The Destructive War: William Tecumseh Sherman, Stonewall Jackson, and the Americans.* New York: Vintage, 1991.

Scobey, David. "Anatomy of the Promenade: The Politics of Bourgeois Sociability in Nineteenth-Century New York." *Social History* 17 (1992): 203–26.

Smith, Adelaide W. *Reminiscences of an Army Nurse during the Civil War.* New York: Greaves, 1911.

Subject-Matter Index of Patents for Inventions Issued by the United States Patent Office from 1790 to 1873, Inclusive. New York: Arno, 1976; original edition, 1874.

11

The Long Arm of Benjamin Franklin

David Waldstreicher

IN 1786 BENJAMIN FRANKLIN invented a device "for taking down Books from high Shelves." He called it "the *Long Arm*" (fig. 11.1). This "simple machine," a wooden pole with a somewhat pliable end-piece, extended not only its inventor's arms but also his legs, since it made mounting a ladder unnecessary. Franklin further anthropomorphosed the machine by referring to its end pieces, which grasped books, as "the *Thumb*" and "the *Finger*," and to the cord pulled taut by its operator as a "sinew." At several stages of conception (or, at least, description) Franklin—a careful writer—chose to explain his mechanical device as a substitute, or additional, limb.[1]

A limb for those in need of one, like the aged inventor himself. The eighty-year-old statesman, scientist, and sage suffered from periodic battles with gout. The causes of gout remained obscure in the late eighteenth century, yet the disease had been identified as somehow circulatory and related to diet. There was no cure. Nevertheless, gout was something to be fought, a disease that called on the patient to heal himself. It always returned, but it did at least go away. Franklin found himself "not sure that it is not itself really a Remedy instead of being a Disease."[2]

Gout for someone like Franklin was an exception that proved the rule of what Elaine Forman Crane has called "the defining force of pain" in the everyday lives of early Americans. Everyone faced bodily necessity; some, like Franklin, optimistically sought to mitigate the facts of life. Everyone faced the constraints of a hierarchical world; some cre-

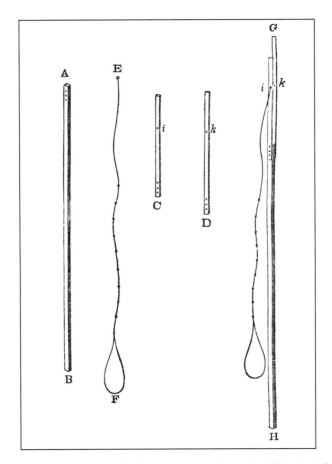

FIG. 11.1. Franklin's diagram for his Long Arm. From Jared Sparks, *The Works of Benjamin Franklin* (Philadelphia, 1840), 6: 563. Reproduced by permission of Franklin Collection, Yale University Library.

atively manipulated selves and appearances, in search of power and autonomy. Gout itself tended to be anthropomorphosed into *the* gout, to be visualized as a small but dextrous monster or described, in the conceit favored by Franklin's nephew, as a "troublesome companion," because it acted like powerful people: an unpredictable and constraining force, yet possibly less a curse than a higher power, a monitor, a warning to heed necessity. Gout had the potential to turn limbs, the servile parts of the body, into not-so-arbitrary rulers, or bearers of punishment for bodily sins, as Franklin described the situation in his "Dialogue between the Gout and Dr. Franklin" (1780). Would good behavior keep the mistress of pain and her "wholesome corrections" at bay? Only careful attention to the gout's whims could turn the twitching, even speaking foot or hand into a silent, cooperative member once again.[3]

Franklin had won fame for his own domestic labor-saving devices and for his efforts to make sense of labor and its costs in the Atlantic political economy. He took neither political nor economic arrangements for granted; indeed, he specialized in the relationship between population (working bodies), the economy, and political regulation. His own particular complaint suggested the connections between increasingly numerous and vociferous bodies in the colonies and a growing imperial body politic. The pain of gout, disease of the extremities, could be seen as a warning sign, an early symptom for what might become more lasting pathologies. Pain of the limbs, in short, was a constitutional disorder, pregnant with meaning for the state of the body as a whole. By the time he invented the Long Arm, and decided that gout was simultaneously a plague and a cure, Franklin had pursued the trope of the distressed colony as diseased limb for more than a third of a century. "Oh let not Britain seek to oppress us," he had written in 1753, "but like an affectionate parent endeavour to secure freedom to her children; they may be able one day to assist her in defending her own—Whereas a Mortification begun in the foot may spread upwards to the destruction of the nobler parts of the body." In notes for a pamphlet against the Stamp Act in 1766, he made the dangers even more explicit: "'The Empire weaken'd, and the Foundation laid of a total Separation. Mortification in the Foot."[4] Colonial complaints were more than a little pain in the toe of the British empire. Like the gout, colonial protests were the limbs, the productive parts of the body, talking back. Well attended, they secured the health and liberty of the entire empire.

After the colonial limbs did separate from the main body of the empire in 1776, Franklin began to compare democratic upheaval within the new American states to cases of disorderly, or at least discoursing, limbs. But the seeds of the actual Long Arm as a practical materialization of his ideas about bodies and politics appear in the documentary record for the first time in two letters of November 1772, when Franklin was a colonial agent in London. On the third of that month Franklin mentioned to his son William the acquisition of a roomful of books that, like his own activities to bring Parliament to its senses on the subject of

American rights, he hoped would be of future use to his countrymen. On the same day, in a letter to the Charleston printer Peter Timothy, he complained that he could not perform personal and diplomatic duties because he had been "gouty of late."[5]

This was neither the first nor the last time Franklin found his activities of moving about and writing on behalf of the colonies complicated by illness in general and the gout in particular. And he was in good company. In 1766–67, William Pitt's relatively pro-American government had nearly ground to a halt because of the pain in the prime minister's lame legs. On that occasion, the relation between cause and effect—between endangered constitutions and pains in the limbs— seemed rather less clear. As Franklin put it at the time, Pitt's own "Constitution is said to be totally destroyed by the gout." Anti-administration cartoonists drew the parallel: corruption itself lay in the manipulation of Pitt's conspicuous crutches. By 1766, that corruption already included the manipulation of "sedition" in places like New York (fig. 11.2).[6]

At the very moment that Americans talked of raising statues to Pitt, his aching feet were bringing him down, not only practically but also rhetorically in the hands of his and the colonies' enemies. Franklin, as governor of Pennsylvania twenty years later, took the lesson to heart. In short, Benjamin Franklin did not invent a new, longer, wooden arm merely because of his age and his pain in a roomful of tall shelves. He also needed a "Long Arm" because he was Benjamin Franklin.

For decades, like the prime minister and the king himself, Franklin had been projected, and had learned to project himself, as the quintessential national body.[7] The political as well as personal repercussions of Franklin's body—especially the important place of the arms and hands in this body politic—can be seen in three of the best-known portraits of Franklin, from his Philadelphia period through his London years to his ambassadorship to France. The Robert Feke portrait of 1746, for example, depicts a forty-year-old newly minted gentleman, richly clothed, complete with wig and the commanding hand seen in so many gentry portraits of the era (fig. 11.3). This is not the early-to-bed-and-early-to-rise, wheelbarrow-pushing Franklin of the 1771 *Autobiography*. It is the picture of a provincial gentleman about to retire from his business, who commands and directs with his hands rather than working with them.

The second image, derived from Franklin's time in London as a colonial agent, shows us a diplomat and statesman who is, most of all,

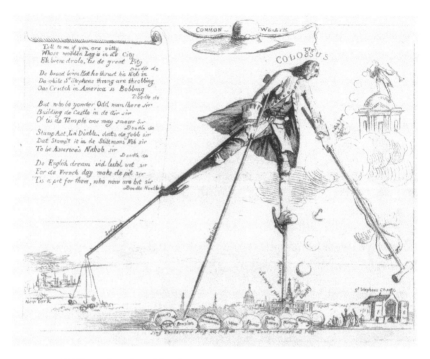

FIG. 11.2. William Pitt the Elder (1766). Reproduced by permission of American Antiquarian Society.

a man of the Enlightenment (fig. 11.4). With his hands he holds his head and his papers, suggesting the ideal grounding of the republic of letters (and the colonists' protests circa 1767) in Reason. Franklin's bifocals—another of his inventions—allow him to grasp his papers at a reasonable distance. By holding on to his inventions and his papers, Franklin keeps his head, and earns his place under the gaze of a bust of Sir Isaac Newton.[8]

The even better known Cochin engraving of 1777 (fig. 11.5) retains the bifocals, though Franklin cheekily looks both through and beyond them. Here, seeking French sympathy for the American revolutionaries, he poses in the idealized Quaker costume he actually wore in France, topped off with a fur hat of "native" origin. Variably identified by scholars as Quaker and Indian garb, the costume perhaps deliberately confused the two, both of which symbolized a rejection of European patterns of consumption.[9] The costume completely covers Franklin's body in this bust shot. The engraving shows no hands, for he is neither gentleman nor working man. A simple Quaker, a natural man of the new world, he commits no machinations.

Franklin tailored all three images to fit his own aspirations and those of America's ruling classes at midcentury, during the controversial 1760s, and during the revolutionary late 1770s. By 1786 certainly, every invention of Franklin's could also serve as public self-invention, even as an ideological statement. The portraits reveal what Ormond Seavey has described as the tendency for Franklin's reinventions of self to merge with his public services, a pattern that emerged early in his life and only intensified as his fame became useful to the nascent American state.[10] There is a paradox here that requires some reflection. Franklin, one of the few Founding Fathers to have worked with his hands, became the preeminent man of the disembodied republic of letters, and a widely circulated visual image to boot (so to speak). Who better, then,

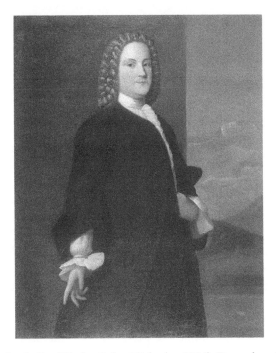

FIG. 11.3. *Benjamin Franklin*, by Robert Feke (ca. 1746). Reproduced by permission of the Harvard University Portrait Collection, Bequest of Dr. John Collins Warden, 1856.

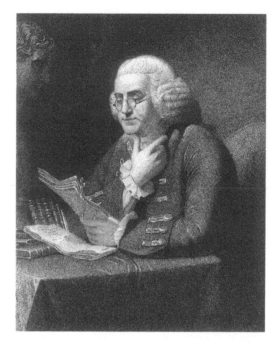

FIG. 11.4. Engraving by T. B. Welch, after David Martin, *Portrait of Benjamin Franklin* (1767). Reproduced by permission of Franklin Collection, Yale University Library.

to mediate the local and international meanings of a representative national body? Who better to resolve the conundrum of the king's two bodies for a republic?

The dialectic of real (or laboring) and imagined (or political) bodies in the founding of the United States, a subject of increasing interest to scholars, suggests a pressing need to consider Franklin's invention of a substitute limb in 1786 in light of his use of images of the limbs, and arms in particular, throughout his career.[11] In doing so, we must entertain not just the deep and continuing meaning making being done with metaphors of the "body politic," but also the simultaneous emergence of a distinctly modern bodily condition, exacerbated perhaps by disembodying forms of media like print. We become obsessed with our bodies precisely to the extent that we are alienated from our bodies. We then produce, in Foucauldian terms, body knowledges, and body-knowledge effects. Alternatively, in the terms advanced by Elaine

Scarry, the "made object is a projection of the live body that itself recip-
rocates the live body" and remakes us in the process: the artifact is a site
not only of "projection" but also of "reciprocation." It seems more than
coincidental that Scarry's rich and nuanced understanding of pain, language, objectification, and embodiment begins in a consideration of the
structure of warfare, from which so many prosthetic innovations would
derive. The insight should be extended to the colonial and imperial politics that first produced warfare in its modern, nationalist forms.[12]

Franklin developed a particular interest in images of mutilated
limbs because that imagery enabled him to identify, explore, allegorize,
and narrate contemporary problems that emerged from the relationship
between directing faculties and working extremities in the colonial context.[13] In late colonial America, two overlapping sorts of relationships

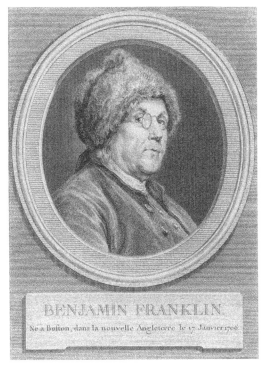

FIG. 11.5. *Benjamin Franklin*. Engraving by Augustin St. Aubin from a drawing
by Charles-Nicholas Cochin (1777). Reproduced by permission of Franklin
Collection, Yale University Library.

between agents and executors came to be discussed through the imagery of heads and hands. The first was that of labor: owners and workers—usually masters and servants or slaves. The second relationship was that of empire: the head here was the metropole, and its limbs the quickly growing colonies. Under these sorts of conditions, it is hard to imagine a prosthesis failing to do political work, especially if the device is invented and publicized by a man whose very fame and fortune derived from his reputation for saving labor and for saving his fellow colonists from the risks of extending the provincial body politic. I do not wish to suggest that Franklin invented his Long Arm solely to do cultural and political rather than actual or manual work. What I wish to accomplish here is to begin to understand the cultural and political, as well as bodily, demands that led to an obsession and an invention. In the process I hope to recover the set of needs and possibilities that led Franklin to describe his library device as an "arm" and to take such evident pleasure in its workings.

Benjamin Franklin was born into a colonial world in which labor was scarce, the most valuable of commodities. Little wonder that at the age of twenty-three he would write, in his first effort at political economy, that "the Riches of a Country are to be valued by the Quantity of Labour its Inhabitants are able to purchase." He knew these conditions intimately; they made possible his rise from runaway to master printer in his youth. The first part of Franklin's *Autobiography*, written in 1771, narrates his rise from apprentice to owner of a newspaper, printer of the colony's money, and moving force behind America's first subscription library by 1731.[14] The text is usually read as a story about self-invention in a new land of opportunity. Less often noted is young Benjamin's near escape from various forms of unfreedom: apprenticeship, indentured servitude, and debt (which for people of Franklin's class often meant repayment by servitude). In Benjamin Franklin's America, the labor shortage meant not only opportunity but also danger for the youngest son of a Boston tallow chandler.

Franklin did get ahead, though, and according to his memoir there were two ways he managed to rise into the owning class of artisans by the 1730s. The first was his attention to self-improvement and efficiency. Second, and really prior, was mobility itself. Benjamin Franklin ran away from his brother to New York and then to Philadelphia, where he gradually negotiated better labor terms for himself. Later he traveled to

England, where he learned the most up-to-date methods of writing and printing in the exciting hothouse of publication that was London in the 1720s. Upon his return he profited from both skills, which he would describe in the *Autobiography* as abilities of the arms and hands. As a young apprentice (and a useful "Hand") he "disguise[d] [his] hand" to write for his brother's newspaper.[15] In Samuel Keimer, his boss in Philadelphia, he found a compositor with nimble fingers but weak arms, so Franklin became the pressman, a skill he continued to develop in his London stint. During that time he was known as the "water-American," in part because of his quaffing of water instead of beer, but also because of his prodigious abilities as a swimmer. (One of Franklin's first inventions, as a boy, had been a set of paddles for swimming.)[16] By his early twenties he had developed powerful arms as well as a skilled pair of hands.

Printers like Franklin knew all too well that the potentially leveling, disembodied cultural world of print relied on the back-breaking (as well as arm-broadening) work of people like themselves. One of Franklin's printer protégés would later remark that printers were "obliged to work like Negroes, and in general are esteemed little better."[17] Franklin himself went so far as to broadcast his own strength of body as well as character by theatrically wheeling his purchases of paper through the streets of Philadelphia, lest his customers miss how hard he had earned their shillings. When Franklin pushed his own paper he did more than display his diligence: he saved money that would have been paid to someone else for doing the job. This was the context for his early elaboration of a labor theory of value, which Karl Marx would call "the first conscious, clear, and almost trite analysis of exchange value into labor value."[18] Franklin worked out this analysis of political economy because he saw, from the distinct position of one of the laborers, the commodification of work and workers occurring at an innovative, new pace.

As a master printer, Franklin made a point of doing much of his own work, but he also began to think about the conditions under which the purchase and use of others' labor would be profitable. In a society in which "hands" referred simultaneously to body parts and to servants and slaves, the problem of the hand was the problem of mobilizing labor, gaining control over personal and political economies, and over other people as well as oneself. The ambiguities that resulted are apparent in successive editions of Franklin's *Poor Richard's Almanack* during the 1730s and 1740s. Franklin's aphoristic recommendations to tradesmen and farmers promoted self-reliance, efficient labor, and bodily self-control. He also counseled the master class on how to handle the servant problem. "Never intreat a servant to dwell with thee," urges Richard: keep surrogates at an objective, though observable, distance. Husbandmen are urged to keep working on their own farms "[t]ho' his collected rent his bags supply,/ Or honest careful slaves scarce need his eye." Land itself was worth little unless labor costs stayed low: hence the productive ambiguity in the cry of another farmer in the almanac: "Help, Hands; For I have no Lands."[19]

Which hands are being begged to work harder? Is a body part being personified, or are workers themselves an extension of the patriarch's body, alternatives to other kinds of property? Reliance on "hands" seemed both problem and solution in the booming middle colonies. At a time of expanding trade and of labor imports, when Franklin was himself profiting from the sale, rent, and recapture of "hands" through the medium of the advertisements in his newspaper, Poor Richard seems surprisingly ambivalent about the commodification of human labor as practiced in contemporary Pennsylvania. Franklin, seeking to speak for and to the majority, urged his audience to retain a hands-on approach, without getting so close as to conflate the head of the family with the hands that labor.

The available evidence suggests that Franklin had mixed feelings about depending on others' labor. He was not confident in real-life surrogates, but he required them if he was to become, and remain, Benjamin Franklin. In his own later account, most of his working associates let him down until he took on David Hall as a partner in 1748. By then Franklin had long since set up a system of silent partnership in printing shops all up and down the western Atlantic, from Newport to Antigua.[20] He had extended himself at some risk. But he took care to construct elaborate contracts that gave him significant profits but limited liability. The best way to extend oneself was to convince people to do what he would have them do. Thus, as he tells us in the *Autobiography*, "I put my self as much as I could out of sight" when proposing the first subscription library in Philadelphia. As an economic actor as well as a writer and politician, Franklin faced the problem of how to mobilize people without exploiting them, or at least not seeming to exploit them, for his own gain.[21]

After 1748 Franklin devoted himself full-time to politics, science, and the republic of letters that connected those realms. His specialty, insofar as a philosophe could have a specialty, was political economy. In *Observations Concerning the Increase of Mankind* (1751), he objected to the English government's restrictive regulation of colonial manufactures and of labor supply, casting the problem of such regulations in terms of the loss to the colonies of free, value-producing, white people-commodities. The powers in London had it backward: the increase of a well-governed people in a new land not hemmed in by war or by slavery's discouragement to "white" settlement would mean great wealth to the home country because of the laws of natural increase. There would be more and more consumers for English manufactures with each passing year. For Franklin, the interest of the colonists and that of the home country were the same. Britain's extremities, its working colonial hands, were vital organs to be grown, not jealously girded or amputated:

> In fine, A Nation well regulated is like a Polypus; take away a Limb, its Place is soon supply'd; cut it in two, and each deficient Part shall speedily grow out of the Part remaining. Thus if you have Room and Subsistence enough, as you may by dividing, make ten Polypes out of one, you may of one make ten Nations, equally populous and powerful; or rather, increase a nation ten fold in Numbers and Strength.[22]

The brilliance of the *Observations* lies in its enunciation of physiocratic principles, with all their scientific inevitability, from the perspective of the colonies. Franklin called not for free trade but for better regulation. Better regulation would guarantee the growth of one powerful Anglo-American nation, instead of the independent growth of the colonies: a threat never made explicitly but raised nonetheless as a scientifically provable fact derived from natural law. The threat of division—the alternatives of rebellion by hands or extension of the entire imperial body politic—loomed already for Franklin at midcentury.

Early and consistently, the problem of the regulation of the empire, and thus the problem of colonial identity, appeared to Franklin as the problem of hands growing—and growing out of control. The difficulty was that it was not exactly clear who were the hands. Who were the people-commodities who labored for the good of the whole? The colonists? Or the colonists' hands, their laborers? Already in 1740, during the War of Jenkins' Ear, Franklin complained vociferously on behalf of Pennsylvania masters when the British navy impressed their indentured servants. The colonial wars over trade and expansion provided opportunities for the colonists' human investments to run away and serve higher-bidding agents of the British body politic. Worse, more and more of the empire's problem, pain-inducing, violent hands were being intentionally retailed to the less profitable mainland colonies. During the 1750s Franklin led the way in arguing against the English practice of transporting convicts. He took on a distinctive American identity for the first time in a 1751 essay on the subject, which he signed "Americanus." England showed "Contempt" for the colonies by creating and subsidizing the trade in old world reprobates. In this stunning example of early American gothic, Americanus relates a news story about a Maryland servant who cut off his own hand rather than killing his mistress with it, only to throw down the bloody gauntlet and cry, *"Now make me work, if you can."*[23]

"Hands" amputating themselves to spite their masters' faces: for Franklin there could be no more telling symbol for corruption in the Anglo-American body politic. Even a casual reading of Franklin's productions of this period makes it apparent that he developed a remarkable repertoire of—if not an obsession with—images of mutilation, of lopped-off limbs.[24] If the empire was a healthy body politic, the empire in distress contained, or actually was, a body mutilated, unable to work. Twenty years later Franklin still employed the trope: in the disease of imperial controversy, "harsher treatment may increase the inflammation, make the cure less practicable, and in time bring on the necessity of an amputation; death indeed to the severed limb, weakness and lamentation to the mutilated body." During the decades between these examples, the rapidly growing British North American empire had become even more vulnerable at the extremities thanks to frontier warfare and the competition for Indian allies. For a time, Native Americans successfully manipulated the British and French empires into creating a market for enemy scalps—a situation in which, as Peter Way has argued, bodies and body parts were explicitly commodified as part of the battle for control of North American trade.[25]

Franklin's representations of the arms, then, mediated the complex relationship between theories of labor and understandings of empire.

They registered simultaneously the real violence between masters and workers and the possibility of conflict between Britain and its colonies. Franklin, the voice of the master class, circulated stories of servants who committed acts of theft, rape, and mutilation as part of his larger political strategy of blaming the British for the discontents of the colonists (and their servants). Subject to impressment of their laborers and a long-standing shortage of cheap labor, the colonial master classes watched fearfully for signs that their superiors in the metropole might ally themselves, not with their fellow men of property, but with Indians, servants, and/or slaves. Franklin, who as printer, political economist, and diplomat spent decades mediating this long conversation, ultimately came to identify the British themselves with the "hands" who would not be controlled. By identifying the British ultimately with the unruly hands, Franklin projected the two-sided anxieties of members of a colonial master class: their insecurity vis-à-vis both the workers they owned and the British politicians and merchants who exercised power over them.

In the search for colonial autonomy within the empire and, eventually, independence, this projection proved strategically crucial. For to see colonies as the limbs was to present the colonies as what they were in British mercantilist theory: laborers in the empire, and thus analogous to the servants and slaves employed by Franklin and those who advertised in his newspaper. Such a subordination justified the very regulations Franklin had been moved to protest. Images and stories of mutilation were so charged, and thus effective, because of their very ambiguity. They simultaneously evoked servant rebellion and masters' violence, identification on the one hand with the (English) master class and, on the other hand, with unfree (foreign) servants and slaves. After comparing transported felons to snakes—animals that bite and poison limbs—Franklin in another essay suggested that since American snakes are native "felons-convict since the beginning of the world," they should be sentenced to transport . . . to England! Who is a snake? asked Franklin, much as Melville's Ishmael would later ask, much more directly about the Atlantic world, "Who ain't a slave?" In the context of a political debate, Franklin attacked both the snake-servants and those who would poison the body politic by sending them over. Americans, ideally, were the happy, middling sort: neither tyrannical masters nor tyrannized slaves. Meanwhile, knowing that some Britons had come to see the North American colonies as quarrelsome, backbiting

FIG. 11.6. "Join, or Die." *Pennsylvania Gazette*, May 9, 1754. Reproduced by permission of Library Company of Philadelphia.

extremities, Franklin seized upon the iconography of the snake to illustrate his call for intercolonial unity (fig. 11.6).[26]

Beginning in 1757, Franklin spent most of the next twenty-eight years serving Pennsylvania, other colonies, and eventually the United States as an agent in London and Paris. There he not only represented America in his person and through widely distributed visual images, he also represented the American people allegorically in pseudonymous newspaper essays and, eventually, in chapbooks printed on his own press at Passy, France. He repeatedly resisted the tendency of British supporters of the colonial regulations to wave off American complaints as the carping of servant-children who should mind their labors or, worse, as the hypocritical rantings of paranoid slave drivers.[27] Rather, it was the mother country that was cutting off its colonial limbs, in part by sending over dangerous slaves and servants who ruined productivity and good trading relations. In "Magna Britania Her Colonies Reduced" (1766), Franklin's second influential and widely reprinted political cartoon (which he first sent around as a calling card), he accused the empire, as he had earlier accused convict servants, of self-mutilation (fig. 11.7). His home colony of Pennsylvania is the amputated right hand, which can no longer even grasp the laurel branch next to it in the foreground. The maimed empire's ships have brooms on their masts, "denoting," Franklin wrote, "their being on sale."[28]

Increased trade and population growth made the relationship between the imperial head and the colonial hands only more charged after the Seven Years' War. Franklin experienced personally a similar sense of expansion and frustration, garnering both acclaim and attacks during these years as his reputation continued to grow. The sheer volume of his scientific and political correspondence made it harder and harder for him to keep tabs on his far-flung network of printers and post officers. His political influence at home in Pennsylvania seemed to decrease with distance, yet other colonies began to appoint him as their representative at Whitehall. Meanwhile, he suffered episodes of physical debility. For months after a series of injuries in 1763–64 he found himself more dependent than ever on servants, including a slave who helped him put on his shirt.[29]

During the late 1760s and early 1770s Franklin found himself treated simultaneously as an icon and "as a Snake in the Grass." He was dressed down before Parliament as akin to a "cruel African" for criticizing the administration's colonial policies.[30] These were the years when the gout began to plague Franklin, and especially badly during some moments of acute political crisis (e.g., early 1765, June 1770, June 1776).[31] When Franklin had to be carried into the Continental Congress on a litter by convict laborers during the summer of 1776, the irony of his longtime fame and his sometime weakness, his historic self-sufficiency and his current dependence, appeared in yet another kind of public display.

Despite his advanced years and his infirmities, Franklin became only more important as a symbol of Americanness and, not coincidentally, as an actor on the stage of international politics. His participation in the salons and state dinners of the Revolutionary era, especially during the war on his mission to France, has often been described as a delightful respite from a life of labor, a cosmopolitan fulfillment for a man of the world finally surrounded by his intellectual equals. Yet while abroad once again Franklin fought for his own and America's reputation, desperately trying to spin his fame into a more positive interpretation of the proper relationship of formerly colonial limbs to the bod-

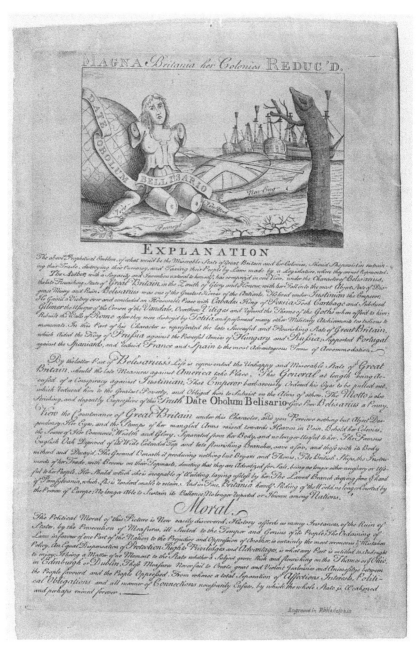

FIG. 11.7. "Magna Britania Her Colonies Reduced" (Philadelphia, 1766). Reproduced by permission of Library Company of Philadelphia.

316

ies of Atlantic empires. During the diplomatically crucial French mission, there was no denying that Franklin himself had become a tool of great use in a battle of empires. In one French cartoon, "Doctor" Franklin was an enema, a distinct pain in the posterior of the British empire, a presence felt by the patient to be worse than the disease (fig. 11.8).

This print gets, fundamentally we might say, to the heart of Franklin's role as an *agent* of the new United States. The French had allied with the Americans to weaken their enemy—Britain. So the agent Franklin, seemingly an Anglo, was also a kind of double agent, in the service of others. If the British bum is gleefully portrayed here in its position of greatest vulnerability, it is revealing that "Doctor" Franklin is portrayed as a tool, rather than as a person. Being a representative American had its Parisian pleasures to be sure, but it did not, and could not, solve for Franklin the ongoing problem of colonial (now American) self-determination. The sexual violation *cum* medical intervention suggested in "L'Anglais a toute extrémité" may, from a French perspective, helpfully distinguish the violating (American) tool from the violated

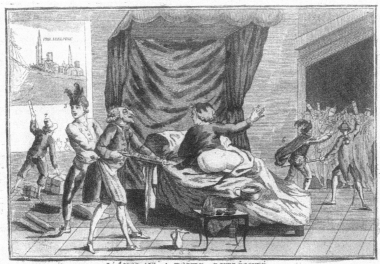

FIG. 11.8. "L'Anglais a toute extrémité." Reproduced by permission of Bibliothèque nationale de France, Paris.

British body politic. But it dehumanizes "Doctor" Franklin in the very moment of his international agency. He becomes an extension of someone else's, French hand: rigid, potent, but hardly in control.[32]

As his own Revolution neared a successful military conclusion, Franklin sought to rationalize the disorderly possibilities of the working extremities. In the "Dialogue between the Gout and Dr. Franklin," the eloquent disease wreaks its revenge on the big toe at midnight. The Left Hand, in a fictional petition, objects to its second-class status. During the American 1780s, America's own oppressed hands, inspired by Revolutionary rhetoric, had begun to talk back, in backcountry tax revolts and petitions against slavery. Clearly, for Franklin, the coming to voice of working people was both salutary and dangerous, both what he always proposed when those workers were like himself, and what he most feared, when the persons in question were slaves or servants.

When Franklin returned from France he found the United States (and his home state of Pennsylvania) in a postrevolutionary state of local ferment and federal disempowerment that historians long referred to as "the critical period." Both state and national constitutions were said by many to be unsound, or in "flux"—another eighteenth-century medical and juridical term—and some began to discuss constitutions in a highly charged architectural language that called upon expert builders and "framers." Both the Revolutionary Pennsylvania constitution and the Articles of Confederation came under attack for being too democratic, too much subject to the whims of ordinary, nonpropertied people. Artisans and working people in places like Philadelphia had taken a distinct interest in the framing of new political systems; gentlemen responded in part by talking of themselves, and each other, as innovative manipulators of wood, as manufacturers of political houses. Not only body politics of monarchy, but also the spontaneous, immanent, embodied democracy of Revolutionary action were being revised into a materialized republicanism, in which there was no substitute for a sound "foundation" and frame.[33]

As young America's most famous statesman, businessman, and cultural hero, Franklin had to keep his books, his furniture, and his body in good working order. At the time he invented the Long Arm, he was busy publishing his scientific papers as well as serving as president of Pennsylvania's executive council under its controversially democratic state constitution. At this time "he studiously read even while taking the long hot baths which were his relief from the [kidney] stone."[34] In the Long Arm essay Franklin described the problem of getting around his own library at a time when he was America's best-known man of letters: a printer, a maker of books, who became a writer and subject of them; a founder of libraries who had become a patron of them. If the library is a microcosm of the republic of letters, being able to get around its perimeters is a necessary precondition for stability and for continuing upward mobility. The descriptive essay itself shows off the literal ascent of Franklin's shelves, and thus of Franklin himself, even as it seeks to solve the problem of his declining mobility or "activity." The prosthesis comes in to solve the problem not just of infirmity but of success. The more books Franklin has, the more arm and leg he needs. The more power he has, the more he finds himself potentially dependent on other arms, or the arms of others.[35]

Like Franklin's protests against the political sins of the empire, and like the invention of American nationality itself, the gesture of inventing the Long Arm was at once empowering and alienating. The arm, as a machine, was an extension of its inventor's body and yet it keeps us—and him—at a distance. A facsimile now leans against a corner in the Benjamin Franklin Court Museum in Philadelphia. Grouped with an assortment of the great man's more costly household artifacts, it is an oddly stiff, rather large limb, akin to Tiny Tim's crutch in Dickens's *Christmas Carol* (fig. 11.9). It appears almost lonely, even reproachful, apart from any shelves or books: an arm wrenched out of context, despite the brief label on the railing. In the sequence of the Franklin Museum's tour, relief was (until very recently) provided by a film in which an aged, gouty, proud but egalitarian Franklin himself, played with such gusto by Howard DaSilva, limps energetically with us around his house and his Philadelphia. DaSilva's Franklin speaks directly to us in the late twentieth century, showing off his political and practical inventions, sharing his successful designs for upward mobility and American nationhood. Franklin thus lives and walks the streets of Philadelphia in his material, political, and literary inventions. He limps, but leaves the Long Arm behind.[36]

The Long Arm in the museum reminds the public that Franklin always kept his feet on the ground. His inventions and self-inventions exist for our benefit, and should inspire us to love him as we love an ancestor: less a father (for fathers tell us what to do) than a founding grandfather, a figure from whom we inherit our favorite characteristics.[37]

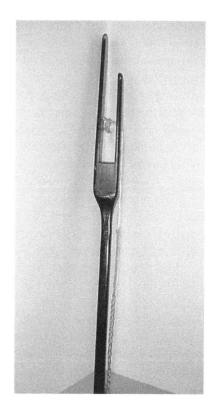

FIG. 11.9. Franklin's Long Arm device. Courtesy of Independence National Historic Park.

Franklin's legacy becomes recoverable insofar as we can see his inventions as the invention, the dream, of *us*, of our technologies, our priorities, and perhaps most of all our relationship to that which we would transcend. The film and the museum let us into Franklin's house and make that house, much as Franklin made his inventions and self-inventions, a mythic template for how Americans should behave and think about themselves. Like the Arm itself, what they encourage us to think about—and to not think about—is of more than antiquarian significance.

The "Description of an Instrument" is a narrative of saving labor, and when seen in light of Franklin's life and his earlier writings on empire, labor, and bodily extremities, it seems a desperate as well as a principled attempt to do without *laborers*. It is easy to take for granted this desire, for we are so much the product of Benjamin Franklin's America; but it is the key to understanding Franklin's Long Arm and the hold it has on us. A nation on the move has required a "hand" turned inventor and statesman to help us forget our colonial, and unfree, origins, and to remember, in a less painful fashion, the work of Revolution. Men cannot choose their grandfathers, wrote Horace Kallen, but we do—every day. In doing so we forget the other Founding Fathers and the work they did, much as Americans repeatedly (one might say systematically) forget that there are hardworking poor people in our country, some of whose ancestors also fought for their freedom—but on the other side of the Revolution.[38]

The problem of mobility and stability in the republic of letters and the republic of America is the problem of who will do the work when more work needs to be done. The Long Arm, if it works, allows Franklin to remain both the humble petitioner and the gentleman. It allows him to have high shelves, but also to keep his feet on the ground. The Long Arm does not speak; it does not cause pain; it does not rebel. Its sound construction allows its owner to re-join the American republic and the republic of letters. The Long Arm was a dream of order on the part of a man whose body had long since become abstracted yet painful, spectacular but all too real. In its creation of self-sufficiency, its design for library use, its special attention to the extension of the arms, its artful effacement of its own political resonances, and its written description inviting us to do it ourselves, Franklin's Long Arm desires, and deserves, to stand alone: a self-made prosthesis for the self-made man.

NOTES

This essay is dedicated to Kate M. Ohno—scholar, editor, material culture maven, and friend—who provided key sources, inspiration, and ample encouragement. Special thanks also to Karie Diethorn, David Serlin, and Kariann Yokota for advice and provocations.

1. Benjamin Franklin, "Description of an Instrument for Taking Down Books from High Shelves," in *Benjamin Franklin: Writings*, ed. J. A. Leo LeMay (New York, 1990), 1116–18. The description was not published during Franklin's lifetime. Franklin considered it a "philosophical Paper." When he sent it, along with three others, to Jonathan Williams to be forwarded to fellow scientist James Bowdoin, he specifically stated that although none of the four papers might be important enough to be presented to the American Philosophical Society, the "Description of the long Arm," unlike the others, contained

something of "practical Utility." Albert Henry Smyth, ed., *The Writings of Benjamin Franklin* (New York, 1906), 9: 483–86.

2. Roy Porter and G. S. Rousseau, *Gout: The Patrician Malady* (New Haven, 1998), 4–5, 13, 73, 77–78; Franklin to Benjamin Vaughan, May 4, 1779, in *The Papers of Benjamin Franklin*, ed. Benjamin W. Labaree et al. (New Haven, 1958–), 29: 437–38. For Franklin's illnesses of the 1780s, see Claude-Ann Lopez and Eugenia W. Herbert, *The Private Franklin: The Man and His Family* (New Haven, 1975), 236. On the body as an economic system in the eighteenth century, see Roy Porter, "Consumption: Disease of the Consumer Society?" in Roy Porter and John Brewer, eds., *Consumption and the World of Goods* (New York, 1993).

3. Elaine Forman Crane, "'I Have Suffer'd Much Today': The Defining Force of Pain in Early America," in Ronald Hoffman, Mechal Sobel, and Fredrika J. Teute, eds., *Through a Glass Darkly: Reflections on Personal Identity in Early America* (Chapel Hill, 1997), 370–403; Porter and Rousseau, *Gout*, 253, 267; Jonathan Williams Jr. to Franklin, March 9, 1779, Franklin to John Ross, June 8, 1765, *Papers of Benjamin Franklin*, 29: 85, 12: 172; LeMay, ed., *Benjamin Franklin: Writings*, 943–52.

4. Porter and Rousseau, *Gout*, 5–12, 77–78, 86–88; *Papers of Benjamin Franklin*, 4: 486, 13: 83, 22: 361.

5. LeMay, ed., *Benjamin Franklin: Writings*, 1115–16; *Papers of Benjamin Franklin*, 12: 428, 14: 223.

6. For Pitt's popularity and iconographic status (New Yorkers raised a statue to him in 1770), see Lester C. Olson, *Emblems of American Community in the Revolutionary Era* (Washington, DC, 1991), 5, 82–83. The resonances of Pitt's legs and crutches in political imagery drew on, and would again be succeeded by, the "boot" that stood in for Lord Bute. Diana Donald, *The Age of Caricature: Satirical Prints in the Reign of George III* (New Haven, 1996), 50–60; Olson, *Emblems of American Community*, 143.

7. On spectacular political bodies in America and their relation to the tradition of the king's body, see Michael Paul Rogin, *Ronald Reagan, the Movie and other Episodes in American Political Demonology* (Berkeley, 1987). For Franklin's self-conscious projection of his portraits I am indebted to R. Jackson Wilson, *Figures of Speech: American Writers and the Literary Marketplace* (New York, 1989), 21–26, 41–43. See also Charles Coleman Sellers, *Benjamin Franklin in Portraiture* (New Haven, 1962); Ellen G. Miles, "The French Portraits of Benjamin Franklin," and Wayne Craven, "The American and British Portraits of Benjamin Franklin," in J. A. Leo LeMay, ed., *Reappraising Benjamin Franklin: A Bicentennial Perspective* (Newark, DE, 1993), 272–89, 242–71; Brandon Brame Fortune with Deborah J. Warner, *Franklin and His Friends: Portraying the Man of Science in Eighteenth-Century America* (Philadelphia, 1999).

8. Robert A. Ferguson analyzes the rhetoric of grasping in "We Hold These Truths: Strategies of Control in the Literature of the Founders," in Sacvan

Bercovitch, ed., *Reconstructing American Literary History* (Cambridge, MA, 1986), 1–29.

9. Wilson, *Figures of Speech*, 21–22; Michael Warner, "Savage Franklin" in Gianfranco Balestra and Luigi Sampietro, eds., *Benjamin Franklin: An American Genius* (Rome, 1993), 83.

10. Ormond Seavey, *Becoming Benjamin Franklin: The Autobiography and the Life* (University Park, PA, 1988).

11. As a printer-editor, the man at home in the imagined community of print-capitalism, Franklin has rightly been described by Michael Warner as profiting from innovative forms of disembodiment. Precisely for this reason, I will argue, he obsessively commented on the actions of bodies and their surrogates in the marketplace. Recent works according great importance to Revolutionary and post-Revolutionary embodiment include Michael Warner, *The Letters of the Republic: Publication and the Public Sphere in Eighteenth Century America* (Cambridge, MA, 1990); Michael Meranze, *Laboratories of Virtue: Punishment, Revolution, and Authority in Philadelphia, 1760–1835* (Chapel Hill, 1996); Robert B. St. George, *Conversing by Signs: Poetics of Implication in Colonial New England Culture* (Chapel Hill, 1998), chap. 3; Dana Nelson, *National Manhood: Capitalist Citizenship and the Imagined Fraternity of White Men* (Durham, NC, 1998). For the nineteenth and twentieth centuries, see especially Lauren Berlant, *The Anatomy of National Fantasy: Hawthorne, Utopia, and Everyday Life* (Chicago, 1991); Berlant, *The Queen of America Goes to Washington City: Essays on Sex and Citizenship* (Durham, NC, 1997); Robyn Wiegman, *American Anatomies: Theorizing Race and Gender* (Durham, NC, 1996).

12. Scarry, *The Body in Pain: The Making and Unmaking of the World* (New York, 1986), 280.

13. For a rich account of the discourse of head and hands in a later period of transforming workplace and class relations, see Stephen P. Rice, "Minding the Machine: The Language of Class in Industrializing America, 1820–1860" (Ph.D. diss., Yale University, 1997).

14. Franklin, *A Modest Enquiry into the Nature and Necessity of a Paper-Currency* (1729), in LeMay, ed., *Benjamin Franklin: Writings*, 127; Franklin, *The Autobiography*, ed. J. A. Leo LeMay (New York, 1990), 1–68.

15. Franklin, *Autobiography*, 14, 19.

16. On Franklin as a swimmer, see Claude-Anne Lopez, *My Life with Benjamin Franklin* (New Haven, 2000), 17–23.

17. James Parker, *A Letter to a Gentleman in the City of New York* (1759), cited in Jeffrey L. Pasley, *"The Tyranny of Printers": Newspaper Politics in the Early American Republic* (Charlottesville, 2001), chap. 2; David Waldstreicher, "Reading the Runaways: Self-Fashioning, Print Culture, and Confidence in Slavery in the Eighteenth Century Mid-Atlantic," *William and Mary Quarterly*, 3d ser., 56 (1999): 243-72.

18. Karl Marx, *On America and the Civil War*, ed. Saul K. Padover (New York, 1972), 18.

19. *Poor Richard Improved . . . 1748; Poor Richard . . . 1745*, in *Papers of Benjamin Franklin*, 2: 196, 3: 5, 260.

20. Carl Van Doren, *Benjamin Franklin* (New York, 1939), 116-22; *Papers of Benjamin Franklin*, 1: 339, 2: 409 n.7, 3: 263, 322. As Ralph D. Frasca has stressed, Franklin helped a series of other printers rise from journeyman to master. But it is striking that in the *Autobiography* he stresses instead how untrustworthy his early partners and associates could be, and how often they failed. Frasca, "From Apprentice to Journeyman to Partner: Benjamin Franklin's Workers and the Growth of the Early American Printing Trade," *Pennsylvania Magazine of History and Biography* 104 (1990): 229-46.

21. Franklin, *Autobiography*, 77. For Franklin as artful employer of representations and personae, see Warner, *Letters of the Republic*, 73-96; Mitchell Breitweiser, *Cotton Mather and Benjamin Franklin: The Price of Representative Personality* (New York, 1984); Seavey, *Becoming Benjamin Franklin*. For recent historians' accounts of the manipulative Franklin, with less and more critical emphases, see Robert Middlekauff, *Benjamin Franklin and His Enemies* (Berkeley, 1995); Francis Jennings, *Benjamin Franklin, Politician* (New York, 1996); David T. Morgan, *The Devious Dr. Franklin, Colonial Agent* (Macon, GA, 1996); Barbara B. Oberg, "Introduction: The Enemies of Benjamin Franklin," *Pennsylvania History* 65 (1998): 4-5.

22. LeMay, ed., *Benjamin Franklin: Writings*, 373-74.

23. *Papers of Benjamin Franklin*, 2: 288-89; LeMay, ed., *Benjamin Franklin: Writings*, 358.

24. This, perhaps, is the real American "birth of horror," arising from all-too-related conflicts in the macro-patriarchy of the empire and the micro-patriarchy of the colonial household and workplace (which were usually the same place). For rather different interpretations of the origins of the "gothic imagination" in America, see Daniel A. Cohen, *Pillars of Salt, Monuments of Grace: New England Crime Literature and the Origins of American Popular Culture* (New York, 1993); and Karen Halttunen, *Murder Most Foul: The Killer and the American Gothic Imagination* (Cambridge, MA, 1998).

25. Franklin, "Rise of Our Present State of Misunderstanding" (1770), *Papers of Benjamin Franklin*, 17: 273, cited in Andrew Burstein, *Sentimental Democracy: The Evolution of America's Romantic Self-Image* (New York, 1999), 72; Peter Way, "The Cutting Edge of Culture: British Soldiers Encounter Native Americans in the French and Indian War," in Martin Daunton and Rick Halpern, eds., *Empire and Others: British Encounters with Indigenous Peoples, 1600-1850* (Philadelphia, 1999), 131-33.

26. LeMay, ed., *Benjamin Franklin: Writings*, 359-61; Karen Severud Cook, "Benjamin Franklin and the Snake That Would Not Die," *British Library Journal*

22 (1996): 88-111. For this middling sensibility in the following century, see David R. Roediger, *The Wages of Whiteness: Race and the Making of the American Working Class* (New York, 1991).

27. Verner W. Crane, ed., *Benjamin Franklin's Letters to the Press* (Chapel Hill, 1950).

28. *Papers of Benjamin Franklin*, 13: 80-81; Olson, *Emblems of American Community*, 203-9.

29. *Papers of Benjamin Franklin*, 10: 392, 12: 42; David Freeman Hawke, *Franklin* (New York, 1976), 202-3, 205.

30. *New York Gazette or Weekly Post-Boy*, Sept. 18, 1766; Jack P. Greene, "The Alienation of Benjamin Franklin, British American," in *Understanding the American Revolution: Issues and Actors* (Charlottesville, 1995), 248.

31. *Papers of Benjamin Franklin*, 12: 127; 13: 83, 17: 168; Hawke, *Franklin*, 231, 356.

32. In a 1780 Dutch version, Franklin himself appears with John Paul Jones, wielding the enema syringe while a Dutchman holds a vomit pan. Donald H. Cresswell, *The American Revolution in Drawings and Prints* (Washington, DC, 1975), 337. Many thanks to Kate Ohno for these references.

33. Franklin, "The Handsome and Deformed Leg," "Petition of the Right Hand," in LeMay, ed., *Benjamin Franklin: Writings*, 951-53, 1115-16. On Philadelphia artisans and politics, see Eric Foner, *Tom Paine and Revolutionary America* (New York, 1976); Gary B. Nash, *The Urban Crucible* (Cambridge, MA, 1986); Steven Rosswurm, *Arms, Country and Class* (New Brunswick, NJ, 1987). For the dense metaphorical context of "framing" in the late 1780s, especially in Philadelphia, see Laura Rigal, *The American Manufactory: Art, Labor, and the World of Things in the Early Republic* (Princeton, NJ, 1998), 3-54. On the relationship between highly visible gentry bodies and their houses, see Rhys Isaac, *The Transformation of Virginia, 1740-1790* (Chapel Hill, 1982); Richard L. Bushman, *The Refinement of America: Persons, Houses, Cities* (New York, 1992); St. George, *Conversing by Signs.*

34. Van Doren, *Benjamin Franklin*, 737.

35. A first-person account from the very moment of Franklin's invention of the Long Arm conveys how important it was to him to remain self-sufficient. When young Andrew Ellicott tried to help him put water on a fire and shave,

> he thanked me and replied he ever made it a point to wait upon himself and although he began to find himself infirm he was determined not to encrease his infirmities by giving way to them—After his water was hot I observed his Object was to shave himself which Operation he performed without a Glass and with great expedition—I Asked him if he never employed a Barber he answered "no" and continued nearly in the following words "I think happiness does not consist so much in

a perticular peices of good fortune that perhaps accidentally fall to a
Mans lot as to be able in his old age to do those little things which he
was unable to perform himself would be done by others with a spar-
ing hand."

Catharine Van Cortlandt Mathews, *Andrew Ellicott: His Life and Lessons* (New
York, 1908), 50-51. Thanks to Kate Ohno for this reference and many others.

36. I visited the Franklin Court, which is part of Independence Hall National Park, in December 1998. In early 2000 the museum replaced the earlier
film (ca. 1975) with the new film produced by the Discovery Channel. Karie Diethorn, Chief Curator, Independence Hall National Park, personal communication, August 23, 2000.

37. My understanding of this cultural grandfather complex is indebted to
Werner Sollors, *Beyond Ethnicity: Consent and Descent in American Culture* (New
York, 1986).

38. For a stunning example of the work of recovering the other Founding
Fathers, see Woody Holton, *Forced Founders: Indians, Debtors, Slaves, and the Making of the American Revolution in Virginia* (Chapel Hill, 1999). On forgetting the
presence of working people, and recasting them as the problem rather than the
victims in the present and recent American past, see Mike Davis, *City of Quartz:
Excavating the Future in Los Angeles* (New York, 1991); and Norman M. Klein, *The
History of Forgetting: Los Angeles and the Erasure of Memory* (New York, 1997).

12

Technology Sits Cross-Legged

Developing the Jaipur Foot Prosthesis

Raman Srinivasan

> The Jaipur Foot is not a foot. . . . not a foot alone. . . . It has become an outlook, a way of looking at the patient both within the world of medicine and in terms of her life beyond the hospital.
>
> —P. K. Sethi, 1986

THE TERM "JAIPUR FOOT" is a convenient way of naming a whole class of prosthetic feet developed in the city of Jaipur, India. It refers to a class of handcrafted, multiple-axis prosthetic devices that evoke the human foot exceptionally well in form and function, and yet are cheaper than a pair of Indian shoes. Nonliterate artisans can fit amputees with a rugged, lightweight, skin-colored lower-limb prosthesis in less than an hour. These artisans are usually able to align the prosthesis accurately by visual examination. The amputee learns to use her new machine almost immediately, requiring little or no training. Furthermore, the Jaipur foot prosthesis is waterproof, abrasion-resistant, and durable. It enables an amputee to resume a normal lifestyle more or less quickly. Amputees who currently use the Jaipur foot prosthesis include a celebrated dancer, a professional cricket player, the leader of a much-feared Tamil terrorist faction, tree climbers and toddy tappers, cycle-rickshaw drivers, farmers, and craftsmen.

The Jaipur foot prosthesis is a significant advancement in the history of rehabilitation medicine and medical technology, affecting the lives of hundreds of thousands of amputees in the developing nations. It is now used and manufactured in Nicaragua, Sri Lanka, Thailand, Cambodia, Vietnam, Kenya, and India. The Jaipur foot is particularly

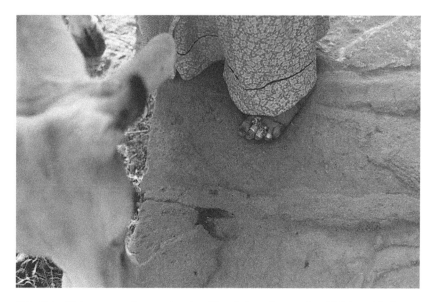

FIG. 12.1. This woman has customized her Jaipur foot to her liking, with decorative rings and painted toenails. Photograph courtesy of the author.

well suited for developing nations because it is cheap, enduring, and efficient. It is also culturally appropriate, by virtue of its design, as it enables its users to squat, sit cross-legged on the floor, and walk barefoot. Most important, however, the technology for making this prosthetic device requires little in the way of start-up capital or cumbersome machinery, uses locally available materials such as rubber and wood, and provides ample scope for the expression of artistic skills and artisanship. As a consequence, it is not protected by intellectual property regimes, thus making it widely available.

The term "Jaipur foot" brings to mind not only the footpiece but also the design and manufacture of lower-limb prosthetics; in fact, it has become a way of talking about a new style of rehabilitation medicine in tropical countries. Dr. Pramod Karan Sethi, professor of orthopedic surgery at the Sawai Man Singh Hospital at Jaipur, is generally recognized as the key individual in the development of the Jaipur foot.[1] He began research on the prosthesis in 1966 and continues to improve it, even today. He is unusual in being able to work readily and easily with a wide variety of collaborators, including Indian rocket scientists, voluntary agencies, students, journalists, filmmakers, professors in engineering colleges, entrepreneurs, philanthropists, as well as both anonymous Indian craftsmen and medical personnel from the West.

Sethi is an inspiringly talented and idealistic orthopedic surgeon, teacher, and entrepreneur. "I grew up hearing about Mahatma Gandhi," he said,

> and that made a deep impact on me. Gandhi was an immensely charismatic person. And once you saw him, it left a deep impression on your life; his ideas of *ahimsa*, nonviolence and *Swadeshi*, indigentality, became real, practicable, and simple. And you were tempted to follow the Mahatma, just keep walking behind him, singing and dancing, and you met others like yourself, and then you and your friends went from town to hamlet, hamlet to town spreading the message of self-rule, self-reliance, and nonviolence. If you could not follow the Mahatma right away, you, at the very least, tried to use your skills to do something for the downtrodden, the *daridranaryaan*, god in the guise of the downtrodden. You changed your life to follow the Mahatma. It was so simple.

Even though Sethi went to England to study advanced surgery and became a member of the Royal College of Surgeons, he returned to his homeland with a firm resolve to put his knowledge in the service of his fellow Indians. He could have quite easily established a lucrative practice in Delhi or Bombay since, in the years after India gained its independence from Britain, surgeons and doctors were few in number, and those who were "England-returned" commanded even greater fees. All one had to do was hang the shingle, and the rupee notes piled up. Instead, the brilliant young doctor returned to Jaipur and quietly began teaching surgery at the S.M.S. Medical College. Unlike those who went around calling themselves Gandhians, he resolved to keep his inspiration quiet, as it is said in the ancient texts.

Each city has a purpose, a destiny. Benares kills death. Delhi corrupts. Paris and the pursuit of pleasure go together. In Philadelphia you declare independence, pray for peace, and count your coins with the Quakers. Here in Jaipur, a pomegranate-pink city, one's sweet dreams alone come true. You may indeed meet the prince riding a white horse, and he, handsome in his polo outfit, may even invite you over to his palace, and you become his *syce* and take care of his noble steeds. It used to be the capital of the erstwhile princely state of Jaipur and is now the capital of the state of Rajasthan. Life shone, even in the feudal fifties, full of royal splendor and Rajput grace. That was before Congress politicians themselves began to imitate the feudal lords and the royal family began to go a-begging for votes from the farmer and the cobbler. Jaipur exuded the charm of a different era. Everybody knew everybody. People stopped on the broad roads to talk to one another. Time ambled along like the graceful royal elephant, with majesty and magic, sure of where it was taking you.

Raja Jai Singh's elephant always knew where he was taking the raja. He, that enormous tusker, memorialized in numerous paintings, ensured Jai Singh's victory, and led him from Man Singh's mountaintop fort to the verdant valley at the foot of the Kali Kho Hill, past the tank of Shiva, and thus was Jaipur born in 1727. Vidyadhar, a Bengali architect of great renown, was invited to plan a new city, worthy of the Solar dynasty. And to build the city, artisans of all kinds were invited: jewelers, gem cutters, silversmiths, goldsmiths, carpenters and stonecutters, sculptors and architects, priests and potters, coppersmiths, blacksmiths and bards, wheelwrights and weavers, painters, musicians, dancers, drummers, courtesans and cooks, from as far away as Bengal and Bihar, Agra and Andhra, Gujrat and Gowd, from Awadh and Magadh, Delhi and Dakkan, Mysore and Travancore. Each caste settled in its own alley and did its duty. Charitable Jain merchants bought and sold their wares. Sometimes they charged too much in interest, but then they didn't ask their clients to sign a thousand papers. To amuse the public on holidays, city planners built playgrounds where boys could fly multicolored kites and play *kabbadi* and *gilli danda*. Sometimes elephants were brought to the grounds for exhibition fights. The great *koncanada*, the conch-like trumpeting of the bull elephants, echoed off the amber mountains and the hairs on your forearms stood erect in involuntary attention.

Jaipur abounds in splendid chariots, and if one speaks kindly to the charioteer as one mounts his splendid vehicle, he may share his wisdom during the ride: "Sir, Jaipur is an enchanted city. It is said, even now, sometimes, on a full moon night, one can hear divine beings, demigods play music all along the ridge at the north end, and the moon seems to shine there with a bluish tinge, unseen elsewhere. But Jaipur has been growing fast, very fast. Its population doubled every ten years since independence (don't get me wrong, it is good for my business), that is, if you believe the government reports. How does the government know, I ask you, brother, that there were 744,225 camels in all of Rajasthan in 1972 and that, of those, 20,621 camels lived in Jaipur? How did they find that out? Do they have nothing better to do, in any case? Now everyone seems to have a moped, or a motorcycle, or motorscooter, and there are too many of them, hooting and tooting, and crashing into you all the time. No good. Any surprise more and more people get crippled? They, the motorized monsters, ghastly beasts, run around too fast and there is just not enough room on the road to stop and talk, if you see your second cousin from the other side on his way to the temple. You are sure to get hit by one of those phat-phatis farting around crazily on three wheels." The cycle-rickshaw driver took me to Sethi's house.

When I first visited him in 1986, Sethi lived in a newer part of town, outside the walled city. It was the nice, upper-middle-class home of a college professor in a provincial capital. "There are two kinds of cultures in the world, chair-sitting and floor-sitting," he said. I was sitting on a well-cushioned couch. So was he. On the wall behind him was a three-by-four-foot abstract oil painting with an Anglo-Saxon name signed in the righthand corner. "We in India are floor-sitters," he was saying. "We eat seated on the floor, we work sitting cross-legged or squatting on the ground." My dangling feet were playing with the thick ply of the DuPont carpet on the floor.

Sethi became a celebrity after he got the Magsaysay Award for his role in the creation of the Jaipur foot in 1981. The Rockefeller Brothers Fund, which had instituted this prize in the early 1950s to combat communism in southeast Asia after the tragic death of Ramon Magsaysay, a charismatic president of the Philippines, wanted people to think of the Magsaysay Award as the Asian Nobel Prize. Ever since, Indians have been among the honored, and the Magsaysay alumni tended to look out for prospective awardees in their countries. In order to keep the communists away, the fund gives awards annually to a number of "do-gooders" (that is what one of the Rockefellers called them, in a private moment), which are heavily publicized all over Asia by the Magsaysay Foundation.

After Sethi was honored with the award, he was feted and adored like a Nobel laureate. And, for a period, he was infected by cultural studies. Stress does strange things. The award brought a steady stream

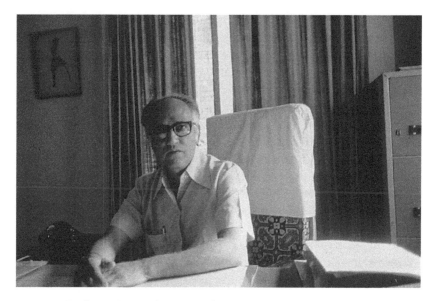

FIG. 12.2. Professor Pramod Karan Sethi, Jaipur, 1986. Photograph courtesy of the author.

of journalists, celebrity worshippers, immature and arrogant graduate students, slick social scientists, missionaries, doctors, and amputees to his doorstep. Sethi himself was invited to address meetings all over the world and traveled a great deal. The award rudely transformed a quiet and intense life of research, teaching, and surgery. All the adulation abroad automatically brought more and more honors at home as the burden of fame grew heavier and heavier. "As soon as my friend, the playwright Vijay Tendulkar, heard that I got the award, he warned me, 'Now you'd better be careful.' I now understand what he meant then. The award provoked a lot of jealousy and bitterness that I could have done without."

Even though I was one of the many irritants at Sethi's door because of all the publicity that the Jaipur foot had generated in the Indian media, he was extraordinarily patient and generous with me. He told me how the Jaipur foot came to be developed. Sethi readily acknowledged that he could not have done anything without the help and support of numerous artisans, philanthropists, and amputees, and the governments of Rajasthan and India. His former students and colleagues, anxious that someone should write the history of the Jaipur foot in an unbiased fashion, were eager to tell me their own roles in its history. But while many, many people played a part in the development of the Jaipur foot and associated prostheses, Sethi was undoubtedly the prime mover.

Sethi was the first to perceive the problem and think of a possible solution. He found the financial resources, introduced institutional innovations, and implemented a radical departure in the design, production, and fitting of lower-limb prostheses. He spearheaded a significant evolution in rehabilitation medicine in India and successfully persuaded several tropical and semitropical countries to adopt his methods. In addition, he has theorized about the sociology of medicine, physical rehabilitation, management of traumatic injuries, and rural development. His work in no way undermines, negates, or belittles the contributions made by his colleagues, who for the most part have been extraordinarily broad-minded and generous. Everybody involved in the development of this technology unanimously agreed to forgo his or her intellectual property rights, a rare phenomenon in the history of twentieth-century medicine and technology. All parties involved could have significantly improved their material prospects had they chosen to patent the prosthesis. Such is the archaic idealism that Mahatma Gandhi inspired and India sustains. As the great scholar Ananda Coomaraswamy has frequently said, "There is no private property in ideas, because these are gifts of the Spirit. Ideas are never made, but can only be 'invented,' that is, 'found,' and entertained."

The story of fitting tens of thousands of Indian amputees with the Jaipur foot actually begins in the late nineteenth century. A daring smuggling operation, conducted at the urging of Sir Clemens Markham in June 1876 by the British buccaneer Henry Wickham, brought 70,000 caoutchouc (rubber) seeds from Brazil to the Kew Gardens in London. As a young civil servant, Sir Markham had originated and directed the successful movement of quinine from Peru to India. Now he wanted to cultivate the caoutchouc seeds in India. Of the 70,000 seedlings Henry Wickham brought from the Amazon, only 1,900 seeds germinated. In August 1876, thirty-eight cases of seeds, under the charge of a royal gardener, were shipped by steamer to Ceylon, where it was hoped they would find a more hospitable climate than Calcutta, where earlier attempts to cultivate rubber had failed.

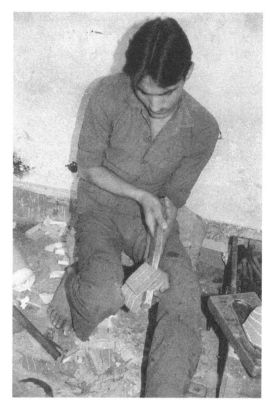

FIG. 12.3. Artisan carving laminated rubber insert for the Jaipur foot, July 1986. Photograph courtesy of the author.

Ceylon, the Isle of Serendipity, had become a colony of coffee planters, as coffee fever had gripped the island in the 1840s. But by 1869, coffee blight opened the way for other plantation crops. Rubber came along at the right time. (Tea and Cinchona too were looked at more favorably after the great coffee blight.) Sir Markham had secured for the empire a safe and reliable source of an important strategic material. Almost a century later, in 1955, G. M. Muller, a British orthopedic surgeon living in Ceylon, outlined the need for a rubber foot prosthesis that was waterproof, rugged, and cheap for use in the monsoon-drenched climate of Ceylon. Sethi remembered reading the note in the *Journal of Bone and Joint Surgery*: "Muller described a below-knee prosthesis that looked like a rubber galosh. The stump fit into the long neck of the galosh, and the bottom part was solid rubber. It struck me as being a good idea."

Sethi tried to duplicate Muller's prosthesis.

> I looked for someone who knew how to work with rubber. There were numerous vulcanizers and tire retreaders in town, and I approached them. One finally agreed to make a rubber foot. A mold was made. We packed the rubber in, and put it in the furnace to vulcanize it. The first time, the mold broke and all the rubber came out. It was a mess. I was so discouraged that I stopped working on it for a while. Then my students came looking for thesis topics. And I suggested to one of them to follow up on Muller's idea. So we tried again. This time it worked and we fitted this solid rubber foot to an amputee. It was too heavy.

The amputee who wore Sethi's newly designed foot felt the rubber foot dance to its own tune. It seemed to have a life of its own because its weight was distributed differently from a human limb. But while the gait was abnormal and the foot ugly, it was rugged and waterproof. And unlike the imported Solid Ankle Cushioned Heel (or SACH) foot, the Jaipur foot did not require an amputee to wear an external shoe. Sethi felt he had taken a small, if uncertain, step forward.

During the time that Sethi worked in a teaching hospital, the population of Jaipur multiplied like the rabbits of Fibonacci. As the patient load at the hospital grew and grew again, there was no time for research. "I operated almost every day," he said. The royal roads of Jaipur got congested. Camels looked down, with supreme indifference, at honking cars as they mingled uneasily on the city streets.

> We began to see more traumatic injuries. Our operating theaters were impossible to keep sterile. I tried my best. But it was simply not possible. We began to encounter more sepsis. More amputations. It was causing great concern. Cripples found no work. They became beggars. So I tried to send as many as I could to the Army Limb Fitting Center in Pune. At first, they did not want to deal with anyone who was not a veteran. The British army had set it up during World War II to help Indian soldiers wounded in the war. Their technology and approach to rehabilitation medicine dated back to the war. And you see, Jaipur is a small town and soon I began to recognize many of my patients, the

ones I had sent to Pune for artificial limbs, on the streets hobbling on crutches, begging. I asked my colleagues about this. "Oh! they just like to beg. They are lazy." Somehow, I could not accept that. So when one of them came back to the hospital, I asked him why he did not use his army limb. He mumbled something. I asked him again. "Who will wear those heavy army boots all the time. I am no soldier," he replied. So I started to stop on the streets and ask other patients of mine why they were back on crutches.

Slowly, I was persuaded that the shoe was the villain. So I went back to Muller's note and wondered if we could make a rubber foot that just looked like a human foot. By then, we had a man with a diploma in prosthetics and orthotics working for us, and I asked him if he could make a rubber foot prosthesis. He was really unwilling to do anything not in the textbook. Schooling had sealed his mind shut. Masterji heard of my need and things began to move.

Who is Masterji?

"I am an artist," Masterji said simply. He remembers when Sethi approached him with the idea for the rubber prosthesis. "'Can you make me a foot that looks like a foot?' Doctor Sahib asked, and I said, 'Sure I can,' and so here I am making what they all call prosthetics and orthotics. I am not a prosthetist or orthotist. I am not educated like yourself. I am just an artist."

Masterji was sitting on the floor, leaning against a bolster. In that busy room, once you saw him, sitting like a Rajput prince of a bygone era, your eyes kept returning to his form. He seemed vast, and his body shone as if it were a mountain of silver, reminding me of Hanumanji. He was broad-shouldered, barrel-chested, and imposing, even in his yellowed white undershirt and off-white *dhoti*. His face was calm and confident, his eyes large and compassionate. He rarely smiled. His hair was just beginning to turn gray and cut very short, and when he turned his head to give instructions, you saw a slim tuft of hair tied into a jaunty topknot. A large low workbench with an electric drill mounted on a cast iron stand sat, like an obedient elephant, in front of Masterji. On it was a shiny black high-density polyethylene pipe, a long elephant trunk being transformed into a full-leg prosthesis. He caught my eye and winked. "Research," he said.

"Did you see the statue of the amputee at the entrance?" he asked me. "I made it. I wanted to give back the hospital something. I made it

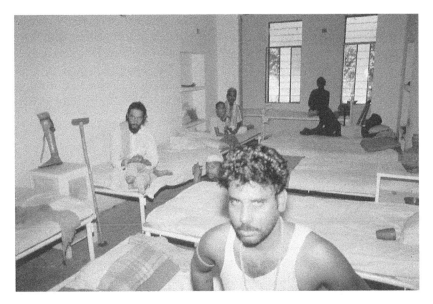

FIG. 12.4. Amputee ward at the Sawai Man Singh Hospital, Jaipur. Photograph courtesy of the author.

entirely from sheet metal, beaten aluminum. Not one part was cast in a foundry. That's who I am, an artist," he reiterated.

At the end of the day, as Masterji drove home on his tiny moped, I wandered toward the Regional Rehabilitation Center to look at the statue of the Unknown Amputee. As I neared it, I saw an extended family of Rajasthani villagers, tall and handsome, their faces shining, their bright clothes looking like gold, eyes intently drinking in the statue. Then I saw one of the women lift up the fringe of her *sari* ever so slightly, and step upon the low cement platform on which the Unknown Amputee stood with immense dignity. As she went up, I glanced shamelessly at her feet. They were covered with intricate designs done with henna and bejeweled with silver toe-rings and anklets. Since her feet were dusty, she washed them under a faucet. I continued to stare, and I noticed that her right foot was a Jaipur foot. Who would have thought of putting toe-rings and henna patterns on a prosthesis?

Masterji was how everybody addressed him. He was known as Ramachandra Sharma, but only in the dust-covered government files. He was born in a very poor home, an undistinguished adobe hut, in an impoverished desert hamlet. "When I was about ten," he said, "I helped my father carve a banana tree in green stone. You can still see it, it is by the gate of Devi temple in the fort at Amber. And on a bright day, at a certain hour, when the light is just right, the banana leaf turns translucent green, and it then seems to have just sprouted that morning." Masterji learned a number of trades, stonecarving, carpentry, woodcarving, blacksmithy, wheelwrighting, ivoryworking, and sandalwood work, and later still, he mastered jewelry making.

> Once a customer came to me with a gold chain whose design I could not duplicate. This had never before happened to me. So I found out the address of the man who made it. He lived all the way in Gaya, a Bengali. So I went there, to Gaya, from Jaipur. I found him and waited, and waited and waited every day, at his threshold for two months— Nachiketas waited only three days, you know—and then the Bengali decided to teach me his secret. Those were the days when people had a passion and a commitment to what they did. It was a *tapasya*, a fervent and ardent discipline, to be a craftsman. And thus there was joy, too, in being one.

I could not help but admire his story. He seemed deep as the Indian Ocean. All I saw was the wave.[2]

And then having passed through the stations of life, Masterji was ready to retire to teach what he knew. When the maharaja of Jaipur had opened a School of Arts and Crafts, Ramachandra Sharma became a master, and since then people have called him Masterji. Even the erudite Professor Sethi calls him Masterji. After Indian independence, the maharajahs gave way to democracy-shamocracy, elections, and MPs. Patronage suffered. In 1966 the School of Arts and Crafts shut down for lack of funds, and Sethi hired Masterji as an instructor for the disabled. Sethi hoped that Masterji could help in their vocational rehabilitation by teaching them some "weaving-sheaving." And so Masterji came to spend time at the hospital. He heard of the need to make a prosthetic foot that looked like a foot, and set out to make it.

"'If you can imagine it, you can make it,' my guru used to say," said Masterji.

> "How do you think airplanes and cars came into being?" he would ask. He was a wise man, my guru, he was a wise man, indeed. He used

to say, "*You* have to keep thinking about what more *you* can do with all that you have learned in a different situation. Don't think that wood-carving is all you'll be doing in a lifetime. The world is always changing. What I have taught you will not be enough. What we know is but a fistful of beach sand, what we know not is vast as the ocean itself."

Masterji spoke of his teacher with reverence and infinite gratitude. The teacher-student relationship is the most intimate, mysterious, intense, and sacred relationship in all of India.

Tradition evokes different connotations in India than it does, perhaps, in the West. Masterji clearly saw himself belonging to a tradition of Indian art. "Tradition is a method, a compendium of laws, laws of solving equations, and that there is no way to the answer, to the Truth, but through that inherent method by which we humans have recognized . . . the way of finding proper solutions to a problem." When Sethi speaks of Masterji as a traditional craftsman it is high praise, an acknowledgment of Masterji's innovative and inventive gifts. When Masterji speaks of a tradition of gurus, he is talking of the freedom to reach across centuries of clock-time; of the freedom to leap, like Hanuman, across seas and mountains, to unlock the mystery, to find the answer. Masterji, with ample help from the visible and the invisible, the manifest and the unmanifest, made an artificial foot that looked like a human foot, and worked nearly as well as a human foot, and yet cost less than a pair of shoes. "It had to cost less than a pair of shoes because many of our villagers, you do know, don't you, cannot afford a pair of shoes." Now the amputee in the village can get on with his or her life. Sethi began to take the Jaipur foot on the road. The foot moved far and wide.

Ramoji Rao was no ordinary Indian entrepreneur. He established his own film company, Usha Kiron Movies, in Hyderabad. It was going to be the first ray of dawn in a brave new Indian film world. He began boldly, moving away from the familiar mythological dramas and fantasies of the Indian cinema. He made provocative films about real politicians. His movies were neither fiction nor fact, but they were true. They were real. The people saw his films, the critics loved them. Coins of gold filled his treasury.

But soon he was tired of depicting demonic politicians. "I was looking for something positive, something inspiring. I heard of this young Tamil dancer of Bharatanatyam, from Bombay, who had lost her leg and performed with an artificial leg." The story intrigued him. He investigated. Sudha Chandran was born dancing, so to speak. She made her debut as a classical dancer in Bombay when she was not quite eight years old. By the time she was seventeen, she had given close to one hundred solo performances all over India. She practiced daily, like an ascetic in *tapasya*, immersed in mobile meditation. Like a true devotee of Shiva Nataraja, the cosmic dancer, she perfected her art; her discipline was fervent and arduous.

One scorching midsummer day, in May 1981, the planets and stars aligned themselves malevolently, and Sudha's car crashed. She survived, but gangrene soon set in. On June 6, 1981, her right leg was amputated three inches below the knee. Emptiness reigned. "For six months, I was obsessed with walking again—but not with crutches," Sudha said. While in the hospital, she read an article in the newspaper about one Dr. Sethi, who had won the Magsaysay Award for having designed an artificial leg suited to Indian conditions. Sudha Chandran wrote to Sethi and met him in December 1981. "I asked him if I could dance again. His reply was 'Why not?' That was all I needed to hear." Sethi, his colleague Masterji, and others worked hard to make her a special prosthesis that would withstand the high-energy movements of Bharata's dance.

Initially, they put a spring in the ankle, but it jammed during practice. She decided to bring her dance teacher, her guru, with her to Jaipur. "For twenty days, Dr. Sethi watched me work with my guru because he wanted to study the footwork involved in the dance to decide what sort of limb to give me." The doctor and Masterji decided to fit her with a custom-made Jaipur foot that matched her skin color. To match skin tone was itself a minor medical revolution for, even in 1981, multinational drug companies were selling millions of Band-Aids in India that matched only Caucasian skin. Sudha Chandran soon resumed her dance practice. "I danced like a three-year-old. It was painful, too. The stump would bleed, my mother was in tears all the time, and my guru almost gave up hope." But she was bound to dance. The doctors and artisans in Jaipur worked hard to make it easier on her.

On January 28, 1984, Sudha Chandran made a second debut, a grand debut, at the South Indian Welfare Society in Bombay, the very same small hall where she had first performed thirteen years earlier. Sixteen hundred people packed a hall designed for eight hundred. "I was nervous," she remembers. So was the crowd, and she could sense the anxiety in the audience. "I paid obeisance to the Lord of Dance and started." Two and a half hours later, the auditorium broke into a thunderous applause, and it was absolutely electrifying. The gods showered flowers from the heavens, or so it seemed. She created a great sensation in Bombay.

Ramoji Rao decided to make a film about Sudha, and he persuaded her to play herself. Rao and Chandran agreed to fictionalize part of her story. Sethi, Masterji, and the artisans in Jaipur made guest appearances. The film was first made in Telugu, and was released early in 1986. *Mayuri* was an instant box office hit. People demanded that it be dubbed into Tamil and Hindi. The film grossed "megabucks," some say as much as forty-five million rupees. The film launched Sudha Chandran into an international orbit, and inspired thousands of amputees to come to Jaipur. Jaipur could cope with that kind of upsurge because Jaipur is that kind of city. The Vardhamana Mahavira, the twenty-fourth of the great Jaina beings who attained perfection in 526 B.C., had ensured that.

Although most of India suffered terribly under Mrs. Gandhi's tyrannical dictatorship, 1975 was a good year in the history of the Jaipur foot. It was an important year for the Jains, an ancient religious sect of India. They celebrated the 2,500th anniversary of their teacher, the Mahavira, the Great Courageous One. The Mahavira is the one and only one in all of Indian history to be called a Mahavira, a meta-brave, in a manner of speaking, not because of his heroic deeds done on the battlefield but because he embodied absolute nonviolence. It takes greater courage not to hurt. Realizing this, the founder of the greatest ancient Indian empire, Chandragupta, became a Jain monk.

Jain doctrine espouses an utterly uncompromising pursuit of non-violent asceticism. Even today, Jain monks and nuns take the greatest care to avoid hurting the smallest of bugs. Many cover their mouths with a square piece of white cloth to avoid accidentally ingesting microscopic creatures. Strict is their adherence to nonviolence, and their asceticism is extraordinarily severe, even by Indian standards.

Unlike the orthodox philosophies of India, the Jains consider the manifest world to be very real. As one wag put it, for the Jains the world is real; it only appears to be illusory. None of the Vedantic thinking that "the world is a city seen in a mirror." The whole universe is traced to everlasting, uncreated, independent categories of the sentient and the insentient. The soul, the *anima*, is embodied because of residual action, *karma*. And each embodied soul fights a constant battle to diminish these residual actions to zero by extinguishing old traces and creating new positive actions. The soul, it is said, is like a gourd stuck at the bottom of a lotus pond covered by karmic mud and silt. Once rid of karmic junk, the soul naturally floats, like a bubble, to the top of the ocean of existence, becoming absolutely anonymous, buoyant, and free. Another telling image of Jain philosophy is the one of a monk plucking each one of his hairs slowly, deliberately, and painfully in order to depilate himself completely. It is said that one can achieve perfection by similarly pulling away at each residual act that is our inheritance, our history, and the reason for our birth. Hence the Jain obsession with not hurting anything. Why acquire fresh karma and suffer more? Nevermore! the Jains declare.

So the Jains stayed away from most worldly vocations. It is easy to imagine that a farmer may hurt hundreds of earthworms unknowingly when plowing. So reasoning thus, many Jains chose to be merchants, moneylenders, and financiers, and migrated far and wide in order to live truthfully and nonviolently. And by adhering to their beliefs, they succeeded. The Jains are, indeed, one of the wealthiest communities in India and in the Indic world outside India, too. Although constituting only half of 1 percent of India's vast population, they have exerted a significant influence on the development of Indian civilization by the sheer intensity of their faith. For example, Jain culture's strict adherence to nonviolence, *ahimsa*, and thus to vegetarian diet, had a profound formative effect on Mahatma Gandhi. Gandhi wrote, "*Ahimsa* is the farthest limit of humility" and "I must reduce myself to zero."[3]

How to reduce oneself to zero? By being anonymous and self-effacing, a true indicator of a pilgrim's movement. Thus Arjun Agarwaala, the king of the coal-belt in Bihar, a Jain, quietly and anonymously funded Sethi's research and development for many, many years. A man so anonymous that he prefers the silences of history. Not everybody is an Arjun Agarwaala.[4] Jain theologians' mercantilist calculus of karma, deeds, good and bad, makes for a straightforward but difficult solution. Philanthropy aids one to reduce the burden of one's karmic load. And so over the centuries, Jains have promoted social and religious philanthropy. They have been generous patrons of arts and crafts. They have helped the miserable and indigent, maybe more so than most other Indian communities.

When the 2,500th anniversary of the Mahavira was celebrated in 1975, a group of philanthropic Jains in Jaipur decided to constitute the Lord Mahavir Society for Assisting the Disabled. A substantial corpus fund was collected quickly and the society commissions artisans to make Jaipur feet and other prostheses. The society also pays the travel expenses for amputees and their companions, and outfits them with new prosthetics and clothes. When it succeeded in Jaipur, Jains in other parts of India quickly imitated the Jaipur Society and took the Jaipur foot technology all over India.

Philosophically speaking, the Jains are, perhaps, the only realists in India, the only ones truly convinced about the reality of the world. The form is real. But so also is the soul. So they seem to have both feet planted firmly on the ground but soar toward the heavens with their arms uplifted in prayer. Thus the giant statue of Bahubali at Shravanabelagola, in South India, with creepers and other plants carved as if growing on and around a tall, vertical being, a perfected person, Bahubali.

Even after attaining perfection, in Jain stories, people maintain their human physical form, they even get expansive, whereas in Vedanta, especially as expounded by Sankara, once one realizes the Truth, there is no two, just one. The formless is free to be. Freedom from form, space, and time is Bliss. However, the Jains being realists, and thus pragmatic, organized a philanthropy to provide prosthetics. And it is true; no one else does it as successfully or with such ardent belief in the ability of prosthetics to restore reality and normality, not even the foreign Christian missionary doctors. And so with prosthetic foot kissing the earth, the Rajput amputee leaps upwards to the heavens and on to his *Chetak*, his ever-faithful and noble steed, which will bring him back from the battle, wounded but alive, so that he may recover, nursed by the Minas, to vanquish the invaders. So what if it takes a few centuries, as long as one is following one's deepest propensities?

How to dip into the Nothingness, the zero, where one is at one, in atonement, and not two? Gandhi's life, as Erik Erikson observed, was an attempt to institutionalize nothingness. And how can this be done? This is the challenge of post-traditional India.

No amount of reading of Indian philosophies prepared me to face the nothingness institutionalized in the courtyard of the Lord Mahavir Society for Assisting the Disabled. A masterpiece of Sethi and his

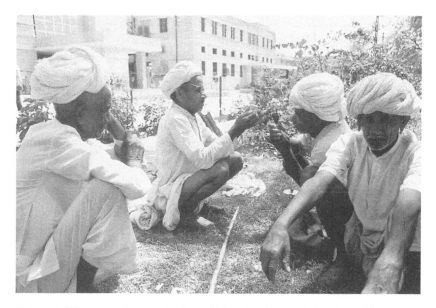

FIG. 12.5. Visitors waiting at the Sawai Man Singh Hospital, Jaipur. Photograph courtesy of the author.

colleagues, it is a place where the genius of India is alive and kicking with both legs, real and artificial: an extraordinary institutional innovation, a rediscovery of an Indian way of doing rehabilitation medicine. As Sethi told me, "It is the colonized mind set free."

As soon as I started toward the compound, I saw its two big welded steel gates. The strong white light that the sun cast in Jaipur was hitting the left gate like a thousand halogen lamps. Countless disembodied limbs, smooth and shiny like the legs of young American women sunning at the beach, leaned against the gates. Multifarious odors enveloped me like a pashmina shawl. The aromas of *dal, sabji,* and slightly burned *phulka rotis* overlaid with acrid *mirchi* competed vigorously with more industrial odors of burning rubber, molten metal, and singed foundry sand. Sounds of many kinds clamored for recognition. Human voices, some melodious, some raucous, plaintive, and bullying, different cadences of different regions, walloping sound patterns of different languages rolled like waves. I could even spot the difficult sounds of my native Tamil flowing effortlessly from throats born in Tirunelveli. Mellifluous Telugu mixed merrily with much harsher Punjabi. However, the overwhelming sounds were the *tang! dang! kadang badaang* of steel hammers beating the thin and softer aluminum. The horrific screeches of electric grinding wheels rose above all irregularly like a demon squealing in pain.

The interior courtyard was vast and crowded, more so than the cramped markets of Jaipur, more so than the most crowded temple processions, more so than the entrance to the central station, more so than the exits at the airports in India. Most of the people, men, women, and children, in the courtyard were missing at least one lower limb. To be a biped seemed strange, a bewildered bystander in the country of the disabled. Yet there was none of the ill air of a hospital. On the contrary, there was the incredible vitality of the weekly village shandy. Men hobbled musically, sure and quick like tabla players. Women with the saris covering the absent limbs were graceful, even more normal looking than the men. Some of the children were practically racing through the courtyard. Numerous cycles adapted for use by amputees lay strewn in the courtyard. One of them looked like an early motorcar. It was empty but for a pair of legs resting regally on the seat. Under a tree, on a raised cement platform, a small group of men were debating. Under another tree, a couple of women were cooking, while in another corner some men were washing clothes. In another corner, a young man was repeatedly climbing a short sickly tree and jumping off its lowest branch.

Across the courtyard, by the acrid foundry, a newly fitted amputee was tremulously planting her feet on the ground. She walked slowly, at first, then after a few steps, she walked quickly. She tried to squat, but then she began to complain loudly to Masterji in her dialect: "How do I do my business, how do I shit, man, if I can't squat comfortably, you tell me, c'mon!" She pleaded, she harangued, and she cajoled Masterji and his assistants until they fitted her with a perfect prosthesis. I had never before witnessed anything like this. She refused to be satisfied with a prosthesis that did not work for her, and she forced Masterji and his assistants to improvise. No one seemed to mind. The urban, educated, middle-class amputees were the ones who displayed bovine resignation on their faces and limped away.

When medicine moves out of febrile concrete cages called hospitals and into the open courtyard, under flowering trees, technology, too, learns to sit gracefully, cross-legged on the floor. Many amputees have stayed on to become prosthetists and orthotists at the courtyard, banging metal against metal, sitting on the earth, making more body parts.

Such is the rehabilitation of medicine and technology in India, their transformation and liberation. And if you stay there long enough, amidst all the voice and noise is such silence that you can hear yourself hearing it. From the origin comes originality, and thus we are all Bharata's children, chiding the mother lioness to play with the cubs. And thereafter, just as the great Buddhist philosopher Nagarjuna said, *tasmad, gatis ca ganta ca gantavyam ca na vidyate*, "Neither motion nor mover nor the space to be moved in is evident."[5]

This is the meaning of the Jaipur foot.

NOTES

The author is deeply grateful to Professor P. K. Sethi, Masterji, Mr. Santosh Zacharia, and Shri Ganga Ram for their patience and generosity. Thanks also to Dr. David Iglehart of Applied Science Fiction of Austin, Texas, for his help in restoring images of the Jaipur foot used in this volume.

In this essay, I let the historical narrative succumb to the tropological temptations of India. I found no other satisfactory alternative. I found the data recorded in the files of P. K. Sethi's office of little help in reconstructing the history of the Jaipur foot, although they did assist me in interviewing various participants in the history of the prosthesis. As the noted anthropologist and historian Gananath Obeyesekere has written, in the context of doing research on the South Asian Pattini, "[a] historiography that relies exclusively on well-documented and incontrovertible historical evidence, such as evidence from inscriptions, must surely be wrong, since it assumes that the *recorded* data must be the *significant* data shaping history and controlling the formation and transformation of a people."

1. All quotations taken from interviews conducted by the author with Professor P. K. Sethi and his colleagues, Masterji, other residents of the city, and visitors to the prosthesis center, between March 1986 and January 1990.

2. *Tapas(ya)* belongs to the pre-Aryan, non-Vedic heritage of archaic Indian asceticism. It is among the most ancient non-Brahmanic elements of the old Indian yoga. It is a technique for the winning of complete mastery over oneself through sustained self-inflicted sufferings to the utmost limit of intensity and time; also, it is the way to conquer the powers of the universe itself, the macrocosm, by subduing completely their reflection in the microcosm, one's own organism. See Heinrich Zimmer, *Philosophies of India*, ed. Joseph Campbell (Princeton: Princeton University Press, 1951), 400. "The gods gained their divine rank through tapasya." *Taitriya Brahmana* 3.12, 3.1.

3. Mahatma Gandhi, *Gandhi's Autobiography: The Story of My Experiments with Truth* (Washington, DC: Public Affairs Press, 1948), 371.

4. Ambalal Sarabhai, the father of Vikram Sarabhai, made an anonymous contribution to Mahatma Gandhi's ashram in Ahmedabad at a critical time. Ambalal Sarabhai, it is said, had a passion for anonymity in his philanthropy. In the Indic traditions, it is held that one who follows the dharma is anonymous and self-effacing. Zimmer, *Philosophies of India*, 152–53.

5. See, for instance, David J. Kalupahana, *Nagarjuna: The Philosophy of the Middle Way* (Albany: State University of New York Press, 1986).

Contributors

ELSPETH BROWN is an assistant professor of history at the University of Toronto, Canada, where she teaches courses in American social and cultural history. Her essay is drawn from her recently completed dissertation, "The Corporate Eye: Photography and the Rationalization of American Culture, 1884–1929."

ALEX FAULKNER is a research fellow in the School of Social Sciences at the University of Wales in Cardiff, and coordinator of the Health and Social Care Research Support Unit, a joint venture between Cardiff University and the University of Wales College of Medicine. His research interests include the sociology of health, health technology policy, and issues in the history, innovation, and regulation of medical devices.

KIRSTEN E. GARDNER is an assistant professor of history and gender studies at the University of Texas at San Antonio. She is currently working on a history of female cancer awareness programs in the United States, 1910s–1970s.

ELIZABETH HAIKEN is the author of *Venus Envy: A History of Cosmetic Surgery*. She received her Ph.D. from the University of California at Berkeley in 1994 and has taught at the University of Tennessee and the University of British Columbia. She now lives and works in the San Francisco Bay area.

STEVEN KURZMAN is a doctoral candidate in anthropology at the University of California at Santa Cruz. He is currently completing his dissertation based on ethnographic fieldwork in the American prosthetics field, and has also done research on prostheses in India and Cambodia.

JENNIFER DAVIS McDAID is an archives research coordinator at the Library of Virginia, where she has worked since 1991. She earned a master's degree from the College of William and Mary.

STEPHEN MIHM is a doctoral candidate in the History Department at New York University. He is presently writing a cultural history of counterfeiting in antebellum America.

KATHERINE OTT is a curator in the Science, Medicine, and Society Division of the National Museum of American History, Smithsonian Institution. She is the author of *Fevered Lives: Tuberculosis in American Culture since 1870*. She has taught university courses on the history of the body and sexuality, material culture and museums, and has developed exhibits on maxillofacial surgery, the disability rights movement, and other topics in American culture.

HEATHER R. PERRY is a doctoral candidate in history at Indiana University. She is currently working on a dissertation entitled "Re-Arming the Disabled: Medicine, Masculinity and Social Organization in World War I Germany." She has also served as a research fellow at the Zentrum für interdisziplinäre Frauenforschung at the Christian-Albrechts-Universität zu Kiel, Germany, where she conducted research for this essay.

DAVID SERLIN is an assistant professor of history and American studies at Albright College. He is the author of the forthcoming *Replaceable You: Engineering the American Body after World War Two*, and an editor and columnist for the journal *Cabinet*. He lives in Reading, Pennsylvania, and Brooklyn, New York.

RAMAN SRINIVASAN earned his B.S. in materials science at the Indian Institute of Technology in Madras, and completed his Ph.D. at the University of Pennsylvania. In 1994 he returned to India and cofounded one of India's first Internet portals. A former Warren Weaver Fellow at the Rockefeller Foundation, Srinivasan is currently the director of strategic alliances at Ramco Systems, one of India's leading software companies. He is also deeply involved in the study of Asian elephants.

DAVID WALDSTREICHER is the author of *In the Midst of Perpetual Fetes: The Making of American Nationalism, 1776–1820*, and is now working on *Runaway America: Benjamin Franklin, Slavery, and the American Revolution*. He teaches history at the University of Notre Dame.

Index

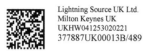